MEDICAL RADIOLOGY
Diagnostic Imaging

Softcover Edition

Editors:
A. L. Baert, Leuven
K. Sartor, Heidelberg

Springer

Berlin
Heidelberg
New York
Barcelona
Hong Kong
London
Milan
Paris
Tokyo

Javier Lucaya · Janet L. Strife (Eds.)

Pediatric Chest Imaging

Chest Imaging in Infants and Children

With Contributions by

R. Agid · J. Bar-Ziv · A. S. Brody · A. Castellote · T. Chung · P. A. Daltro · L. F. Donnelly
H. Ducou Le Pointe · G. F. Eich · G. Enriquez · D. P. Frush · P. García-Peña · D. Gilday
L. Grover · J. O. Haller · S. C. Kaste · C. Kellenberger · B. Koplewitz · J. Lucaya · J. Mata
K. McHugh · E. Nunez-Santos · X. Serres · J. L. Strife · U. V. Willi

Foreword by
A. L. Baert

With 303 Figures in 578 Separate Illustrations, Some in Color

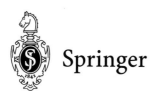 Springer

JAVIER LUCAYA, MD
Director, Division of Diagnostic Imaging
and Institute for Diagnostic Imaging
Vall d'Hebron Hospitals
Autonomous University of Barcelona
Ps. Vall d' Hebron, 119–129
08035-Barcelona
Spain

JANET L. STRIFE, MD
Radiologist-in-Chief
Children's Hospital Medical Center
3333 Burnet Avenue
Cincinnati, OH 45229-3039

MEDICAL RADIOLOGY · Diagnostic Imaging and Radiation Oncology
Series Editors: A. L. Baert · L. W. Brady · H. P. Heilmann · F. Molls · K. Sartor

Continuation of
Handbuch der medizinischen Radiologie
Encyclopedia of Medical Radiology

ISBN 3-540-43557-3 Springer-Verlag Berlin Heidelberg New York

Library of Congress Cataloging-in-Publication Data
Pediatric chest imaging : chest imaging in infants and children / J. Lucaya, J. L. Strife
(eds.) ; with contributions by J. Bar-Ziv ... [et al.] ; foreword by A. L. Baert.
      p. ; cm. -- (Medical radiology)
      Includes bibliographical references and index.
      ISBN 3540675272 (hard cover; alk. paper) ISBN 3540435573 (soft cover; alk. paper)
      1. Chest--Imaging. 2. Pediatric diagnostic imaging. I. Lucaya, J. (Javier), 1993- II.
Strife, Janet L. III. Bar-Ziv, Jacob. IV. Series.
      [DNLM: 1. Lung Diseases–diagnosis--Child. 2. Lung Diseases--diagnosis-Infant. 3.
Diagnostic Imaging--methods–Child. 4. Diagnostic Imaging--methods--Infant. 5.
Radiography, Thoracic--Child. 6. Radiography, Thoracic--Infant. WS 280 P36635 2002]
RJ433.5.D5 P43 2002
618.92'240754--dc21   2001020500

Springer-Verlag Berlin Heidelberg New York
a member of BertelsmannSpringer Science+Business Media GmbH

http://www.springer.de

Cover-Design and Typesetting: Verlagsservice Teichmann, 69256 Mauer

SPIN: 108 771 24   21/3130 – 5 4 3 2 1 0 – Printed on acid-free paper

We dedicate this book to

our wonderful families,
who mean everything to us,

and to the outstanding teachers
we both have had the great fortune to have,

Dr. Frederic N. Silverman
and the late *Dr. Benjamin Felson.*

Foreword

I am grateful that Dr. J. Lucaya and Dr. J. L. Strife, both leading and internationally recognized specialists in the field, accepted the challenging task of editing this volume on recent advances in pediatric chest imaging.

In this book primary attention is given to the great potential of the new cross-sectional techniques. Indeed, their role in pediatric chest imaging is becoming increasingly important and this volume sets out to provide the indispensable knowledge in this area as it has evolved from our actual clinical experience.

It is now well accepted that in conjunction with the standard chest radiograph, still a primary tool in the management of children with lung diseases, the new cross-sectional techniques ensure complete and appropriate assessment of these conditions and may frequently provide better guidance for optimal conservative or surgical management.

The editors have been inspired and successful in their selection of an impressive group of international experts in the field of pediatric chest imaging. It is my great pleasure and privilege to congratulate the editors and the contributing authors on the excellence and topicality of the material that has been brought together in this latest volume in our series "Medical Radiology".

Their combined efforts have resulted in an outstanding book that will provide a solid learning base as well as efficient guidelines for general and pediatric radiologists in their daily working environment. But it is evident that pediatricians and pediatric surgeons interested in enlarging their knowledge on the pediatric chest will also find a wealth of up-to-date information herein.

I am convinced that this book will be well received by all of them and that it will meet the same success as many other volumes previously published in this series. I welcome any constructive criticism that might be offered.

Leuven   ALBERT L. BAERT

Preface

Remarkable advances have taken place in both technology and knowledge in imaging of the pediatric chest. Of all examinations ordered for children, chest radiographs are the most common; however, the editors have elected not to focus on information provided by conventional radiographs as this is available in most pediatric radiology textbooks. Instead, we have given priority to describing the imaging features provided by new techniques. Since one image is worth a thousand words, we have decided that the illustrations for this book are of utmost importance, not only in quantity but also in quality. We believe that the extensive collection of figures will be of great value to the reader.

One of the priorities of imaging in children is to obtain the maximum diagnostic information with the least possible radiation to the patient. For this reason, this book emphasizes the use of techniques such as ultrasonography and MRI, which, though seldom used in the study of pediatric chest disorders, can provide a wealth of information without the use of ionizing radiation. In addition, we have included data on technical parameters of CT studies that can be used for diagnostic examinations with significantly less radiation exposure than is still common practice.

We are grateful for the expertise and knowledge of our invited authors. Some authors were asked to dedicate their chapter to a specific technique, such as the chapters on cardiac MR, high resolution CT, chest ultrasound, and nuclear medicine. On the other hand, several authors were asked to present their knowledge of specific pediatric diseases. These include chapters on pulmonary manifestations of AIDS, controversies in imaging in lymphoma, and thoracic manifestations of systemic diseases. In editing this book, we received the collaboration of a large group of internationally recognized pediatric radiologists who have presented their extensive experience and practical know-how on each particular topic.

We hope that this volume of Medical Radiology - Diagnostic Imaging (Chest Imaging in Infants and Children) will meet the needs of radiologists in updating their knowledge concerning chest imaging and will increase their knowledge of pediatric diseases. We express our gratitude to Ursula Davis of Springer for her editorial assistance and support during its preparation.

Barcelona   JAVIER LUCAYA
Cincinnati   JANET L. STRIFE

Acknowledgements:
The editors thank their departmental staffs for continuing support during the preparation of this book, Ms. Celine Cavallo for editing advice, and Ms. Ursula Davis and Mr. Kurt Teichmann from Springer-Verlag for their superb management and guidance.

Contents

1 Chest US

GOYA ENRIQUEZ, XAVIER SERRES

CONTENTS

1.1
Introduction

Ultrasound (US) has been underused in the study of chest pathologies in children. Initially the technique was applied mainly to detect pleural fluid, but in recent years the applications of US for the chest have been widely extended (YANG et al. 1992b; PAN-CHYR et al. 1992; CIVARDI et al. 1993; BEN-AMI et al. 1993; GEHMACHER et al. 1995; SEIBERT et al. 1998; KIM et al. 2000; WERNECKE 2000). Although air in healthy lungs and calcium in bony structures hinder transmission of the US beam, chest lesions involving the lung, mediastinum and pleura can be studied through ana-

GOYA ENRIQUEZ, MD
Department of Pediatric Radiology, Vall d'Hebron Hospitals, ps. Vall d'Hebron 119–129, Barcelona 08035, Spain
XAVIER SERRES, MD, PhD
Department of Radiology, Hospital General de Granollers, Avda. Francesc Ribas s/n, Granollers 08400, Spain

tomical "acoustic windows" (supraclavicular, suprasternal, parasternal and intercostal spaces), and by the transdiaphragmatic (subxiphoid and subcostal) approach. Furthermore, the lack of costal cartilage ossification and low bone mineral content in infants allows transosseous (trans-sternal and transcostal) scanning.

Technological advances in the geometry of the transducers have facilitated access to the chest through these acoustic windows. Color and power Doppler abilities permit study of vascular structures without the use of intravenous contrast material. Improvements in the resolution of the equipment provide images of excellent quality, which facilitates recognition of parenchymal, pleural and extra-pleural lesions (WEINBERG et al. 1986; MULLER 1993; WERNECKE 2000).

The technique has several advantages that are particularly beneficial in children: unlike computed tomography (CT), US does not use ionizing radiation or require administration of contrast material to identify vascular structures, most patients do not require sedation and examination can be performed at bedside. Furthermore, sonography is the only technique that permits visualization of the lesions in real time in different planes.

We have divided this chapter into: lung parenchyma, pleura, mediastinum and diaphragm.

1.2
Lung Parenchyma

1.2.1
Examination Technique

Ultrasound examination of the lung parenchyma should be performed following careful evaluation of chest X-rays. According to the location of the lesion, the patient is placed in the supine, prone or lateral decubitus position, and the appropriate transducer and acoustic window are selected. Longitudinal, transverse or oblique views can be obtained as required. The transdiaphragmatic approach using the liver and spleen as acoustic windows is recommended to study lesions located at the base of the lung. The supraclavicular, parasternal and paravertebral approaches are indicated for evaluating apical and paramediastinal lesions. The remaining lung parenchyma should be approached intercostally.

The type of transducer used depends on the capabilities of the instrument and the operator's preferences; however, we can offer some general guidelines. We recommend sector or convex transducers for the transdiaphragmatic approach. When the patient is studied through the parasternal and intercostal windows, linear or convex transducers provide better identification of the pleuro-pulmonary interface. Sector transducers are not recommended with these two approaches since they produce reverberation artifacts in the near field that preclude identification of anatomical structures. When using the supraclavicular window, sector or small linear probes are highly appropriate. Transducer frequency varies with patient age and depth of the lesion. High-frequency transducers (5–10 MHz) are best for imaging neonates and infants and for superficial lesions.

Color and power Doppler are very useful for complementing conventional studies in certain situations, e.g. when identifying vascular supply in pulmonary sequestration, assessing vascularity of lung consolidation and studying flow patterns within lung masses.

Sedation is seldom required for US exams performed in neonates and small children. In this regard it helps to warm the gel and to avoid examining hungry infants. It may be a good idea to show the children toys or movies to hold their attention during the study.

1.2.2
Normal US Appearance and Artifacts

The normal aerated lung produces echogenic images with characteristic posterior comet-tail reverberations behind the visceral pleura. These echogenic structures are induced by the air flowing in the alveoli and their intensity depends on their distance from the probe. When using a subcostal approach the comet-tail reverberations related to the aerated lung bases are observed adjacent to the diaphragm (Fig. 1.1). During respiration the normal lung exhibits

in real time a characteristic to-and-fro movement against the visceral pleura, known as the "gliding sign" (BEN-AMI et al. 1993; SEIBERT et al. 1998).

The main *artifacts* produced on US study of the aerated lung parenchyma are the so-called mirror image artifacts, caused by sound wave reflection when the ultrasound beam strikes the lung surface. Depending on the angle at which the US beam is directed during transdiaphragmatic scanning of the lung base, a dual image of the liver or spleen can be displayed above the diaphragm, simulating parenchymal consolidation. This artifact, known as "pseudo-consolidation" (BEN-AMI et al. 1993) is indicative of

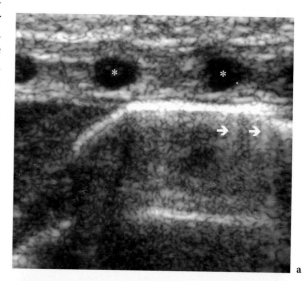

a

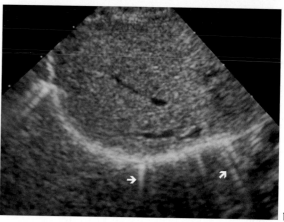

b

Fig. 1.1a,b. Normal lung in a 3-month-old boy. a Parasternal longitudinal US scan shows comet-tail artifacts (*arrows*) evoked by alveolar air-flow. Non-ossified costal cartilage (*asterisks*) allows visualization of the lung and pleura (upper echogenic line). b Transdiaphragmatic transverse view of the right lower lobe. Comet-tail reverberations are seen adjacent to the diaphragm (*arrows*)

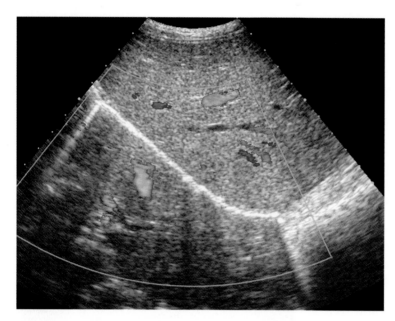

Fig. 1.2. Mirror image artifact. Transdiaphragmatic longitudinal US scan in a 2-month-old boy shows "duplication" of the liver and its Doppler signals, projecting over the right lung base

normal air-filled lung. Mirroring of the image can also occur when using color Doppler, resulting in duplication of vascular structures (Fig. 1.2).

1.2.3
Indications for Lung US

US of the lung parenchyma is indicated for the initial evaluation and follow-up of pulmonary congenital malformations discovered by prenatal ultrasound and to study pulmonary consolidations and masses. It can also be used to guide biopsies of superficially located lung tumors.

1.2.4
Pulmonary Lesions

1.2.4.1
Congenital Malformations of the Lung

Pulmonary sequestration and cystic adenomatoid malformation, which probably result from maldevelopment of the primitive foregut, are the most common congenital malformations of the lung. Some authors consider these two entities to be part of a single spectrum since the histological changes of cystic adenomatoid malformation and sequestration can coexist in the same lesion (MAY et al. 1993).

1.2.4.1.1
Sequestration

Pulmonary sequestration is a congenital malformation composed of pulmonary tissue, which lacks normal connection to the tracheobronchial tree and the pulmonary arteries. The tissue is usually supplied by a systemic artery that arises from the thoracic or abdominal aorta. There are two types: intralobar and extralobar. Intralobar sequestration is contained within the normal visceral pleura, and its venous drainage is through the pulmonary veins. Intralobar sequestration usually occurs in older infants and

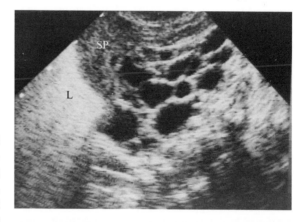

Fig. 1.3. Extralobar cystic sequestration in a 2-week-old boy. Transdiaphragmatic longitudinal view of the upper abdomen depicts multilocular mass in the left suprarenal region. *SP*, spleen; *L*, echogenic lung due to hyaline membrane disease

some authors consider it to be an acquired lesion (FRAZIER et al. 1997). Extralobar sequestration has its own pleural covering and venous drainage is into the systemic circulation (azygos–hemiazygos system, portal vein or inferior vena cava) (MAY et al. 1993; Ko et al. 2000).

Most cases of extralobar sequestration occur in the left hemithorax and are usually discovered prenatally in countries where obstetric sonography is performed routinely. The sequestration typically appears as a solid mass, with echogenicity superior to the normal lung. Visualization of the systemic arterial blood supply to the mass confirms the diagnosis and can be demonstrated with color Doppler sonography. Partial resolution of the echogenic lung mass has been reported on sonograms obtained late in gestation and many of these children are asymptomatic at birth (WINTERS et al. 1997).

At US study, extralobar sequestration is seen as a homogeneous or inhomogeneous echogenic mass usually located in the juxtadiaphragmatic and sometimes in the suprarenal region. Exceptionally it may have a multicystic appearance (Fig. 1.3). Collateral air drift can produce small hyperechogenic nodules within the mass. Enlargement of the azygos–hemiazygos system has been described as an imaging finding of extralobar sequestration (Ko et al. 2000). We recommend a subxiphoid approach to study the mass, to search for an anomalous vessel arising from the aorta and to demonstrate the systemic venous drainage (Fig. 1.4).

1.2.4.1.2
Cystic Adenomatoid Malformation of the Lung

Cystic adenomatoid malformation of the lung is a hamartomatous lesion that results from the arrest of bronchiolar maturation and the overgrowth of mesenchymal elements. Sonographic findings vary depending on the type of malformation (MAY et al. 1993). Type 1 is the most common form and appears as single or multiple large cysts, often involving the entire pulmonary lobe. In Type 2, the mass has an echogenic appearance with numerous small cysts. Type 3 malformations appear as homogeneous echogenic masses without cysts. Sonographic differentiation between cystic adenomatoid malformation and pulmonary sequestration may not be possible. A systemic vessel arising from the aorta has been also described in patients with adenomatoid malformation of the lung (WINTERS et al. 1997).

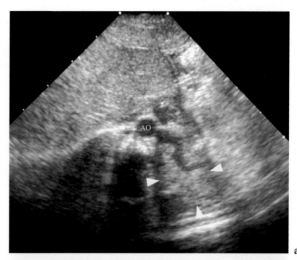

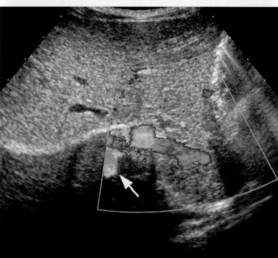

Fig. 1.4a,b. Extralobar solid sequestration in a 2-month-old boy. **a** In this subxifoid transverse scan an echogenic mass (*arrowheads*) can be seen behind the left lobe of the liver. Note tortuous vessel arising from the aorta (*AO*). **b** Color Doppler shows the abnormal vessel arising from the aorta and supplying the mass. Venous drainage is inferred to be through the enlarged azygos (*arrow*)

1.2.4.1.3
Bronchogenic Cyst

Bronchogenic cysts, which result from abnormal budding of the embryonic foregut, are usually located in the subcarinal region and occasionally within the pulmonary parenchyma. Depending on their content, intrapulmonary cysts are seen as unilocular anechoic or weakly echogenic lesions. US is particularly helpful in cases where CT is inconclusive about the solid or cystic nature of the lesion (see Chap. 5, Fig. 5.4c).

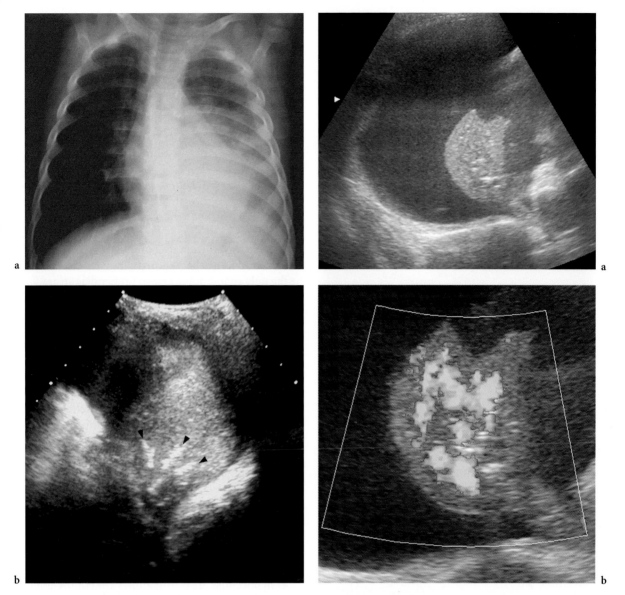

Fig. 1.5a,b. A 6-year-old girl with left-sided pneumonia and pleural effusion. **a** Increased opacity of the left lung base associated with pleural fluid is seen in the chest X-ray. **b** Intercostal oblique US scan with the patient in a prone position shows multiple bright, linear, branching structures (*arrowheads*) corresponding to air sonobronchograms

Fig. 1.6a,b. A 10-year-old boy with pleural effusion. a Transverse US scan of the right hemithorax shows profuse pleural fluid and atelectatic lung. b Crowded pulmonary vessels, characteristic of pulmonary collapse, are demonstrated by power Doppler

1.2.4.2
Lung Consolidation

The two most common lung lesions characterized by a decrease in or absence of pulmonary air are pneumonic consolidation and atelectasis. Pneumonic consolidation refers to filling of the normal air spaces with fluid and inflammatory cells, thereby converting the highly reflective lung into a solid structure through which sound is easily transmitted. Air-filled bronchi can be identified in the consolidated lung as echogenic branching images converging towards the lung root. This feature is known as "sonographic air bronchogram" (WEINBERG et al. 1986; ACUNAS et al. 1986; YANG et al. 1992b; SEIBERT et al. 1998; KIM et al. 2000) and is equivalent to the air bronchogram observed on chest X-rays (Fig. 1.5). The loss of lung volume in atelectasis produces a characteristic crowding of the air-filled bronchi and pulmonary vessels (Fig. 1.6) (WEINBERG et al. 1986).

In patients with asthma, cystic fibrosis or severe inflammatory processes, the bronchi contain mucus or secretions. In these cases, US demonstrates anechoic tubular branching structures known as "sonographic fluid bronchogram" (KIM et al. 2000). The fluid-filled bronchi have imperceptible walls and may contain

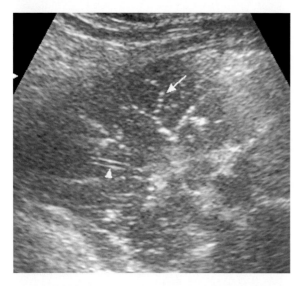

Fig. 1.7. Sonographic fluid bronchogram in a 6-year-old boy with asthma. Intercostal transverse scan shows bright dots that moved in real time over a hypoechoic background (*arrow*). The well-defined walls of the pulmonary vessel are clearly seen (*arrowhead*) while the bronchus wall is imperceptible

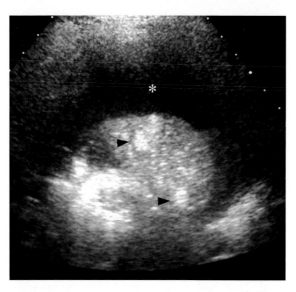

Fig. 1.8. A 12-year-old patient with pneumonia and pleural effusion. Intercostal transverse scan discloses consolidated lung with small echogenic nodules, representing sonoalveolograms (*arrowheads*). The hypoechoic pleural effusion (*asterisk*) delineates the boundary of the lung

air bubbles. On conventional US these features differentiate fluid bronchograms from pulmonary vessels (Fig. 1.7). Definitive differentiation is made by color Doppler. In resolving pneumonia, some air-filled alveoli may produce echogenic nodules within the area of consolidation, a finding that is termed "sonographic air alveologram" (Fig. 1.8) (SEIBERT et al. 1998).

The presence of a sonographic air bronchogram, fluid bronchogram, or air alveologram, or recognition of pulmonary vessels within the lesion are the characteristic features of lung consolidation and are never seen in pleural effusion or tumors. In peripheral lung consolidation, visualization of pulmonary vessels may be the only sonographic clue to proper diagnosis.

In a prospective US study including color and power Doppler in 19 patients with lobar pneumonia, we were able to classify lung consolidation into three groups according to sonographic findings and degree of vascularization:

1. *Well-vascularized pneumonia* (nine patients). In these cases the consolidation presented a homogeneous appearance (similar to the echogenicity of the liver parenchyma) with multiple vascular structures (Fig. 1.9).
2. *Poorly vascularized pneumonia without necrotic areas* (four patients). In contrast to the first type, the number of vessels in the consolidated lung was scant, but the lesion remained homogeneous (Fig. 1.10).
3. *Poorly-vascularized pneumonia with necrotic areas* (six patients). Very few vessels were visible on color Doppler. Consolidation was usually heterogeneous with peripheral areas of cavitation seen as hypoechoic areas, sometimes containing internal echogenic debris (Fig. 1.11).

This last type, known as necrotizing pneumonia, results from necrosis of the lung parenchyma due to occlusion of alveolar capillaries following severe lung infection. *Streptococcus pneumoniae* is one of the most common microorganisms causing this complication in children (KEREM et al. 1994; HEDLUND et al. 1999). In fact, *S. pneumoniae* was the causal agent in four of our six patients with Type 3 pneumonia. In adults, the outcome of necrotizing pneumonia is generally poor and early surgical excision of the gangrenous lung is indicated. However, children can recover completely with medical treatment, although their clinical evolution is long and may require extended hospitalization (BEN-AMI et al. 1993).

The mean hospital stay was 5.6 days for the Type 1 cases, 8.2 days for the patients with Type 2 and 23

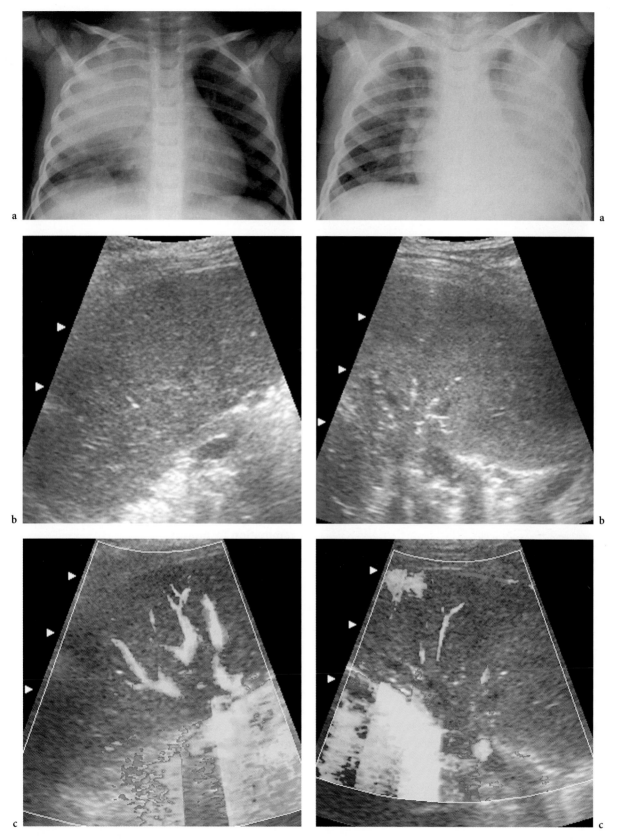

Fig. 1.9a–c. An 8-year-old boy with well-vascularized lobar pneumonia. **a** Chest radiograph shows opacification of the right upper lobe. **b** The consolidated lung has a homogeneous echogenicity (similar to the liver) in this intercostal oblique US scan obtained with the patient in a prone position. **c** Numerous pulmonary vessels are seen at power Doppler

Fig. 1.10a–c. A 6-year-old girl with poorly-vascularized pneumonia. **a** Chest radiograph evidences opacification of the left lung. **b** Intercostal oblique US scan with the patient in a prone position shows homogeneous appearance of the affected lung base with central air sonobronchograms. **c** Very few vessels are seen within the consolidation

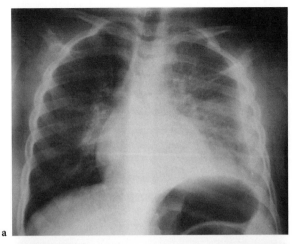

a

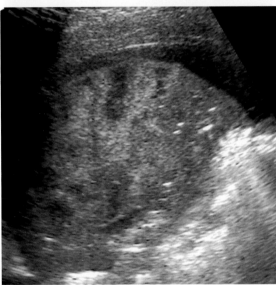

b

Fig. 1.11a,b. Pneumonia with necrotic areas in a 7-year-old boy. **a** Increased opacity in the left lower lobe and pleural effusion is visualized in the X-ray. **b** US scan discloses very heterogeneous appearance of the left lung base with peripheral hypoechoic areas representing necrosis. The sonolucent band corresponds to pleural fluid. High resolution CT (not shown) confirmed the diagnosis of necrotizing pneumonia

days for the patients with Type 3. Thus, in our experience, US provides diagnostic and prognostic information which may influence therapy in children with lobar pneumonia.

Contrast-enhanced chest CT in children with lobar pneumonia can provide information similar to that obtained with chest US (DONNELLY and KLOSTERMAN 1997).

Chest X-ray is the initial imaging procedure used in cases of suspected pneumonia. According to our

experience we recommend complementary chest US studies in patients with pneumonia and associated pleural fluid, in those with lobar pneumonia and severe clinical symptoms and in patients who do not respond well to antibiotic therapy.

When studying consolidation, the radiologist should be aware of the inability of US to determine the extent of a deep lesion. Acoustic reverberation artifacts, caused by areas of aerated lung interposed between the transducer and the area of interest, can hinder visualization of the entire lesion.

1.2.4.3
Lung Tumors

Primary lung tumors, including blastoma, muco-epidermoid carcinoma, hemangiopericytoma and rhabdomyosarcoma, are rare in children. The most common of these is pulmonary blastoma. It usually has a complex echogenic appearance and is located in the periphery of the lung. Due to the peripheral location of this lesion, sonography can be used to guide percutaneous biopsy of the mass.

1.3
Pleura

1.3.1
Examination Technique

The pleura is located very superficially and is therefore easily evaluated by sonography. Most of the pleural surface can be imaged through intercostal and subcostal approaches. However, the mediastinal and the apical pleurae require scanning through the parasternal or supraclavicular approaches, respectively (BEN-AMI et al. 1993; WERNECKE 2000).

Excellent visualization of the pleura–lung interface is obtained with high frequency (8–10 MHz) convex or linear transducers applied at the intercostal, parasternal and supraclavicular spaces. Sector or convex transducers are recommended when using the subcostal approach. While performing the study, certain ultrasound features that are of great diagnostic value should be carefully observed. In real-time sonography, the visceral pleura moves with the respiratory excursions and recognition of this movement provides clues to the diagnosis of several pathologies, such as pneumothorax and pleural infiltration by pulmonary or extrapleural tumors. The absence of visceral pleura movement is a useful finding for sonographic diagnosis of pneumothorax. Similarly, observation of a fixed pulmonary tumor during respiration indicates that the pleura is infiltrated (WERNECKE 2000).

1.3.2
Normal Sonographic Appearance and Artifacts

The pleura is composed of two membranes, the visceral and parietal pleurae. They are separated by a potential space, which can be inferred as a thin hypoechoic band during the respiratory excursions of the visceral pleura in real-time. On the intercostal longitudinal scan, the pleura is visualized as an intensely echogenic linear structure that acquires a curving configuration at the transverse view (Fig.1.12). On subcostal studies the diaphragm, seen as a bright, curving, echogenic line, cannot be differentiated from the parietal pleura covering its thoracic side.

Mirror artifacts are often seen when studying the pleura. These consist in a "duplication" of structures external to the pleura projected over the lung and are caused by reflection of the sound waves at the pleural surface when the US beam strikes it at certain angles (see Figs. 1.2 and 1.36). As a consequence, intercostal muscles of the chest wall can be projected over the lung, simulating pulmonary pathology. This physical phenomenon can also produce a double image of the diaphragm. The two sonographic diaphragms (the anatomic diaphragm and the duplicated image) are separated by a hypolucent band, probably corresponding to the liver, which can be misinterpreted as pleural effusion.

1.3.3
Indications for Pleural US

We believe that ultrasound should replace decubitus chest radiographs as the routine imaging technique to confirm suspected pleural effusion. Massive pleural effusion is one of the main causes of opaque hemithorax seen on chest X-ray films. Ultrasound is extremely useful for studying children with this radiologic finding, which can also be due to other entities, such as pulmonary masses or consolidation. US easily identifies the cause of the opaque chest X-ray and avoids unnecessary invasive procedures (Fig.1.13).

US can also be used to provide imaging guidance for pleural drainage procedures, particularly when the pleural fluid is loculated. With US one can determine the depth of the collection and decide on the safest manner and approach to drain it (SHANKAR et al. 2000). Pneumothorax, the most common complication of pleural taps is exceedingly rare when the procedure is performed under US control (RAPTOPOULOS et al. 1991). In patients with malignant intrathoracic or extrathoracic tumors, pleural implants may "hide" behind pleural fluid collections and go unnoticed on chest X-rays. In these patients, sonography can be

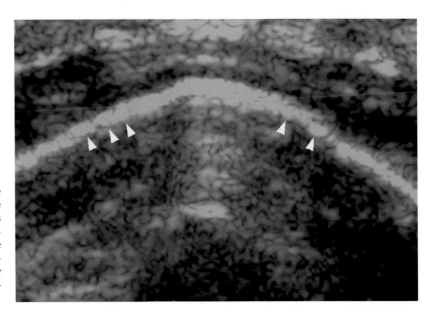

Fig. 1.12. Intercostal transverse view of the normal pleura. The curving pleura-lung interface is well visualized. The small echogenic dots superimposed on the linear interface (*arrowheads*) represent air in the alveoli as they glide against the pleura with respiratory motion

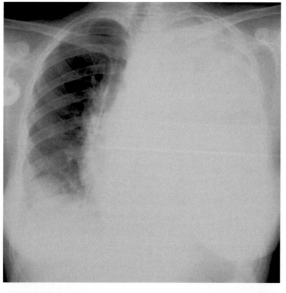

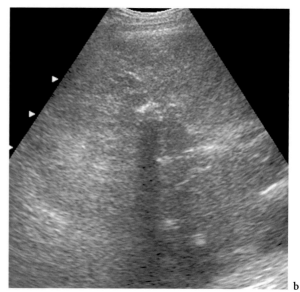

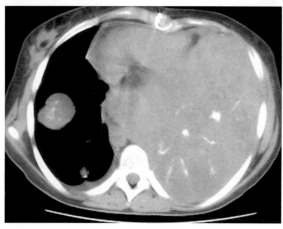

Fig. 1.13a–c. Opaque left hemithorax in a 17-year-old boy with osteogenic sarcoma of the left femur. a Chest X-ray shows opaque hemithorax with increased volume, suggesting massive pleural effusion as well as a nodule in the right lower lobe. b Intercostal transverse US scan rules out pleural fluid and demonstrates that the left hemithorax is occupied by a huge solid mass with echogenic areas and acoustic shadowing, suggestive of calcifications. c Unenhanced CT demonstrates a huge, partially ossified metastasis on the left and the right pulmonary nodule

useful to indicate the origin of the pleural collection and to guide pleural biopsy (SHETH et al. 2000).

1.3.4
Pleural Abnormalities

1.3.4.1
Pneumothorax

Small pockets of air in the pleural space appear as bright, echogenic lines or points. In contrast to what is seen in the normal aerated lung, the image of air in the pleural space does not show comet-tail artifacts, always evoked by air flow in the alveoli (Fig. 1.14). A large pneumothorax can impede visualization of visceral pleura movement, an important indirect sign of air in the pleural space. The presence of air and fluid in the pleural space (hydropneumothorax) results in an air-fluid level on US that can produce a particular movement in real time known as the "curtain sign" (BEN-AMI et al. 1993).

Chest X-ray remains the method of choice for the diagnosis of pneumothorax, but several projections may be required to reveal its presence. In severely ill or traumatized patients who cannot be easily moved, pneumothorax can be confirmed or ruled out using US without changing the patient's position.

1.3.4.2
Pleural Effusions

Sonography is much more sensitive than the supine X-ray for establishing the diagnosis of pleural effu-

fibrin strands, septations (Fig. 1.18), or a honeycomb appearance (Fig. 1.19). Recognition of the septated nature of the pleural collection, information that influences patient management, is not usually provided by chest CT scans (Fig. 1.20).

The sonographic appearance of pleural effusion can be related to the classical division of pleural fluid into exudate or transudate according to its protein content, pleural/serum lactate dehydrogenase (LDH) ratio and other biochemical parameters. On sonography, both transudates and exudates can be anechoic; however, collections presenting some of the complicated features mentioned above are always exudates.

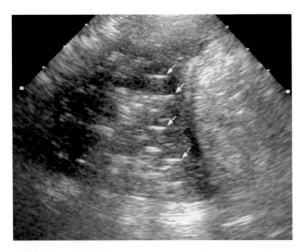

Fig. 1.14. Longitudinal transdiaphragmatic US scan of the lung base in a 7-year-old girl. Air bubbles within the pleural effusion are seen as linear echogenic images without comet-tail artifacts (*arrows*)

sion (EIBENBERGER et al. 1991). On US imaging through an intercostal approach, pleural fluid is identified as a band-like collection separating the parietal and visceral pleura surfaces. When scanning through the abdomen, the collection is seen just above the diaphragm, blurring the costophrenic angle (Fig. 1.15).

There are several sonographic signs typical of pleural fluid that help to distinguish it from ascites. The three most important are: (1) presence of septa within the collection that move with respiration, (2) the "crus sign", and (3) the "bare area sign" (Seibert et al. 1998). The crus sign, pathognomonic of pleural collection, results from displacement of the diaphragmatic crus away from the spine due to interposition of fluid between this structure and the vertebral column (Fig. 1.16). The posterior part of the right lobe of the liver is known as the "bare area" because it is directly attached to the diaphragm without the covering layer of peritoneum. Peritoneal fluid cannot extend behind the right lobe at this point; thus, all fluid collections visualized behind the bare area are necessarily located in the pleural space.

The main role of sonography in the study of pleural effusion is to characterize the simple or complicated nature of the fluid (YANG et al. 1992a). Pleural effusion presenting an anechoic appearance on US study is considered to be simple. Complicated effusions are those that present one or more of the following features: weakly echogenic debris with a swirling movement in real time (Fig. 1.17), thick mobile

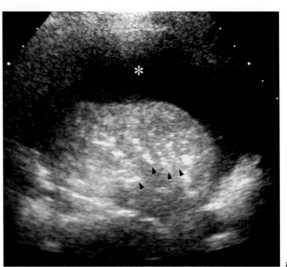

a

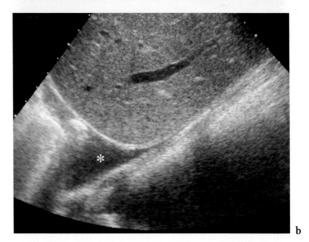

b

Fig. 1.15a,b. Sonographic appearance of pleural effusion. **a** The pleural fluid (*asterisk*) is seen as an anechoic band between the parietal and visceral pleurae in this intercostal, transverse US scan. Note air-bronchograms (*arrowheads*) in the consolidated lung. **b** Longitudinal sector scan through the liver shows the pleural fluid (*asterisk*) occupying the costophrenic angle

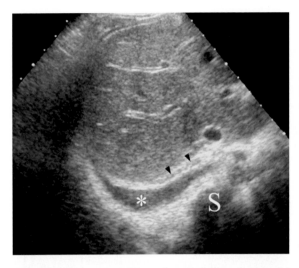

Fig. 1.16. Sector transverse US scan through the liver shows useful sonographic findings that differentiate pleural effusion from ascites. Pleural effusion (*asterisk*) displaces the right diaphragmatic crus (*arrowheads*) away from the spine (*S*) and extends behind the right posterior portion of the liver (*bare area*)

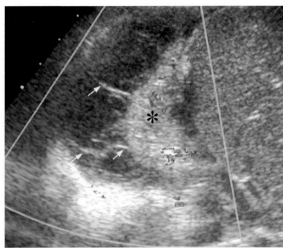

Fig. 1.18. Right sector intercostal longitudinal view demonstrates a collapsed right lower lobe (*asterisk*) surrounded by pleural effusion with multiple fibrin bands (*arrows*)

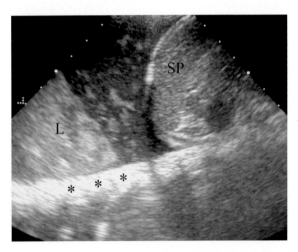

Fig. 1.17. Pleural effusion with floating debris. Longitudinal transdiaphragmatic US demonstrates pleural effusion containing echogenic particles (evidencing its exudative nature) located between the spleen (*SP*) and the consolidated left lower lobe (*L*). The high echogenicity of the ribs (*asterisks*) results from good transmission of the sound beam through the consolidated lung and pleural fluid

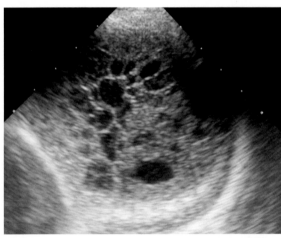

Fig. 1.19. Left transverse, intercostal scan in an 8-year-old boy with streptococcal pneumonia. The pleural space is filled with profuse septations with a honeycomb appearance. This type of collection is not amenable to thoracentesis

Most exudative pleural effusions in pediatric patients are of infectious origin (ALKRINAWI and CHERNICK 1996). These collections are known as parapneumonic effusions, a term that is often used interchangeably with empyema. The diagnosis of empyema is established when pleural fluid is grossly purulent, organisms are identified on Gram stain or culture, pleural fluid has a white blood cell count greater than 5×10^9 cells/L, pH is below 7.0 or glucose level is less than 40 mg/dL.

There is still a great deal of controversy surrounding the clinical management of parapneumonic effusion and empyema (KORNECKI and SIVAN 1997; KRISHNAN et al. 1997; GIVAN and EIGEN 1998; RAMNATH et al. 1998). Two main treatment approaches

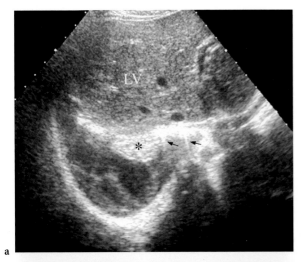

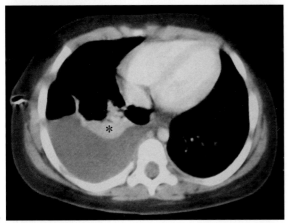

Fig. 1.20a,b. Transverse US scan through the liver (*L*) (**a**) and enhanced CT scan (**b**) of a 5-year-old girl with pleural pneumonia. The compressed, atelectatic lung (*asterisk*) is clearly seen in both studies, but the septated nature of the pleural collection is only evident on the US scan. Note comet-tail artifacts in the normal aerated lung adjacent to the collapse (*arrows*)

lations and septations on US studies, most authors advocate the use of IV antibiotics, together with intrapleural fibrinolytics, mainly urokinase, administered through a thoracostomy tube (PARK et al. 1996; BOUROS et al. 1997). When these measures fail, decortication or video thoracostomy may shorten the lengthy hospital stay (KRISHNAN et al. 1997; KORNECKI and SIVAN 1997). In patients with a severe honeycomb pattern on the initial US scan, early surgical treatment should be considered.

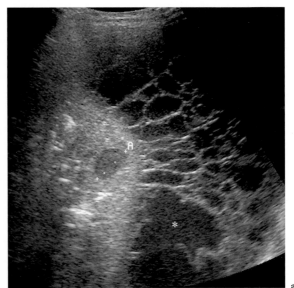

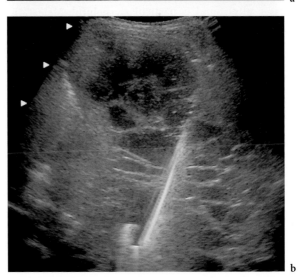

Fig. 1.21a,b. Pleural effusion with multiple septations in a 12-year-old boy with cavitary pneumonia. **a** Caliper measures area of necrosis in the affected lung. The large loculus (*asterisk*) is selected for urokinase instillation by means of an ultrasound-guided pigtail catheter (**b**)

are used: non-surgical, in which patients are treated with antibiotics alone or combined with thoracocentesis or tube thoracostomy; and surgical, consisting of pleural débridement or decortication. The goal of both these methods of treatment is to evacuate infected debris and re-expand the lung, and to reduce hospital stay and morbidity.

Patients who present pleural fluid with few echoes due to debris (low-grade pleural effusion) can be treated with antibiotics alone or antibiotics plus external tube drainage. It has been reported that there is no difference in length of hospitalization between patients treated with either of these options (RAMNATH et al. 1998). In patients presenting locu-

Management of these patients according to the US appearance of pleural collections seems clear-cut; however, in our experience small exudates can rapidly (within 24 h) increase in volume and change their sonographic appearance, despite antibiotic therapy. Thus, close sonographic surveillance of children with pleuro-pneumonia is recommended.

It is clear that sonography has important implications in the management of pleural effusion because of its ability to characterize the internal composition of pleural fluid and monitor the course of the underlying process. Moreover, it is a valuable tool for localizing loculations for thoracocentesis or thoracostomy tube placement (Fig. 1.21). The incidence of pneumothorax is considerably reduced when pleural taps are sonographically guided, particularly in the case of small or loculated collections (RAPTOPOULOS et al. 1991; SHANKAR et al. 2000).

1.3.4.3
Pleural Tumors

Primary tumors originating in the pleura, such as mesothelioma, are very rare in children, and tumoral involvement of this structure is most often due to metastasis. Metastatic disease to the pleura often causes large pleural effusions that are probably due to impaired lymphatic drainage. This secondary pleural fluid, which can be profuse in some patients, may mask the tumoral mass on chest X-rays and in these cases ultrasound is particularly helpful. Metastatic involvement of the pleura can be caused by various intrathoracic or extrathoracic tumors, such as Wilms' tumor, lymphoma, neuroblastoma and rhabdomyosarcoma. These are generally seen as well-delineated, solid echogenic masses (Fig. 1.22).

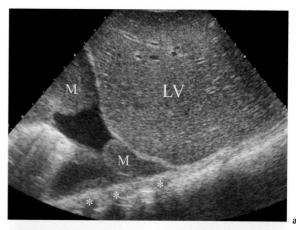

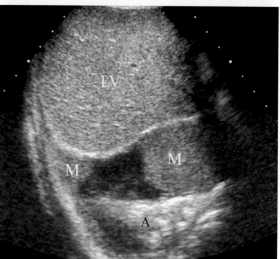

Fig. 1.22a,b. Pleural metastasis in a 5-year-old boy with rhabdomyosarcoma of the biliary tract. **a** Longitudinal view through the liver (*LV*) shows several echogenic nodules (*M*) associated with pleural effusion. The chest wall is delineated by echogenic ribs (*asterisks*). **b** Transverse view additionally demonstrates a crowded bronchogram that differentiates the atelectatic lung (*A*) from the metastatic masses (*M*)

1.4
Mediastinum

1.4.1
Examination Technique

To study the mediastinum in the pediatric population, we recommend small sector or convex multifrequency probes. High-frequency linear transducers are particularly useful in newborns or for studying lesions located superficially. It is advisable to adjust the depth to the region of interest, decrease the number of foci, and reduce the lateral field of vision

in order to increase the frame rate. We recommend including a large vessel or cardiac chamber in the field of study to establish anatomic relationships and to analyze the echogenicity of the lesion to determine if it is cystic or solid.

We divide the mediastinum into anterior, middle and posterior compartments. The anterior mediastinum or prevascular region is found in front of the superior vena cava, aorta and pulmonary artery, and behind the sternum. The middle mediastinum can be further divided into four anatomic regions: paratracheal, supra-aortic, aortopulmonary and subcarinal.

The paratracheal region refers to the right paratracheal area. The supra-aortic refers to the upper portion of the left paratracheal region, above the aortic arch. The aortopulmonary region includes the area below the aortic arch and above the right pulmonary artery and the left bronchus. The subcarinal region is located behind the bifurcation of the pulmonary artery, above the left atrium in front of the esophagus and below the carina. The posterior mediastinum comprises the pre- and paravertebral spaces.

The anterior and middle mediastinum can be well accessed with the following approaches: suprasternal, supraclavicular, parasternal, subxiphoid, and subcostal; the most important of these are the suprasternal and the left parasternal. When using the suprasternal approach, the patient should be in a supine decubitus position with a cushion under the back and the neck slightly extended. The transducer is placed above the sternal manubrium and tilted caudally. To obtain an oblique sagittal view, the probe is displaced laterally to encounter the space between the trachea and sternocleidomastoid muscle. For the parasternal approaches, a right or left lateral decubitus position (the examined side down) is recommended to displace the mediastinum downwards and increase the acoustic window.

The supraclavicular approach is useful for increasing the field of view of the paratracheal regions. The subxiphoid and subcostal approaches are used to visualize the cardiophrenic and retrocrural regions, which will be discussed in Sect. 1.4.5.3. If the sternum is not completely ossified, the trans-sternal approach can be used to study the prevascular and subcarinal regions. The latter region can also be visualized in young children using the thymus as an acoustic window. In older children the subcarinal area can be accessed through the cardiac chambers, placing the transducer at the fifth intercostal space, in an oblique position. The posterior mediastinum is accessed through a paravertebral approach.

1.4.2
Normal US Appearance, Artifacts and Pitfalls

Sonographic study of the mediastinum requires a meticulous technique and extensive knowledge of the mediastinal anatomy. We recommend the use of five standard sonographic slices (three obtained with the suprasternal approach and two with the left parasternal) to visualize the complete anterior and middle regions of the mediastinum. We stress that these standard US slices differ from those obtained with CT. The majority are obtained in oblique, coronal or sagittal planes and, therefore, the same slice may show structures corresponding to more than one anatomic region.

Oblique Coronal View Through the Suprasternal Approach. This section is used to visualize the paratracheal region, located between the right upper pulmonary lobe and the trachea. It is also useful for studying the aortopulmonary region, which is seen in this view as an echogenic triangular image. The probe is placed almost perpendicular to, and slightly compressing, the right sternocleidomastoid muscle. The anatomic reference for this region is the innominate artery and the scan should include the pleural surface of the right upper lobe, the trachea and the upper margin of the left bronchus. The paratracheal region is a virtual space and is considered normal when the pleural surface of the upper lobe abuts the trachea. Pathology in this region is recognized by a separation of these two structures (Fig. 1.23).

Coronal View Through the Suprasternal Approach. This scan is not used to study a specific mediastinal region, but is very useful for visualizing the vessels, particularly the superior vena cava. The view should include the right pulmonary artery and its bifurcation, located within the mediastinum (Fig. 1.24). It is particularly helpful to confirm or rule out superior vena cava thrombosis in patients with a central venous catheter.

Oblique Parasagittal View Through the Suprasternal Approach. This view is used to visualize the aortopulmonary region, which has a characteristic ultrasound appearance and should be identified in all patients submitted to mediastinal exams. The probe is placed above the sternal manubrium between the trachea and left sternocleidomastoid muscle. Due to the presence of mediastinal fat at this level, the aortopulmonary region is seen as a highly echogenic, half-moon-shaped image. The anatomic reference for this region is the aortic arch and the section should also include the origins of the left carotid and subclavian arteries (Fig. 1.25).

Axial View Through the Left Parasternal Approach. This section is used to study the subcarinal and prevascular regions and is similar to the CT slices obtained for this area. The transducer is placed at the second intercostal space. The anatomic reference for this view is the pulmonary artery bifurcation (Fig. 1.26).

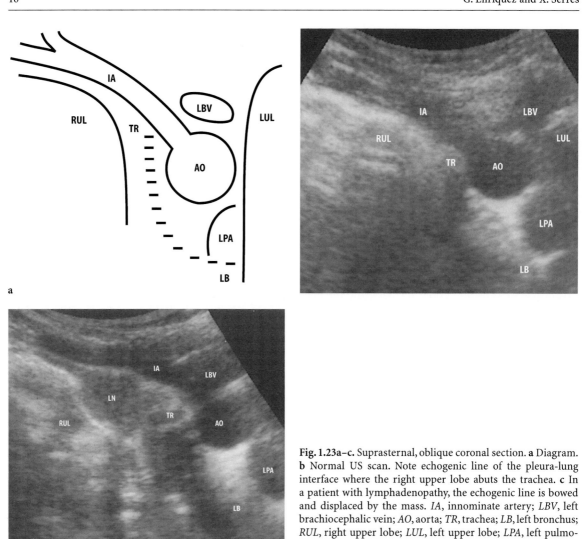

a

b

c

Fig. 1.23a–c. Suprasternal, oblique coronal section. **a** Diagram.
b Normal US scan. Note echogenic line of the pleura-lung
interface where the right upper lobe abuts the trachea. **c** In
a patient with lymphadenopathy, the echogenic line is bowed
and displaced by the mass. *IA,* innominate artery; *LBV,* left
brachiocephalic vein; *AO,* aorta; *TR,* trachea; *LB,* left bronchus;
RUL, right upper lobe; *LUL,* left upper lobe; *LPA,* left pulmonary artery; *LN,* lymph node

a

b

Fig. 1.24a,b. Suprasternal coronal section. **a.** Diagram. **b.** Normal US scan. *RBV,* right brachiocephalic vein; *LBV,* left brachiocephalic vein; *AO,* aorta; *RUL,* right upper lobe; *LUL,* left upper lobe; *RPA,* right pulmonary artery; *VC,* vena cava. The *dot*
indicates a mirror artifact of the vessels adjacent to the pleura, mimicking pleural effusion

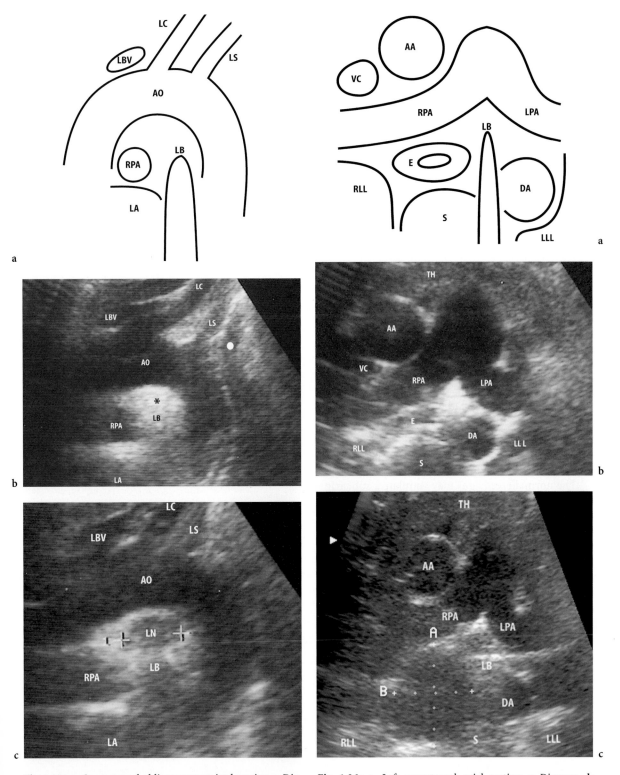

Fig. 1.25a–c. Suprasternal oblique parasagittal section. **a** Diagram. **b** Normal US scan. Note the normal hyperechoic appearance of the aortopulmonary region (*asterisk*). **c** US scan in a patient with lymphadenopathy in this region. *LBV*, left brachiocephalic vein; *AO*, aorta; *RPA*, right pulmonary artery; *LC*, left carotid artery; *LS*, left subclavian artery; *LA*, left atrium; *LB*, left bronchus; *LN*, lymph node; *dot*, vessel mirror artifact

Fig. 1.26a–c. Left parasternal axial section. **a** Diagram. **b** Normal US scan. **c** US scan in a patient with lymphadenopathy (*A*, *B*, calipers) in the subcarinal space. *TH*, thymus; *AA*, ascending aorta; *DA*, descending aorta; *E*, esophagus; *RPA*, right pulmonary artery; *LPA*, left pulmonary artery; *VC*, vena cava; *LB*, left bronchus; *RLL*, right lower lobe; *LLL*, left lower lobe; *S*, spine

Parasagittal View Through the Left Parasternal Approach. Also used to study the subcarinal and prevascular regions, the references for this section are the ascending aorta, the trachea and the esophagus (Fig. 1.27). It is important to identify the esophagus by making the patient swallow saliva or water. For the two parasternal approaches, the patients should be placed in a left decubitus position to increase the size of the anatomic acoustic window.

A number of artifacts are generated during mediastinal sonography. Among the most common are "mirror artifacts" consisting in duplicated images of vessels or normal and abnormal structures adjacent to the mediastinal pleura. Vascular "duplication" in this location can simulate a pleural fluid collection. The tracheal and bronchial cartilage can interrupt the air column in these structures and produce multiple parallel echogenic images with a step-ladder appearance that we refer to as "stair artifact" (Fig. 1.28).

Some normal anatomic structures, such as the pericardial recesses and the esophagus can have a misleading sonographic appearance and simulate pathology. For example, the superior pericardial recess can mimic adenopathy in the aortopulmonary region (Fig. 1.29). The location, triangular shape, changes in size with the heartbeat, and anechoic appearance are the clues that differentiate the pericardial recess from lymph nodes.

The normal esophagus may simulate a subcarinal solid mass, but can be properly identified by making the patient swallow during the exam (Fig. 1.30).

1.4.3
Indications for Mediastinal US

Scanning of children with mediastinal widening, evaluation of vascular anomalies and the search for lymph nodes are the main indications for mediastinal US in children. It can also be used to assess possible complications in patients with indwelling catheters and to perform biopsies.

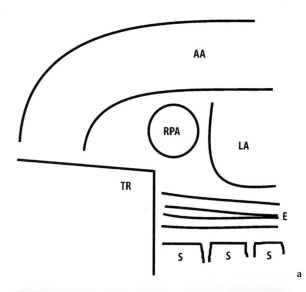

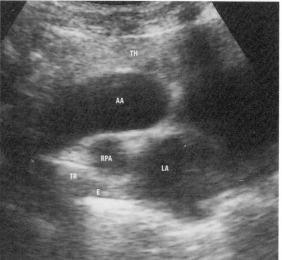

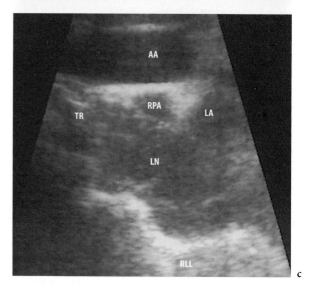

Fig. 1.27a–c. Left parasternal parasagittal section. **a** Diagram. **b** Normal US scan. **c** US scan in a patient with lymphadenopathy in the subcarinal space compressing the right pulmonary artery. *AA*, ascending aorta; *RPA*, right pulmonary artery; *LA*, left atrium; *S*, spine; *TR*, trachea; *TH*, thymus; *E*, esophagus; *LN*, lymph node

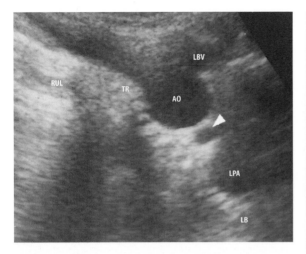

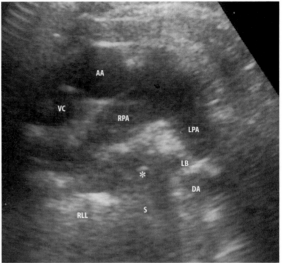

a

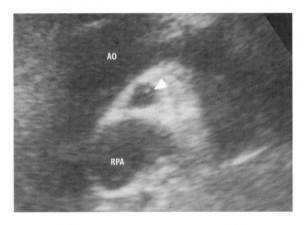

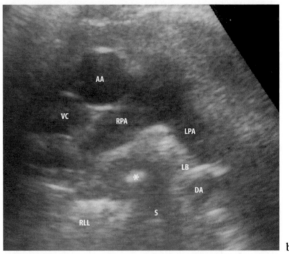

b

Fig. 1.28. Suprasternal oblique coronal view shows a stair-step artifact caused by tracheal (*TR*) and left bronchial (*LB*) cartilage. *Arrowhead* shows superior sinus of the pericardium. *RUL*, right upper lobe; *LBV*, left brachiocephalic vein; *LPA*, left pulmonary artery

Fig. 1.29. Suprasternal oblique parasagittal section shows the superior pericardial recess (*arrowhead*) simulating adenopathy in the aortopulmonary region. Its typical triangular shape and anechoic echotexture permit proper identification. Compare with Fig. 1.25c. *AO*, aorta; *RPA*, right pulmonary artery; *LA*, left atrium

Fig. 1.30a,b. a Esophagus (*asterisk*) simulates a mass in the subcarinal region in this axial view through the left parasternal approach. **b** After the patient swallows, an echogenic image (*asterisk*) corresponding to saliva identifies the esophagus. *AA*, ascending aorta; *DA*, descending aorta; *RPA*, right pulmonary artery; *LPA*, left pulmonary artery; *LB*, left bronchus; *RLL*, right lower lobe; *S*, spine; *VC*, vena cava

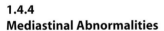

1.4.4
Mediastinal Abnormalities

For illustrative purposes, we have organized mediastinal pathologies according to the region (anterior, middle and posterior) where they most frequently occur.

1.4.4.1
Anterior Mediastinum

Anterior mediastinum pathology in children is commonly related to the thymus; thus, knowledge of the normal US appearance of this organ is essential to recognize lesions in this compartment. On chest X-rays the thymus is identified by characteristic radiological signs, such as the "sail" and "thymic wave" signs. However, it often has a misleading appearance on plain films and simulates a mediastinal mass. In this situation US can clarify the doubtful findings and avoid the practice of more invasive explorations.

On US, the normal thymus has a bilobulated appearance and a homogeneous echotexture with some echogenic strands (KIM et al. 2000). It is hypoechoic relative to the thyroid gland and has a smooth, well-defined margin due to its fibrous capsule. It is a soft organ that does not compress neighboring vascular structures, a characteristic that can help the radiologist to differentiate it from mediastinal masses (Fig. 1.31). The normal thymus can vary considerably in position, extension, size and configuration. In small children the organ can extend from the cervical region to the diaphragm (SWISCHUK and JOHN 1996). During respiration and particularly when the child is crying, the thymus can displace to above the sternal manubrium and simulate a cervical mass (Fig. 1.32).

One important characteristic of the thymus is its tendency to vary in size in response to acute stress. Rapid and severe involution of the gland, a process mediated by endogenous corticosteroid production, occurs in numerous clinical situations (e.g. burns, chemotherapy, severe disease). Weeks to months after cessation of the stress, the thymus can regenerate and even enlarge by "rebound growth". This enlargement

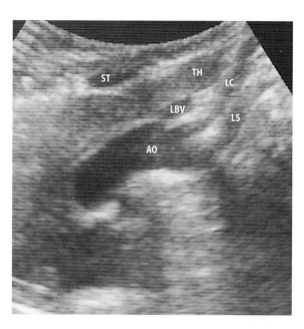

Fig. 1.32. Oblique suprasternal sagittal view in a 2-month-old boy evidences cervical extension of the thymus (*TH*), which is seen anterior to left carotid (*LC*) and left subclavian (*LS*) arteries. *AO*, aorta; *ST*, sternum; *LBV*, left brachiocephalic vein

of the thymus affects both the cortex and medulla and must be differentiated from thymic growth associated with autoimmune diseases. Thymic growth in these cases is known as lymphoid follicular hyperplasia and affects only the medulla. It is a frequent finding in children with HIV infection.

Thymic aplasia and hypoplasia are two congenital anomalies generally associated with immunologic deficiency syndromes, such as DiGeorge's syndrome, Nezelof's disease, and ataxia telangiectasia. Other congenital alterations of the thymus include position anomalies, which are classified as ectopic or aberrant (KOUMANIDOU et al. 1998). Ectopic thymus refers to thymic tissue located in any position except the normal pathway of embryologic descent of the gland. It is occasionally a life-threatening condition due to airway compression. US can detect this anomaly, but is not helpful in patients with ectopic tissue located behind the trachea or in the posterior mediastinum. Aberrant thymus refers to thymic tissue located anywhere along the normal pathway of embryologic descent of the gland. This condition is predominantly asymptomatic and presents as a cervical or suprasternal mass, which can be easily characterized by US. Aberrant thymus should be suspected when the mass presents the same echogenicity as normal thymus (Fig. 1.33).

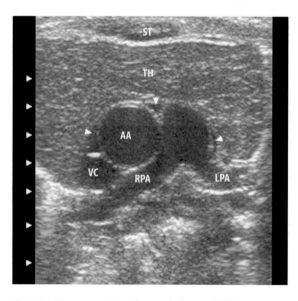

Fig. 1.31. Transverse view of normal thymus (*TH*) in a 4-year-old boy. Vascular structures are not compressed by the gland, which has a rounded configuration. *AA*, ascending aorta; *VC*, vena cava; *RPA*, right pulmonary artery; *LPA*, left pulmonary artery; *ST*, sternum; *arrowheads*, superior pericardial recesses

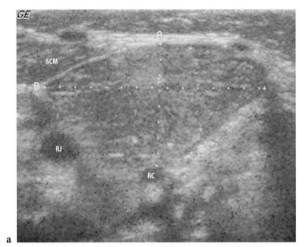

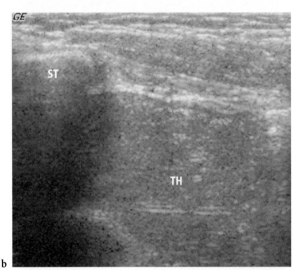

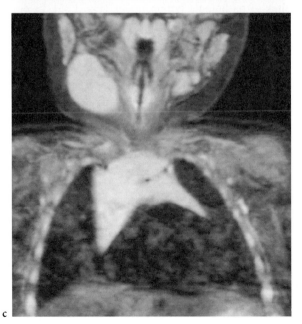

With the use of sonography, thymic cysts are now increasingly detected. They are seen as well-defined uni- or multilocular anechoic lesions, which can have peripheral calcifications (RUDICK and WOOD 1980). Multilocular thymic cysts are seen in approximately 1% of pediatric patients with HIV infection (AVILA et al. 1996) and, since this entity does not require specific treatment, US is recommended for serial follow up.

Primary tumors of the thymus (thymolipoma and thymoma) are exceedingly rare in children. Most thymic tumors in the pediatric age group are secondary to lymphoma or leukemia. The affected gland enlarges and appears as a hypoechoic, heterogeneous, fixed mass compressing the adjacent anatomic structures (LEMAITRE et al. 1987; HAMRICK-TURNER et al. 1994; KIM et al. 2000). All thymic masses that are heterogeneous on US should be further examined by CT or MRI.

Germ cell tumors include a wide spectrum of histological types (teratoma, seminoma, endodermal sinus tumor, choriocarcinoma and embryonal carcinoma) and 94% are located in the anterior mediastinum. The most common germ cell tumor is mature teratoma. On US the tumor may be mostly cystic or have a complex appearance with echogenic fat, soft tissue components and calcifications. In contrast to normal thymus, these tumors often compress the neighboring anatomic structures (Fig. 1.34). CT and MRI are superior to US for delineating the extension of the tumor and for detecting spread to the pericardium or pleura in cases of tumor rupture, a common occurrence in mediastinal teratoma (SASAKA et al. 1998). Lipomas and lymphangiomas are benign tumors that often extend from the cervical area to the anterior mediastinum through the thoracic inlet. Although they can be detected with US, MRI better delineates the entire tumor, including the cervical extension (CASTELLOTE et al. 1999).

Fig. 1.33a–c. Aberrant thymus in a 1-month-old boy with a right cervical mass. **a** US axial view shows the mass (between calipers *A, B*) located in front of the right jugular vein (*RJ*) and right carotid artery (*RC*) and medial to the right sternocleidomastoid muscle (*SCM*). **b** The mass presents the same echogenicity as the normal retrosternal thymus (*TH*); *ST*, sternum. **c** On coronal frequency-selective saturation (FATSAT) MRI, T2-weighted image the cervical mass presents a signal intensity identical to normal thymus

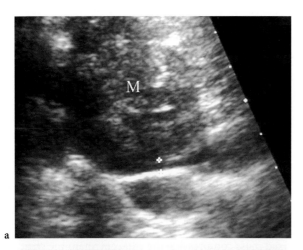

a

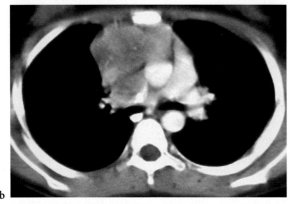

b

Fig. 1.34a,b. Germ cell tumor of the anterior mediastinum in a 4-year-old girl. **a** Transverse US scan obtained with a parasternal approach shows a mass (*M*) with heterogeneous echotexture compressing the superior vena cava (between calipers). **b** Enhanced CT scan reveals the same findings as US. Note compression of the superior vena cava

1.4.4.2
Middle Mediastinum

The lesions usually found in the middle mediastinum are congenital malformations (including vascular anomalies) and lymphadenopathy. The most common congenital malformations are bronchogenic cysts, esophageal duplication cysts and neuroenteric cysts. Bronchogenic cysts, generally located in the subcarinal region, are usually seen as solitary thin-walled anechoic masses with a serous content that can vary in shape during respiration. In some cases fatty material or mucus within the cysts causes internal echoes that simulate a solid mass. Swirling of internal debris seen on real-time examination, the rounded shape, and well-defined wall are the clues

that differentiate bronchogenic cyst from a solid mass. Patients are usually asymptomatic, but internal bleeding or infection can produce a sudden increase in size and associated symptoms of airway compression (DAVIS AND UMLAS 1992).

Most esophageal duplication cysts are found along the lower third of the esophagus. Neuroenteric cysts are the least common type of congenital cysts and are due to incomplete separation of the notochord from the foregut. Although they may be found in the middle mediastinum, they are more common in the posterior mediastinum (paravertebral region) and are often associated with congenital defects of the spine. Due to the different growth patterns of the spine and the thoracic cage, the level of the cyst may not coincide with that of the associated spinal defect. The sonographic features of both esophageal and neuroenteric cysts are identical to those of bronchogenic cysts.

Vascular malformations, including double aortic arch, aberrant left pulmonary artery and anomalous venous return, can also be detected by US. However, MRI is the technique of choice for the study of these malformations.

Lymphadenopathy, secondary to infectious, neoplastic, immunologic, toxic or metabolic processes is the most common mass found in the middle mediastinum. At US lymphadenopathy is seen as scattered or clustered nodules with varying degrees of echogenicity. These clusters are more easily identified by US than CT, where they can simulate a simple solid mass. The right paratracheal region, pulmonary hilum and subcarinal space are the most common sites of pathologic lymph nodes (Fig. 1.35). In our experience most mediastinal lymphadenopathies are of infectious origin. We have observed them in 83% of children with pneumonia of undetermined cause, 94% of children with tuberculosis disease [positive protein purified derivate (PPD), clinical symptoms and abnormalities on chest X-ray] and 50% of children infected by tuberculosis (positive PPD, no respiratory symptoms and normal chest X-ray). The US appearance of tuberculous nodes can change following treatment and present a hypoechoic center and echogenic halo, probably due to internal caseous material (Fig. 1.36). Mediastinal lymphadenopathy can also be found in patients with immunologic processes, such as Kawasaki disease (BOSCH et al. 1998), Castelman disease and autoimmune thyroiditis.

Leukemia and lymphoma are the most frequent neoplastic processes in children that result in lymphadenopathy, which when massive, can extend to the anterior mediastinum. In an attempt to distinguish

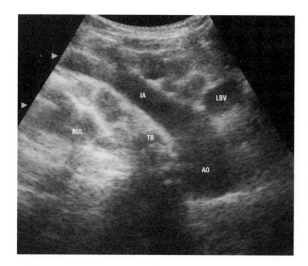

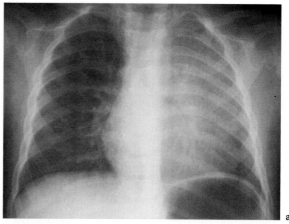

Fig. 1.35. Mediastinal lymphadenopathy in a 6-year-old boy with lymphoma. Oblique coronal view through the suprasternal space shows multiple, enlarged, hypoechoic lymph nodes at both sides of the innominate artery (*IA*). *AO*; aorta; *LBV*, left brachiocephalic vein; *RUL*, right upper lobe; *TR*, trachea

benign or reactive from malignant adenopathy, color and power Doppler has been recently applied to study the perfusion patterns within the nodes (TSCHAM-MLER et al. 1998). Although good results have been obtained in individual cases, more experience with this method is required to obtain conclusive data as to its value for this purpose.

1.4.4.3
Posterior Mediastinum

Among the three mediastinal regions, the posterior mediastinum is the least suitable for study by ultrasound. The majority of lesions located in this region are neurogenic tumors, which frequently extend to the spinal canal, a region that is better studied by MRI or CT. However, lesions located in the lower part of the posterior mediastinum (juxtaphrenic or paravertebral masses) can be studied with ultrasound using a subxiphoid or transdiaphragmatic approach. These approaches may be particularly helpful for examining children with paravertebral soft tissue widening (DONNELLY et al. 2000) in order to differentiate normal patients from those with tumor, atelectasis in the area of the pulmonary ligament, or azygos continuation of the inferior vena cava. In neurogenic tumors, US demonstrates a solid mass with frequent granular or fleck-like calcifications. In atelectasis one will encounter typical signs described for lung consolidation. The vascular nature of the lesion is readily

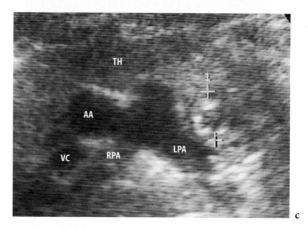

Fig. 1.36a–c. Mediastinal lymphadenopathy in an 8-year-old boy with tuberculosis. **a** Chest radiograph shows opacity and loss of volume due to left upper lobe collapse. **b** US left parasternal axial view demonstrates enlarged lymph nodes (*LN*) anterior to the left pulmonary artery (*LPA*). The atelectatic left upper lobe (*LUL*) and left pulmonary fissure (*arrowheads*) are also seen. Note mirror artifact showing the echogenic collapse on both sides of the fissure. **c** On follow up US study after 2 months of treatment, the node (between calipers) presents a multilayered appearance. *AA*, ascending aorta; *VC*, superior vena cava; *DA*, descending aorta; *TH*, thymus

assessed by color Doppler without administration of intravenous contrast material.

1.5
Diaphragmatic Lesions

A common US study requested in clinical practice is assessment of diaphragmatic motility, which before the development of US, was performed with fluoroscopy. Diaphragmatic paralysis is not uncommon after cardiac surgery or liver transplantation, and US evaluation of this condition can be performed at bedside in the intensive care unit. Since the paralysis is usually unilateral, the movement of the affected diaphragm can be compared to the normal contralateral one by real-time observation in the coronal plane. Use of M-mode allows spectral representation of the impaired and normal diaphragmatic movement.

Congenital and traumatic diaphragmatic hernias can present a misleading aspect on plain chest X-ray and simulate pulmonary consolidation when located on the right side, with the liver being the main component of the hernia. In traumatic liver herniation, the echogenicity of the intrathoracic liver may be different from that of the intra-abdominal liver. This finding represents the sonographic manifestation of the so-called collar sign (AOKI et al. 1998) (Fig. 1.37).

1.6
Conclusion

Sonography is a useful technique for evaluating pediatric chest diseases related to the lung, pleura, and mediastinum. It is especially helpful for rapid assessment of patients with complete opacification of a hemithorax on chest X-ray. Due to its Doppler capabilities, the technique permits noninvasive identification of vascular structures in many congenital and acquired lesions. US is superior to CT for characterizing pleural fluid collections as simple or complicated, thus providing important information for establishing proper treatment. It is the method of choice for screening patients with mediastinal widening, thereby avoiding more invasive study of a normal thymus. Sonography can characterize the solid versus cystic nature of a mediastinal mass in doubtful cases and detect the presence of lymphadenopathy in the paratracheal, aortopulmonary and subcarinal regions.

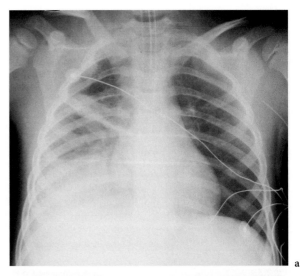

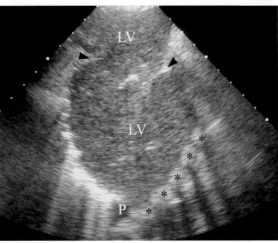

Fig. 1.37a,b. Diaphragmatic hernia in a 5-year-old girl with a motor vehicle injury. **a** Chest X-ray shows opacification of the right lung base and linear atelectasis in the right upper lobe. **b** Longitudinal view of the right hemithorax reveals that the opacity corresponds to herniation of the liver (*LV*) through a diaphragmatic rupture (*arrowhead*). *P*, pleural effusion. The chest wall is delineated by the ribs (*asterisk*)

References

Acunas B, Celik L, Acunas A (1986) Chest sonography. Acta Radiol 30:273–275

Alkrinawi S, Chernick V (1996) Pleural fluid in hospitalized pediatric patients. Clin Pediatr 35:5–9

Aoki AA, Mock CK, Talner LB (1998) Traumatic rupture of the right hemidiaphragm in an automobile accident victim. AJR 171:386

Avila NA, Mueller BU, Carrasquillo JA et al (1996) Multilocular thymic cysts: imaging features in children with human immunodeficiency virus infection. Radiology 201:130–134

Ben-Ami TE, O'Donovan JC, Yousefzadeh DK (1993) Sonography of the chest in children. Radiol Clin North Am 31:517–531

Bosch J, Serres X, Peñas M et al (1998) Mediastinal lymphadenopathy: a variant of incomplete Kawasaki disease. Acta Paediatr 87:1200–1202

Bouros D, Schiza S, Patsourakis G et al (1997) Intrapleural streptokinase versus urokinase in the treatment of complicated parapneumonic effusions. A prospective, double-blind study. Am J Respir Crit Care Med 155:291–295

Castellote A, Vazquez E, Vera J et al (1999) Cervicothoracic lesions in infants and children. Radiographics 19:583–600

Civardi G, Fornari F, Cavanna L et al (1993) Vascular signals from pleura-based lung lesions studied with pulsed Doppler ultrasonography. J Clin Ultrasound 21:617–622

Davis SD, Umlas SL (1992) Radiology of congenital abnormalities of the chest. Curr Opin Radiol 4:25–35

Donnelly LF, Klosterman LA (1997) Pneumonia in children; decreased parenchymal contrast enhancement – CT sign of intense illness and impeding cavitary necrosis. Radiology 205:817–820

Donnelly LF, Frush DP, Zheng J-Y et al (2000) Differentiating normal from abnormal inferior thoracic paravertebral soft tissues on chest radiography in children. AJR 175:477–483

Eibenberger K, Dode W, Metz V et al (1991) Value of supine thoracic radiography in the diagnosis and quantification of pleural effusions: comparison with sonography. Rofo Fortschr Geb Rontgenstr Neuen Bildgeb Verfahr 155:323–326

Frazier AA, Rosado de Christenson ML, Stocker JT et al (1997) Intralobar sequestration: radiologic-pathologic correlation. Radiographics 17:725–745

Gehmacher O, Mathis G, Kopf A et al (1995) Ultrasound imaging of pneumonia. Ultrasound Med Biol 21:1119–1122

Givan DC, Eigen H (1998) Common pleural effusions in children. Clin Chest Med 19:363–371

Hamrick-Turner JE, Saif MF, Powers CI et al (1994) Imaging of childhood non-Hodgkin lymphoma: assessment by histologic subtype. Radiographics 14:11–28

Hedlund GL, Navoy JF, Galliani CA et al (1999) Aggressive manifestations of inflammatory pulmonary pseudotumor in children. Pediatr Radiol 29:112–116

Kerem E, Bar Ziv Y, Rudenski B et al (1994) Bacteremic necrotizing pneumococcal pneumonia in children. Am J Respir Crit Care Med 149:242–244

Kim OH, Kim WS, Kim MJ et al (2000) US in the diagnosis of pediatric chest diseases. Radiographics 20:653–671

Ko SF, Ng SH, Lee TY et al (2000) Noninvasive imaging of bronchopulmonary sequestration. AJR 175:1005–1018

Kornecki A, Sivan Y (1997) Treatment of loculated pleural effusion with intrapleural urokinase in children. J Pediatr Surg 32:1473–1475

Koumanidou CH, Vakaki M, Theophanooulou M et al (1998) Aberrant Thymus in infants: sonographic evaluation. Pediatr Radiol 28:987–989

Krishnan S, Amin N, Dozor AJ et al (1997) Urokinase in the management of complicated parapneumonic effusions in children. Chest 112:1579–1583

Lemaitre L, Leclerc F, Marconi V et al (1987) Ultrasonographic findings in thymic lymphoma in children. Eur J Radiol 7:125–129

May DA, Barth RA, Yeager S et al (1993) Perinatal and postnatal chest sonography. Radiol Clin North Am 31:499–516

Muller LM (1993) Imaging the pleura. Radiology 186:297–309

Pan-Chyr Y, Dun-Bing CH, Chong-Jen Y et al (1992) Ultrasound-guided core biopsy of thoracic tumors. Am Rev Respir Dis 146:763–767

Park CS, Chung WM, Lim MK et al (1996) Transcatheter instillation of urokinase into loculated pleural effusion. Analysis of treatment effect. AJR 167:649–652

Ramnath RR, Heller RM, Ben-Ami T et al (1998) Implications of early sonographic evaluation of parapneumonic effusions in children with pneumonia. Pediatrics 101:68–71

Raptopoulos V, Davis LM, Lee G et al (1991) Factors affecting the development of pneumothorax associated with thoracentesis. AJR 156:917–920

Rudick MG, Wood BP (1980) The use of ultrasound in the diagnosis of a large thymic cyst. Pediatr Radiol 10:113–115

Sasaka K, Kurihara Y, Nakajima Y et al (1998) Spontaneous rupture: a complication of benign mature teratomas of the medistinum. AJR 170:323–328

Seibert JJ, Glasier CHM, Leithiser RE (1998) The pediatric chest. In: Rumack CM, Wilson SR, Charboneau JW (eds) Diagnostic ultrasound, 2nd edn. Mosby-Year Book, St Louis, pp 1617–1644

Shankar S, Gulati M, Kang M et al (2000) Image-guided percutaneous drainage of thoracic empyema. Eur Radiol 10:495–499

Sheth S, Hamper UM, Stanley DB et al (2000) US guidance for thoracic biopsy: a valuable alternative to CT. Radiology 210:721–726

Swischuk LE, John S (1996) Normal thymus extending between the right brachiocephalic vein and the innominate artery. AJR 166:1462–1464

Tschammler A, Ott G, Schang T et al (1998) Lymphadenopathy: differentiation of benign from malignant disease. Color Doppler US assessment of intranodal angioarchitecture. Radiology 208:117–123

Weinberg B, Diakoumakis EE, Kass EG et al (1986) The air bronchogram. AJR 147:593–595

Wernecke K (2000) Ultrasound study of the pleura. Eur Radiol 10:1515–1523

Winters WD, Effmann EL, Nghiem HV et al (1997) Disappearing fetal lung masses: importance of postnatal imaging studies. Pediatr Radiol 27:535–539

Yang PC, Lutz KT, Chang DB et al (1992a) Value of sonography in determining the nature of pleural effusion: analysis of 320 cases. AJR 159:29–33

Yang PC, Lutz KT, Chang DB et al (1992b) Ultrasonographic evaluation of pulmonary consolidation. Am Rev Respir Dis 146:757–762

2 The Contribution of Nuclear Medicine to Pulmonary Imaging

David L. Gilday

CONTENTS

2.1 Introduction

One of the oldest nuclear medicine tests is perfusion lung scintigraphy. It was introduced to diagnose pulmonary embolism. Until recently, pulmonary embolism was considered rare in pediatrics. The main indication for lung scintigraphy is to evaluate pulmonary perfusion in children with either congenital or acquired pulmonary artery stenosis. Quantifying the distribution of ^{99m}Tc MAA is especially useful in following up the results of stenting or dilation of a pulmonary artery. Even pulmonary artery branch narrowing can be followed-up with this technique. It has the advantage of being simple and easy to perform even with the most uncooperative young child or infant. Using ventilation techniques, bronchial obstructive diseases can be evaluated, although computed tomography (CT) has largely supplanted this technique.

Investigation of respiratory problems using nuclear medicine techniques involves assessing the perfusion (Q) and ventilation (V) of the lungs. Ventilation and perfusion studies (V/Q) are used together to better

David L. Gilday, MD, B.Eng (EE), FRCPC, ABNM
Professor of Radiology, University of Toronto, Department of Nuclear Medicine, Hospital for Sick Children, 555 University Ave., Toronto, ON, M5G 1X8, Canada

detect lung abnormalities. Multiple views are obtained in both the ventilation and perfusion portion of the study. The ventilation study can be done with either a noble (inert) gas such as 81mkrypton or 133xenon, or with 99mTc diethylenetriaminopentoacetic acid (DTPA) aerosol.

2.2 Scintigraphy

2.2.1 Aerosol

Aerosol imaging is the commonest technique for imaging pulmonary ventilation. It also the easiest and cheapest and is widely available. The equipment needed to perform an aerosol study consists of a commercial nebulizer, which produces droplets that will be deposited on the surface of the bronchioles. This results in a very accurate picture of the pattern of ventilation. These droplets are produced from a liquid containing 555 MBq (15 mCi) ^{99m}Tc DTPA that is placed in the nebulizer.

A mouthpiece is used to connect the nebulizer tubing to the child, and it is important to ensure that the child makes a tight seal with its lips. A clip is used to block breathing through the nose. If the child is too small for a mouthpiece, then a mask should be used. It is important to ensure that the patient is breathing through the nose since mouth breathing will result in the droplets being swallowed. An aerosol study is very difficult to perform on infants and young children since they cannot inhale deeply enough to withdraw the aerosol from the nebulizer. Patients on a ventilator can still undergo this procedure, but the ventilation equipment must be modified to adapt to the patients' needs. The oxygen powering the nebulizer is run at 10 l for 5 min. The patient is asked to breathe normally. If the patient is breathing shallowly, then some deep inhalations must be encouraged. The child should be encouraged to rinse his/her mouth with water or take a drink of water after the mouthpiece is removed as the air coming through the mouthpiece if very dry.

Eight images are obtained, each for 2 min, in 256×256 matrix in the anterior, posterior, left lateral, right lateral, 45° left anterior oblique (LAO), left posterior oblique (LPO), right anterior oblique (RAO), and right posterior oblique (RPO) positions. An acquisition zoom should be used in all children, so that the computer recorded images are as large as possible.

2.2.2
Noble (Inert) Gases

The commonly used radioactive noble gases are ^{133}xenon and ^{81m}krypton (a generator-produced radiotracer). The gas is inhaled using a plastic breathing bag equipped with a one-way valve connected to a mouthpiece and another one-way valve connected to a waste collection bag. The process is as follows: the patient breathes in from the bag containing the radioactive noble gas and then exhales into the collection bag. The one-way valves permit breathing in only from the breathing bag and the exhaled air can only go to the collection bag. After equilibrium is attained, the child breathes in room air until all the radioactive gas is washed out.

If ^{133}xenon is used, then imaging can only be done of the wash in, the equilibrium phase, and the washout. If ^{81m}krypton is available, then additional views in each of the eight standard lung views are usually obtained.

2.3
Qualitative Perfusion Scintigraphy

A chest X-ray done within the previous 24 h should be available for review. The presence of lung pathology may interfere with the interpretation of the examination and, in some circumstances, it may be necessary to delay the examination. The child should be lying in a supine position for the injection, otherwise postural hydrostatic pressure will change the usual distribution of pulmonary blood flow. The radiopharmaceutical, ^{99m}Tc MAA, is injected after the child has taken several deep breaths. The dose is 75 MBq (2.0 mCi) per square meter of body surface area, or a maximum dose of 130 MBq (3.5 mCi) with a

minimum dose of 18.5 MBq (500 µCi). It is preferable not to inject through a central venous line as the ^{99m}Tc MAA will adhere to this, which may produce artifacts and interfere with any interpretation of the scan.

Immediately following injection, eight images are obtained in 256×256 matrix, each for 1 min in the anterior, posterior, left lateral, right lateral, 45° LAO, LPO, RAO, RPO positions. Each image is acquired for 2 min using the same acquisition zoom as the ventilation study. There should be a symmetrical appearance of both perfusion and ventilation in both lungs (Fig. 2.1).

2.4
Quantitative Perfusion Lung Scintigraphy

This procedure is carried out on patients with pulmonary artery stenosis to assess perfusion to each lung (GLASS et al. 1991). Follow-up studies are also performed after surgery or balloon dilatation to assess perfusion.

The radiopharmaceutical is injected into the patient using the technique described in Sect. 2.2.2. The amount of ^{99m}Tc MAA is less for this technique and is 37 MBq (37 mCi) per square meter of body surface area to a maximum dose of 65 MBq (1.75 mCi), with a minimum dose of 9.3 MBq (250 µCi). Immediately following injection, 2-min anterior and posterior images are acquired in 256×256 matrix. The relative perfusion to each lung is calculated using comparable regions of interest on both the anterior and posterior images. Although it has been recommended to use a geometric mean of the values determined from the two images, we have found that in children there is no difference from the simple arithmetic mean.

2.5
Salivagram

Initial nuclear medicine attempts to detect aspiration were by imaging the chest after a radiotracer labeled drink (usually milk or formula) (McVEAGH et al. 1987). Although this did detect some cases of aspiration secondary to reflux, it was unable to if reflux was not present. The salivagram was introduced as a means of detecting aspiration secondary to disor-

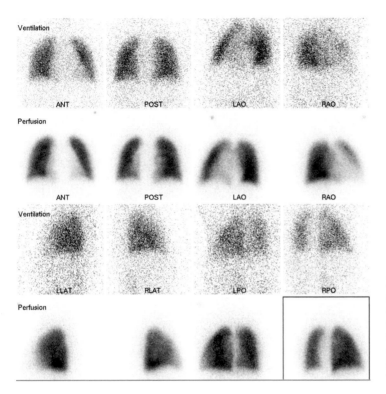

Fig. 2.1. Normal ventilation and perfusion scan. There is a very close match in the distribution of the tracer between the ventilation and the perfusion images. *ANT*, anterior; *POST*, posterior; *LAO*, left anterior oblique; *RAO*, right anterior oblique; *LLAT*, left lateral; *RLAT*, right lateral; *LPO*, left posterior oblique; *RPO*, right posterior oblique

dered pharyngeal motility (HEYMAN 1989; HEYMAN and RESPONDEK 1989).

The patient is placed in a supine position on the imaging table, beneath which the camera is mounted. The infant or child must be well restrained to minimize motion during the study acquisition. Between 1.1 MBq and 2.2 MBq (30–60 µCi) of ^{99m}Tc sulfur colloid is placed under the patient's tongue and allowed to mix with the saliva. Care should be taken that the patient does not spit out the radiopharmaceutical, and that saliva does not run out of the mouth and onto the patient's clothing. Any external contamination will confuse the interpretation of the scan.

A dynamic sequence of images is acquired for 15 s/frame for 5 min (20 frames) in 128×128 matrix. The acquisition is monitored and as soon as the activity clears from the mouth, the acquisition can be stopped. The imaging sequence is repeated twice to optimize the chance of detecting aspiration. At the end of the three series, a single image is acquired in 256×256 matrix for 1 min, using markers on the shoulders.

If activity is seen anywhere in the chest area, the patient's clothing is removed and repeat images acquired to ensure that there is no external contami-

nation. If activity is still seen, a lateral image of the appropriate side is acquired.

2.6
Clinical Interpretation

Although not nearly as common in children as in adults, pulmonary embolism is increasing in incidence. This is in part due to better recognition that pulmonary embolism occurs in childhood, but even more importantly due to increased medical therapies that can cause pulmonary embolism. The increasing use of central venous access catheters and surgery that require children to be bed-ridden for extended periods of time have caused an iatrogenic impetus for the development of pulmonary embolism. The main indication for V/Q imaging is to determine whether pulmonary embolism is present. The incidence of pulmonary emboli is increased with the increasing incidence of thrombosis secondary to medical manipulation and surgery. The diagnosis is usually made according to the PIOPED criteria. However, this was established for adults and does not apply in its entirety to the pediatric population. Even the modifications that was announced in 1995 (Freitas et al. 1995; Stein et al. 1996a,b) do not fully satisfy the requirements of pediatrics. A single segmental or larger abnormality, where there is normal ventilation with absent perfusion is considered as an indica-

tion for pulmonary embolism examination. The typical appearance of a pulmonary embolus is to have a normal chest radiograph and ventilation study with a perfusion scan showing at least one segmental defect. Typically, there are several defects, often involving both lungs. The lower lobes tend to be involved more

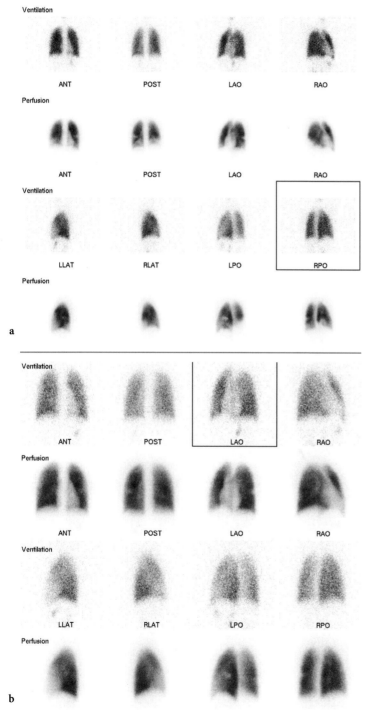

Fig. 2.2a, b. Pulmonary embolism. a In the initial study, there are perfusion defects present in both lower lobes that are not present in the ventilation images. b In the follow up study, the perfusion defects have dramatically decreased in size. *ANT*, anterior; *POST*, posterior; *LAO*, left anterior oblique; *RAO*, right anterior oblique; *LLAT*, left lateral; *RLAT*, right lateral; *LPO*, left posterior oblique; *RPO*, right posterior oblique

frequently due to the greater perfusion (Fig. 2.2). The classic triple match of a ventilation and perfusion defect with a radiographic abnormality is rarely seen in pediatrics. In recent years, there have been several publications indicating that there is a much greater reliance on the V/Q scan by emergency room physicians in an attempt to quickly categorize and triage their patients in the overcrowded emergency units. The overall incidence of pulmonary embolism among this population has gradually increased, but with increased utilization of V/Q scanning, the percentage of patients with pulmonary embolism has fallen significantly. We have found that this is also true in our pediatric population; however, we have also found that there is an increasing incidence of positive V/Q scans for pulmonary embolism.

Children with pulmonary hypertension can be evaluated to see the effect of the hypertension on the lungs. It is a requirement in our hospital that children have a V/Q study prior to lung transplant to determine whether one or both lungs need to be excised.

Quantitative perfusion imaging alone can be used to evaluate the relative perfusion to each lung or lobe due to pulmonary artery stenosis (Fig. 2.3) (GLASS et al. 1991). The technique is especially valuable in following up the effects of intervention for the correction of pulmonary arterial narrowing. This is the most common indication for nuclear medicine imaging in pediatric lung disease.

The diagnosis of aspiration in infants is difficult. Gastroesophageal (GE) reflux imaging and pH studies are done to determine whether GE reflux is present. The "milk scan" was invented to try and see aspiration after reflux (McVEAGH et al. 1987). This technique met with limited acceptance due to the limitation that the only aspiration detectable would be that secondary to GE reflux. A simple study was devised to see if saliva was being aspirated in children with pharyngeal dysfunction (HEYMAN 1989; HEYMAN and RESPONDEK 1989). This proved to be a very sensitive and specific study (Fig. 2.4).

In the past, obstructive airway disease was evaluated using the noble gas ventilation study to determine the nature of a hyperlucent component of the lung. Today CT imaging has largely replaced the role of nuclear medicine in this area of diagnosis.

Percent L upper : 2		Percent R upper : 16
Percent L mid : 12		Percent R mid : 33
Percent L low : 15		Percent R low : 22
Percent LEFT : 29		Percent RIGHT : 71

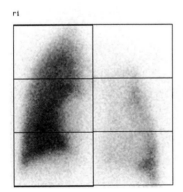
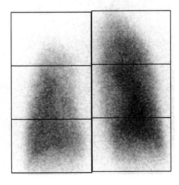

ri

Fig. 2.3. Quantitative lung perfusion. Each lung is quantitated in both the anterior and posterior images

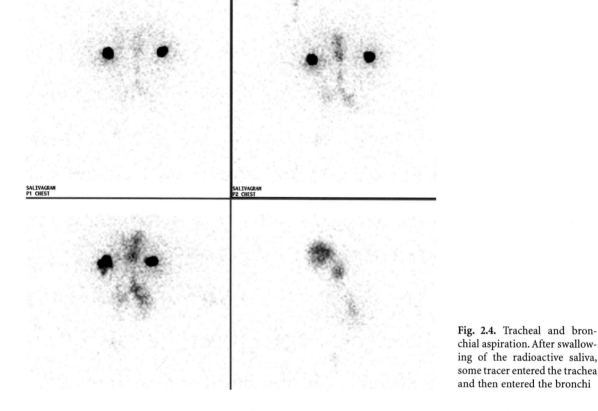

SALIVAGRAM
P1 CHEST

SALIVAGRAM
P2 CHEST

Fig. 2.4. Tracheal and bronchial aspiration. After swallowing of the radioactive saliva, some tracer entered the trachea and then entered the bronchi

References

Freitas JE, Sarosi MG, Nagle CC et al (1995) Modified PIOPED criteria used in clinical practice. J Nucl Med 36(9):1573–1578

Glass T, Heyman S, Seliem M et al (1991) Use of Tc-99 m MAA in determining the etiology of increasing cyanosis following SVC-PA anastomosis for the hypoplastic left heart syndrome. Clin Nucl Med 16(6):410–412

Heyman S (1989) The radionuclide salivagram for detecting the pulmonary aspiration of saliva in an infant. Pediatr Radiol 19(3):208–209

Heyman S, Respondek M (1989) Detection of pulmonary aspiration in children by radionuclide "salivagram". J Nucl Med 30(5):697–699

McVeagh P, Howman-Giles R, Kemp A et al (1987) Pulmonary aspiration studied by radionuclide milk scanning and barium swallow roentgenography." Am J Dis Child 141(8):917–921

Stein PD, Henry JW, Gottschalk A et al (1996a) Small perfusion defects in suspected pulmonary embolism. J Nucl Med 37(8):1313–1316

Stein PD, Relyea B, Gottschalk A et al (1996b) Evaluation of individual criteria for low probability interpretation of ventilation-perfusion lung scans. J Nucl Med 37(4):577–581

3 Helical Chest CT

Pilar García-Peña

CONTENTS

3.1
Introduction

Computed tomography (CT) in children poses unique problems that are not encountered in adults. The relative lack of visceral fat combined with patient motion results in a degradation of image quality that makes the recognition of normal anatomic structures and some pathologies more difficult. The recent major advances in technology in conjunction with meticulous attention paid to CT techniques and better training of radiologists have all improved the sensitivity and specificity of pediatric CT imaging and have

Pilar García-Peña, MD
Department of Pediatric Radiology, Vall d'Hebron Hospitals,
ps. Vall d'Hebron 119–129, Barcelona 08035, Spain

resulted in more precise diagnosis. The introduction of helical CT has further increased the usefulness and extended the indications for CT in the evaluation of pediatric patients. Many of the significant changes in current diagnostic practice are solely related to the introduction of helical CT, which has enabled the study of airway and vascular structures, the development of CT angiography and virtual endoscopy, and improvements in the quality of multiplanar reconstructions.

Helical CT technology has several potential benefits for pediatric patients. The use of IV contrast agents can be optimized, sedation reduced, and radiation exposure to the patient can be decreased by using extended pitch and by eliminating the need to re-scan ambiguous data. Helical CT also improves the image quality of two- and three-dimensional (2- and 3-D) reconstructions, an important factor when analyzing specific diseases in children.

3.2
Technical Considerations

3.2.1
Helical Technique

In contrast to conventional CT, which is based on the collection of data from sequential scans, helical CT data is obtained continuously during table motion and results in a volume of scan data. If direct reconstruction were performed on this data the resulting images would be of poor quality, being compromised by motion artifacts. Thus, to compensate for the problems induced by table motion, the image data is interpolated prior to reconstruction (Brink et al. 1994b; Napel 1995; Siegel and Luker 1995).

When compared to conventional section-by-section CT, helical CT has a number of advantages in the examination of pediatric patients.

By using the reconstruction capabilities of helical CT we can obtain overlapping slices, a fact that improves lesion depiction without increasing radiation exposure. Postprocessing of overlapping slices provides high-quality 2- and 3-D images, extending the diagnostic applications. Image reconstruction can be performed for any slice position along the z-axis interval scanned.

Because of the relatively shorter scanning time (50% or less with some new equipment) there is more precise delivery of contrast medium and enhanced studies can be performed during peak vascular enhancement. This also allows a reduction of up to 25% in the volume of contrast agent needed (COSTELLO et al. 1992b). Since the speed of scanning a particular anatomic area is determined by the collimation thickness and the pitch (defined as the ratio of the table speed, expressed in millimeters per second to collimation thickness, expressed in millimeters multiplied by the time to acquire 360° of data), shorter scan times may help eliminate or decrease motion artifacts (RUBIN et al. 1998). This allows high-quality 2- and 3-D image reconstruction and decreases the use of sedation, a very important consideration in pediatric patients.

Radiation dose can be reduced in helical scanning without compromising diagnostic image quality (TAKAHASHI et al. 1998). As children are more radiosensitive than adults and have a longer life span in which to manifest radiation-related disease, great care must be taken with the use of radiation.

There is essentially no difference in radiation dose in conventional CT (18.3±1.5 mGy) versus 1.0:1 pitch helical CT scanning (17.2±2.1 mGy), obtained using a comparable technique [100 mA, 120 kV(p) 10 mm thickness and 10 mm intervals]. However, dose can be reduced in helical scanning by lowering milliamperes (as in conventional CT) or by increasing pitch (ROGALLA et al. 1999). In our institution we performed a study in two groups of 50 patients maintaining constant parameters of milliamperes, kilovolt (peak) and thickness while varying the pitch. The dose for helical CT performed with 100 mA, 120 kV(p), 10 mm collimation and pitch of 1.0:1 was 18.9±2.2 mGy, while for a pitch of 1.5:1 it was 12.2±1.0 mGy (GARCIA-PEÑA and LUCAYA 1999).

Another potential for dose reduction resides in the fact that re-scanning is rarely necessary when using the helical technique. When two contiguous slices fail to clearly demonstrate a small anatomic structure because of partial volume effects, the intermediate slice can be reconstructed retrospectively without the need to rescan the patient to clarify the problem.

Helical equipment is remarkably silent as compared to conventional scanners. For this reason, pediatric patients are not usually frightened and remain quiet. This in itself reduces the need for sedation and improves image quality.

The quality of multiplanar reformatted images, MPR (coronal, sagittal and curved) and 3-D images is significantly improved with helical CT, which decreases motion-related artifacts and provides a smoothing effect of overlapped image reconstruction, reducing stair-step artifacts. Such 3-D images can be optimally rotated to display specific normal and abnormal structures allowing analysis of selected parts. The most common 3-D image display formats are shaded surface display, maximum/ minimum intensity projection, and volume rendered images.

3.2.1.1
Limitations and Disadvantages of Helical CT Technique

Helical CT does have some technical limitations and disadvantages. These include: (a) heat build-up in the X-ray tube, which limits the milliamperes that can be generated; (b) postprocessing delays related to reconstruction of the images after the data have been acquired; and (c) z-axis blurring (blurring along the longitudinal table axis) with increased pitch because of the faster table speeds. These disadvantages will be overcome by using the new generation of helical scanners. Compared with single multidetector-row helical CT, four multidetector–row helical CT provides a twofold to threefold improvement in volume coverage speed with comparable diagnostic image quality (HU et al. 2000).

3.2.1.2
Pitfalls of Helical CT Technique

A common technical artifact associated with helical data acquisition is the stair-step artifact (WANG and VANNIER 1994). These occur along high-contrast interfaces that are oriented obliquely to the direction of patient travel. Stair-casing causes the edges of longitudinally oriented structures to appear as steps rather than as straight lines (Fig. 3.1). The height of the step longitudinally is proportional to the table increment (pitch) and is independent of the collimation or reconstruction interval.

Another pitfall is related to commencing scanning before organ or vessel enhancement by the contrast

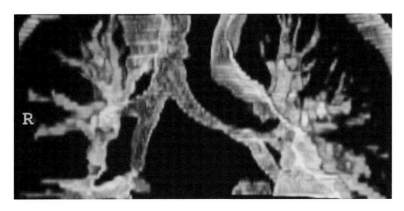

Fig. 3.1. Stair-step artifact in a volume-rendered image (bronchographic anteroposterior view). A 3-year-old boy with bronchiolitis and congenital stenosis in left main bronchus. The artifact occurs along the left bronchus, which is oriented obliquely to the direction of patient travel during data acquisition

agent is homogeneous (SILLVERMAN et al. 1995). These flow artifacts, caused by the mixing of contrast material and non-opacified blood are much more frequent in abdominal studies than in chest CT.

3.2.2
Personnel and Environment Requirements

The optimal team for performing pediatric helical CT includes a pediatric radiologist, a technician and a nurse trained in pediatric care. It is important to ensure a good environment for pediatric patients in the scanning area and every effort should be made to create a warm atmosphere that minimizes anxiety. Soft lighting, silence, toys, a room decorated with children in mind and the presence of a relative can help to comfort a child. It is essential to have immediate access to a resuscitation cart with appropriate drugs and equipment for pediatric patients of all ages.

3.2.3
Previous Exam Evaluation

It is mandatory to check the patient's clinical records and all available imaging studies before performing a helical CT scan. This helps to decide if the indication is correct and allows the exam to be tailored to the specific requirements of the patient. It is particularly important with regard to the need for sedation and IV contrast administration. Careful planning can prevent difficulties during the study and minimize unanswered questions afterward. The radiologist should explain all aspects of the procedure

and the objectives of the study to the parents before obtaining parental consent.

3.2.4
Preparation of the Patient: Fasting Requirements

The patients, parents and nursing staff should be informed of fasting requirements before the day of the procedure. Sometimes, no preparation is required (e.g. when studying pulmonary metastasis). When children need sedation or IV contrast material is to be given during the examination, we use the following fasting regimes before the procedure: In newborns, fasting is decided upon consultation with the neonatologist; infants are kept NPO for 3 h; children for 4 h and adolescents for 6 h.

3.2.5
Immobilization and Other Practical Tips

Sandbags, adhesive bandages, or blankets wrapped around the patient can all be used to immobilize the patient. It is advisable to wrap a lead apron around the child in the regions adjacent to those to be scanned. This protects them from scattered radiation and, at the same time, can help to immobilize the patient. Overlying radioprotective bismuth latex should be placed on a girl's breast to minimize local radiation. Toys hanging from the gantry can be used to attract the attention of the child and help to keep him or her quiet. A system for maintaining body temperature such as warming lamps or heating blankets should be used in infants.

3.2.6
Breath-Holding Information

Children under 6 years of age who cannot follow breath-holding commands are examined under normal quiet breathing. In this age group attempts at breath-holding usually result in exams severely compromised by artifacts. Older children are carefully instructed in breath-holding before the study.

3.2.7
Sedation

Helical CT has reduced the need for sedation (WHITE 1995; KASTE et al. 1997). Since the introduction of silent helical CT in our institution, our overall rate of sedation is only 3% of patients vs. 18% for our previous conventional CT studies. In patients under the age of 6 years, 50% required sedation with conventional CT and only 8% with helical CT. Among the patients in this age group who needed IV contrast, 77% had to be sedated with conventional CT and only 18% with helical CT. Finally, among those who did not need IV contrast material, 24% required sedation with conventional CT and only 2% with helical CT. We believe that the relative silence of the helical equipment more than the speed has determined this reduced need for sedation. However, it has been reported that with multidetector helical CT the rate of sedation can be reduced even further (PAPPAS et al. 2000).

The need for sedation is decided upon depending on the behavior of the child once inside the gantry. In our experience infants under 3 months of age can often be successfully imaged after normal feeding and swaddling. Sleep deprivation the night before the examination has no proven benefit in either decreasing the dose of sedative drugs or the number of sedation procedures and can be disruptive for patients. Before performing an examination with the use of sedation, the radiologist must decide whether its benefits outweigh the associated risks and verify that fasting requirements have been observed. In our institution informed consent for sedation is covered by the standard consent for admission and CT scan examination.

In children under 18 months of age we usually administer oral chloral hydrate at a dose of 50–100 mg/kg (to a maximum dose of 2000 mg) 20 min prior to starting the examination. When using this regimen and if IV contrast injection is contemplated, the intravenous line is placed in the preparation room before the patient is brought to the CT unit.

Patients 18 months of age and older are given intravenous sodium pentobarbital, 6 mg/kg to a maximum dose of 200 mg, diluted in 10 cc saline. The syringe containing the sedation must be appropriately labeled with the drug name. A dose of 2–3 mg/kg should be given initially as slow bolus over 1–2 min. In most children, this dose is adequate and they will fall asleep within the next 4–5 min. If not, an additional dose of 2–3 mg/kg may be given. If the patient still remains awake an additional dose of 2 mg/kg can be given some 30 min later. However, this is rarely necessary. Occasionally, in some patients over 6 months of age who need IV contrast administration, we also use sodium pentobarbital in the above-mentioned doses. Pediatric sedation techniques have been extensively described in the literature (COOK et al. 1992; FRUSH et al. 1996; EGELHOFF et al. 1997).

Every child undergoing sedation in the CT suites should receive oxygen and be monitored during and after the examination (see Chap. 4).

3.2.8
Intravenous Contrast Material Administration

Intravenous administration of a bolus of contrast material for helical CT studies in children can be more complicated than in adults because of the greater variations in vessel size in the pediatric population. Dosage is based on the patient's body weight. Contrast material is administered by hand or power injector, depending on these variations (Frush et al. 1997; Kaste and Young 1996). To avoid the artifact caused by contrast in the axillary vein just after the injection, the syringe is placed vertically downwards and filled with saline solution and contrast. Since saline is less dense than contrast material, it will remain in the syringe until the end of the injection and then flush the vein of contrast. This will help to obtain better images (Hopper et al. 2000).

If contrast material is to be given, a butterfly needle or an intravenous catheter should be placed before the child's arrival in the CT suite. This will avoid the distress associated with venipuncture performed immediately before scanning begins and help to reduce the need for sedation. Local topical analgesics, such as lidocaine cream, can be applied to the intended venipuncture site to minimize the pain from cannula placement. We use 19–25 Gauge butterfly needles, which give injection rates of 4.0–0.5 ml/s. The catheters are 20–26 Gauge, permitting injection rates of 4.0-1.0 ml/s (Table 3.1). One should always use the largest cannula suitable for each patient, though rates as low as 0.5-1.0 ml/s in children can still result in excellent enhanced studies. If the patient already has a central intravenous line in situ, it should be used to gain venous access.

Table 3.1. Rate of contrast media injection depending on needle or catheter gauge

Needle		Catheter	
Gauge	Flow rate	Gauge	Flow rate
25 G	0.5 ml/s	26 G	1.0 ml/s
23 G	0.5-0.8 ml/s	24 G	2.0 ml/s
21 G	0.8-2.0 ml/s	22 G	3.0 ml/s
19 G	2.0-4.0 ml/s	20 G	4.0 ml/s

Non-ionic, low- (240 mg of iodine per milliliter) or high- (300 mg of iodine per milliliter) osmolar contrast media can be used for CT examinations in children (STOKBERGER et al. 1998). In our practice, we use 240 mg/ml in infants and 300 mg/ml in older children.

The usual dose of contrast media is 1-3 ml/kg, to a maximum dose of 100 ml. In newborns the dose used is 2-3 ml/kg, in infants 2 ml/kg, in children 1.5 ml/kg, and in adolescents 1 ml/kg.

In our experience, helical CT has allowed a 20% reduction in the volume of intravenous contrast medium given when compared to conventional CT. Similar findings have been described in the literature (COSTELLO et al. 1992a). Optimal contrast enhancement during helical scanning depends on careful selection of the appropriate time of scanning, as well as on choosing the precise amount of contrast material and the optimal injection rate. The rate of injection depends on the needle or catheter size (Table 3.1). The timing of the onset of scanning is a crucial factor in successful imaging, but is also one of the trickiest aspects of performing pediatric helical CT. In chest examinations scanning is usually initiated after 100% of bolus is administered.

3.2.9
Technical Parameters and Protocols

Helical CT has virtually replaced conventional CT for examinations in which the entire chest is to be evaluated. However, low-dose high-resolution CT remains the technique of choice for the evaluation of the pulmonary parenchyma since it allows scanning at spaced intervals, significantly reducing radiation to the patient while providing excellent definition (Ambrosino et al. 1994; Lucaya et al. 2000b).

Several techniques are used for data acquisition in helical studies of the chest: standard helical CT, high-resolution helical CT, dynamic helical CT and low-dose helical CT.

Standard helical T scanning usually suffices for most helical CT examinations of the chest. When a large area of the chest is to be scanned, such as in a screening examination of the lungs or mediastinum, we use the chest survey protocol (see below), with a section thickness depending on the age of the child. When finer detail and higher-resolution images are required over a smaller area of interest, such as in tracheobronchial stenosis, dehiscences, endobronchial lesions, central airway disease and vascular anomalies, we recommend the airway disease or CT-angiography protocols (see below), using a thinner section to achieve better image quality. Multiplanar and 3-D reconstructions can be useful in the evaluation of airway abnormalities, certain vascular lesions and cervicothoracic or diaphragmatic and peridiaphragmatic lesions. Three-D images can be rotated to optimally display pathologic entities and selected parts of the reconstruction can be analyzed separately.

Helical high-resolution CT scanning of the lung is performed with thin sections (1-2 mm) and a table movement of 2-3 mm, using a high-resolution reconstruction algorithm. This technique is similar to high-resolution CT scanning, but with continuous data acquisition (ENGELER et al. 1994). Lowering the milliamperage setting can reduce radiation dose, but the continuous data acquisition of helical CT still delivers more radiation than the low-dose high-resolution CT technique, in which acquisition is performed with thin collimation and wide sampling intervals. In our institution we prefer low-dose high-resolution CT for the evaluation of pulmonary parenchyma.

Dynamic helical CT has enabled scanning at maximum inspiration and rescanning at maximum expiration. This method has been used to evaluate lung attenuation in patients with air trapping and emphysema. However, it requires cooperative breath-holding by the patient. Recently developed software programs (available on some helical scanners) have enabled dynamic CT densitometry of the lungs (JOHNSON et al. 1998b). Dynamic helical CT can also be used to demonstrate respiratory changes in the cross-sectional area of the central airway, e.g. in patients with tracheobronchomalacia. In our practice, we do not use this technique to evaluate air trapping and emphysema. We prefer expiratory scans with a low-dose high-resolution technique (LUCAYA et al. 2000a).

Low-dose helical CT scanning can be used in many situations. The X-ray tube current should be as low as possible, without compromising image quality (TAKAHASHI et al. 1998). With helical CT technique, a further reduction in radiation dose can be achieved by increasing table speed. Use of a targeted approach to image localized processes can also reduce the radiation dose administered. We use low-dose helical CT (50 mA and pitch 1.5–2) when examining children under the age of 6 years, which in this age group provides diagnostic-quality exams. We also apply this technique for the non-contrast scan in children having both non-contrast and contrast-enhanced exams, and for delayed scans.

The performance of high-quality helical CT requires proper selection of technical parameters, including collimation (section thickness), field of view (FOV), table speed (or pitch), reconstruction intervals, reconstruction algorithms, scan time duration, exposure factors (kilovoltage and milliamperage) and scan initiation (BRINK 1995; FRUSH and DONNELLY 1998). These parameters should be based on the patient's size and the body part to be examined. However, reductions in some of these parameters can lead to problems. Noise increases with decreasing collimation. Scan coverage decreases with reductions in collimation and table speed. Radiation dose increases with reductions in table speed. Decreasing the reconstruction intervals increases processing time. So, the final choice of parameters always involves a balance among these options to achieve diagnostic image resolution. As a general rule, thin collimation and high pitch settings should be selected.

Collimation is usually decided according to the child's body size. We use 5 mm collimation in newborns, infants and children under the age of 6; 8 mm collimation in children 6–12 years old; and 10 mm in children over 12. Thinner collimated sections (2–3 mm) are performed for detailed examinations or high-quality 2-D and 3-D reconstructions, e.g. in airway examinations and CT angiography. Multidetector-row helical scanners facilitate thin collimation, improving volume coverage speed.

The field of view should be as small as possible to achieve optimal image quality. It should match the transverse diameter of the chest or the part being studied. As FOV decreases, pixel size decreases and spatial resolution improves.

The pitch (related to table speed) generally used is 1.5:1. Increasing the pitch will increase scan coverage. This increase should not exceed 2.0:1 when using single-row helical CT. When using multidetector-row helical CT, the most frequent pitches used are 3.0:1–6.0:1.

The image reconstruction interval is usually set at an interval equal to the collimation. If multiplanar or 3-D reconstructions are required, reconstruction with 50% overlap should be performed for better definition. Moreover, overlapping images increase lesion depiction, which is useful in the evaluation of pulmonary nodules.

The most frequent reconstruction algorithm used is the low-spatial frequency (standard) algorithm. The pulmonary parenchyma can also be analyzed with a high-spatial frequency algorithm (bone algorithm).

Scan duration should be tailored as much as possible to the breath-holding ability of the child.

The *exposure factors* include kVp, which is usually set at a fixed level (90, 120–130 kVp) and milliamperage, which is adjusted to body size. High milliamperage should be avoided to reduce radiation exposure. Low mA increases image noise. Helical CT scans in children can be obtained with 100 mA. However, diagnostic quality helical CT scans for the analysis of lung parenchyma and central airways can be obtained with lower exposures, such as 50 mA. The high contrast of these structures allows a reduction in milliamperage. Low mA can also be used in other CT examinations, as mentioned above. A recent study has suggested that unnecessarily high radiation doses are frequently used for CT examination of pediatric patients (PATERSON et al. 2001).

The scan delay time varies with the region of interest and the clinical indication of the study. Enhanced helical CT examination of the chest should be initiated immediately after 100% of the volume of contrast agent has been administered. Longer scan delay times (20–30 s after all contrast has been injected) can be used when tissue enhancement is assessed, as in pulmonary parenchymal consolidation or pleural disease. The scan delay time for CT angiography will be the arterial time, obtained by monitoring the contrast enhancement in the descending aorta. This is done by acquiring very low mA scans at the same level (one scan every 3 s over 15 s) and determining the time of peak contrast. Alternatively, an automated bolus-tracking technique can be used to monitor contrast enhancement and initiate scanning. Scanning begins once an arbitrary threshold level of contrast enhancement is reached (150 CT units in the thoracic aorta). Specific recommendations for the selection of parameters are given in the examination protocols presented below.

3.2.9.1
Protocol: Chest Survey

Indications:	Tumor staging, suspected pulmonary metastasis, pulmonary and mediastinal masses, complex pleuroparenchymal disease, trauma.
Upper limit:	Above lung apices
Lower limit:	Caudal lung bases
Scanner setting:	120 kVp, 50–130 mA
FOV:	As small as possible (180–430 mm)
Slice thickness:	5–8-10 mm
Pitch:	1.5
Reconstruction intervals:	5–8-10 mm, same as thickness, 50% overlap (multiplanar and 3-D reconstructions, lung nodules)
Reconstruction algorithm:	low-spatial frequency and high-spatial frequency (lung)
IV contrast scan delay:	After 100% of bolus given
Phase of respiration:	Single breath-hold (cooperative patients), or quiet breathing (non-cooperative patients)
Comments:	No IV contrast is used in pulmonary metastasis studies. In focal disease the study should include only the area of interest.

3.2.9.2
Protocol: Airway Disease

Indications:	Congenital anomalies, stenosis, dehiscences, endobronchial lesions.
Upper limit:	Thoracic inlet
Lower limit:	Origin of segmental basilar bronchi
Scanner setting:	120 kVp, 50 mA
FOV:	As small as possible (180–430 mm)
Slice thickness:	2–3 mm
Pitch:	1.5

Reconstruction intervals:	1–1.5 mm (50% overlap)
Reconstruction algorithm:	Low-spatial frequency
IV contrast:	None
Phase of respiration:	Single breath-hold (cooperative patients) or quiet breathing (non-cooperative patients)
Postprocessing imaging:	MPR, 3-D images.

3.2.9.3
Protocol: CT Angiography

Indications:	Congenital vascular malformations, pulmonary sequestration, cystic adenomatoid malformation
Upper limit:	Top of the area of interest
Lower limit:	Bottom of the area of interest
Scanner setting:	120 kVp, 100 mA
FOV:	As small as possible (180–430 mm)
Slice thickness:	2–3 mm
Pitch:	1.5
Reconstruction intervals:	1–1.5 (50% overlap)
Reconstruction algorithm:	Low-spatial frequency
IV contrast scan delay:	Arterial time (descending aorta)
Comments:	The automated computer bolus-tracking technique or the arterial timing test protocol (see Sect. 3.2.9.4) can be used to monitor contrast enhancement in the aorta.

3.2.9.4
Protocol: Arterial Timing Test

Indications:	Vascular study
Scanned area (fixed level):	Descending aorta; one scan/3 s
Scanner setting:	90 kVp, 25–50 mA (as low as possible)
FOV:	As small as possible (180–430 mm)
Slice thickness:	2–5 mm
Reconstruction algorithm:	Low-spatial frequency
IV contrast scan delay:	From start of contrast injection
Postprocessing images:	Maximum peak IV contrast curve.

3.2.10
Image Postprocessing

Postprocessing techniques are currently available for generating multidimensional reconstructions of high quality, particularly when the image data has been acquired using thin collimation and axial images have been generated with at least 50% overlapping. The most common multidimensional reconstructions are either 2-D images, such as multiplanar reformations (MPR), or 3-D images, including shaded-surface display (SSD), maximum intensity projection (MIP) and minimum intensity projection (minIP). Additional alternatives include sliding thin slab MIP (STS-MIP) and sliding thin slab minIP (STS-minIP), volume rendering (VR) from an extraluminal perspective and perspective VR from an endoscopic view.

MPR is a 2-D tomographic section that is interpolated along an arbitrary plane (coronal, sagittal, oblique) or a curved surface (Fig. 3.2). Curved MPRs

are useful for displaying serpentine structures, such as blood vessels, airways, and bowel. Clinically they are of great value for evaluating vascular and airway abnormalities and the extent of neoplasms and abscesses. However, the curved MPR technique is highly operator-dependent and lesions can be falsely represented.

SSD generates images with depth and 3-D information. Using binary classification, voxels with attenuation values above a preset threshold are set to white and voxels with lower attenuation values are set to black (Brink 1995). This method first computes a mathematical model of a surface that connects neighboring pixels with CT intensities above a preset threshold. Depth or 3-D perception is created by shading techniques using an imaginary light source that can be arbitrarily positioned. Such data can be then rotated, allowing the image to be viewed from any perspective. Shaded-surface images are used to display the airways, vessels and bone struc-

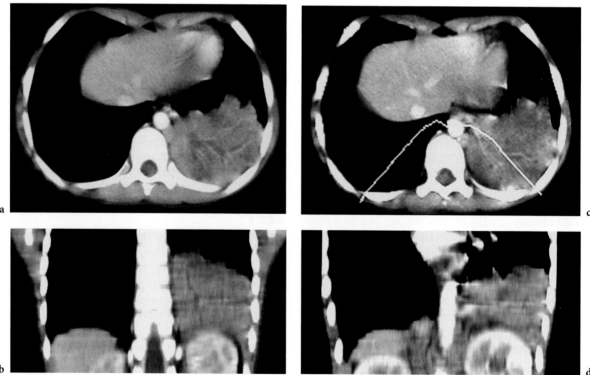

Fig. 3.2a–d. Axial and multiplanar reformation images (2-D images). Pulmonary sequestration in a 7-year-old boy with repeated pulmonary infection in the left lower lobe. **a** Axial image. **b** Coronal multiplanar reformation (MPR) image. The images depict the location and the extension of the heterogeneous mass in the left lower lobe. **c** Axial image with a postprocessing curved line to obtain a curved MPR image. **d** Curved MPR image obtained by processing a series of axial images following a suspected tortuous vessel. This curved image displays the vessel's origin from the aorta and its length better than the axial images and was helpful for diagnosing the pulmonary sequestration

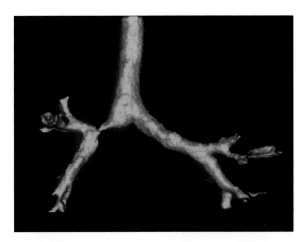

Fig. 3.3. Shaded surface display image of the central airways (anteroposterior view). Right bronchial stenosis in the area of anastomosis in an 11-year-old girl who had undergone lung transplantation for cystic fibrosis

tures (Figs. 3.3, 3.19c). They can provide superb detail on the contours of objects and can be of value in showing overlapping vessels. Because of MIP's transparent nature, SSD is often better for depicting anatomical relationships. However, the threshold must be carefully chosen and should be based on the intensity of the contrast material in the area of interest. The choice of threshold will strongly affect the evaluation of some lesions, such as the degree of stenosis. Choosing too low a threshold may increase noise and also allow the higher density soft tissue to obscure the target vasculature. Choosing a too-high threshold may result in small vessels disappearing and/or stenoses being falsely implied.

Another problem encountered with SSD is that the reduction of CT volume data to a single surface removes the inherent CT quantitative density values, losing gray scale levels. With this threshold technique one cannot differentiate between solid organ intraparenchymal vasculature and enhancing parenchyma, or between high attenuation structures in vessel walls and intraluminal contrast enhancement.

MIP images are generated by mapping the maximum attenuation value along each ray to produce a gray-scale image. Thus, bone and calcified structures are bright and are distinguishable from both iodinated contrast material and soft tissue. In a vascular examination, it will be necessary to postprocess the image to avoid bone images (BRINK 1995).

MIP images are useful for displaying vascular structures and for CT angiography. They reliably display vessel caliber, metallic stents, and wall calcifications, but provide poor separation of overlapping vessels because 3-D relationships are lost. The display of MIP images in a cine loop to simulate a rotating viewing direction improves the lack of 3-D depth. This allows visualization of 3-D relationships and may provide clues to the nature of eccentric stenoses and the crossing or looping of vessels.

MinIP images map the minimal attenuation value to a gray-scale image. MinIP images are valuable in examinations of the central airways (Fig. 3.4).

STS-MIP and/or STS-minIP is a cross-sectional imaging post-processing technique that computes overlapping MIPs of limited depth. The sections are typically thin 2–3-mm sections rendered into approximately 20–30-mm slabs (NAPEL and JEFFREY 1993). STS-MIP can improve the visualization of vessels over greater portions of their lengths. Vascular anatomy is frequently difficult to comprehend from standard cross-sectional images. Blood vessels that are perpendicular or oblique to the section will appear as small circles or ellipses and may mimic the appearance of a pulmonary nodule. With STS-MIP, one can integrate the path of vessels and their connections with other structures into the larger picture of vascular anatomy (Fig. 3.5).

STS-minIP enables airway anatomy to be visualized. It is also useful for displaying the whole volume of parenchymal cysts or bullae (Fig. 3.6).

VR creates 3-D images from information derived from all voxels in the data set. It is not subject to the information loss that is inherent in MIP and SSD images and can be interactively edited at a workstation to optimize the image display. By adjusting vari-

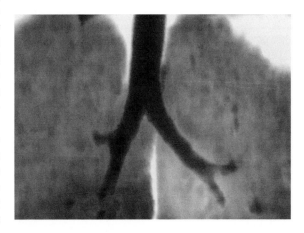

Fig. 3.4. Minimum-intensity projection image of the central airways (anteroposterior view). Normal central airways in a 7-year-old boy with suspected tracheal stenosis

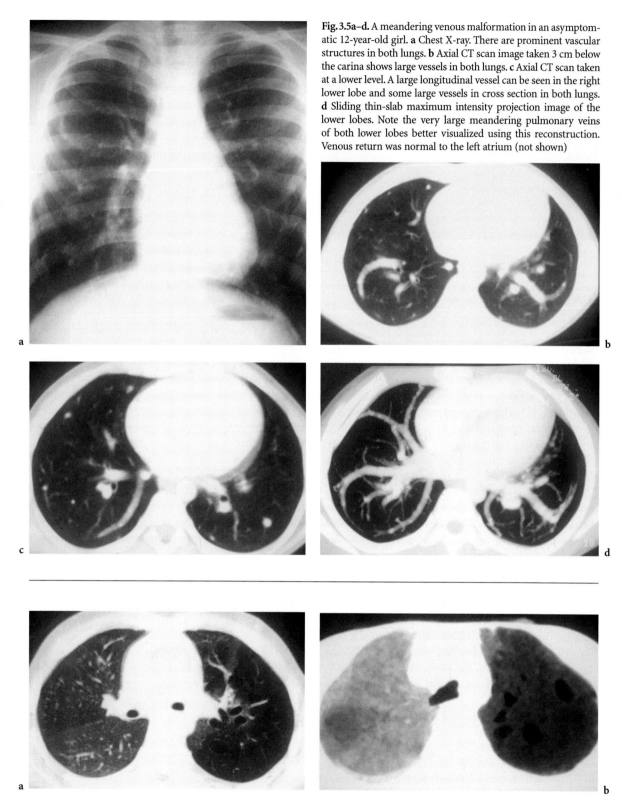

Fig. 3.5a–d. A meandering venous malformation in an asymptomatic 12-year-old girl. **a** Chest X-ray. There are prominent vascular structures in both lungs. **b** Axial CT scan image taken 3 cm below the carina shows large vessels in both lungs. **c** Axial CT scan taken at a lower level. A large longitudinal vessel can be seen in the right lower lobe and some large vessels in cross section in both lungs. **d** Sliding thin-slab maximum intensity projection image of the lower lobes. Note the very large meandering pulmonary veins of both lower lobes better visualized using this reconstruction. Venous return was normal to the left atrium (not shown)

Fig. 3.6a,b. Bronchial atresia of the left upper lobe in a 4-year-old girl with cough. **a** Axial CT image. Hyperlucency of the left upper lobe with suspected cystic lesions. **b** Sliding thin-slab minimum intensity projection image of the upper lobes. Hyperlucency at the same level and very well delineated cystic images better shown with this technique.

ous parameters, such as opacity, brightness, window and level, the data set can be manipulated to display objects of highest attenuation (e.g. bone, enhanced vasculature) or to include lower attenuation structures (e.g. viscera). The parameters can also be manipulated to create transparency of the displayed objects. This technique enables perspective VR of body cavities and hollow viscera from an extraluminal visualization or from an endoscopic viewpoint (virtual bronchoscopy) (Figs. 3.7, 3.8). VR from extraluminal visualization of the tracheobronchial tree creates images similar to conventional bronchograms and is applicable in clinical practice without the concomitant administration of a contrast agent. Other clinical applications include cardiovascular imaging and chest wall disease (JOHNSON et al. 1998a).

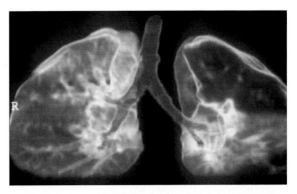

Fig. 3.7. Volume-rendered image using extraluminal visualization (bronchographic volume rendered image) in left upper bronchial atresia. An anteroposterior view with emphysema and absence of the left upper lobe bronchus. The transparency of the image allows visualization of the pulmonary vasculature

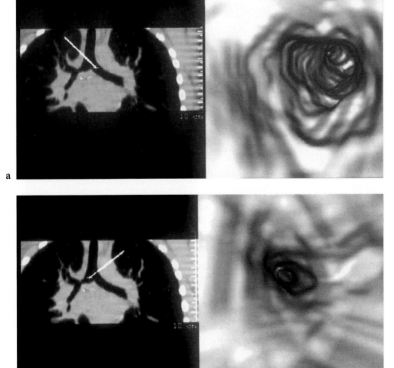

a

b

Fig. 3.8a,b. Virtual bronchoscopy (intraluminal visualization). Coronal multiplanar reformation image at the left shows the direction of view. Right bronchial stenosis in the area of the anastomosis in an 11-year-old boy with lung transplantation. **a** Bronchoscopic view showing left bronchus with normal caliber. **b** Bronchoscopic view of the stenotic right bronchus

3.3
Helical Chest Main Applications

The introduction of helical technology has extended the clinical indications of chest CT.

The most important diagnostic indications in children include evaluation of pulmonary nodules and thoracic masses, lesions located in difficult areas (e.g. cervico-thoracic, diaphragmatic, peri-diaphragmatic or chest wall regions) and in the central airways, definition of vascular anatomy and study of critically ill patients. In our institution, the most common indications for chest studies are the detection and characterization of pulmonary nodules and definition of mediastinal masses in children with known or suspected malignancies (46%). Other indications include infection (31%), congenital malformations (9%), vascular studies (5%) and others (9%).

3.3.1
Evaluation of Pulmonary Nodules and Chest Masses

Several studies have demonstrated that at least 10% more pulmonary nodules can be identified with helical than with conventional CT (COSTELLO et al. 1991; REMY-JARDIN et al. 1993). The ability to obtain overlapping reconstructions at smaller intervals with the contiguous volume data acquired increases the certainty that scans are obtained through the center of any lesion. These images depict the lesion without any volume averaging effect. In the setting of suspected metastatic disease using a single breath-hold technique, helical CT eliminates respiratory misregistration in patients caused by variations in the depth of respiration. This improves its ability to detect small nodules.

In children unable to breath-hold who must be scanned during quiet respiration, helical CT has evidenced no significant loss of accuracy in the detection of pulmonary metastases (COAKLEY et al. 1997a). The problem of variable respiratory excursion is further minimized by volume acquisition and the possibility of overlapping image reconstruction (BUCKLEY et al. 1995; COAKLEY et al. 1997b).

The volumetric data created during helical CT and the coronal and sagittal images reconstructed from them are useful for delineating the anatomy of vascular lesions that appear similar to nodules. It can also clarify the spatial relationships of a nodule to the pleura or diaphragm (BRINK et al. 1994a), a task that is especially difficult with conventional section-by-section CT because of the large excursion of the diaphragm between breaths.

Low-dose helical CT of the chest is highly sensitive for detecting pulmonary nodules, and could be an ideal alternative to conventional-dose helical CT for screening purposes (GARTENSCHLÄGER et al. 1998). Recommendations for the selection of parameters are given in the chest survey protocol (see Sect. 3.2.9.1). It is not necessary to use intravenous contrast agents in the evaluation of pulmonary nodules.

To evaluate solitary pulmonary masses and mediastinal lesions, another indication of helical CT, we recommend the chest survey protocol with IV contrast material (see Sect. 3.2.9.1). The rapid scanning speed facilitates scanning during the time of peak contrast enhancement, permitting optimal definition of anatomic features. This is particularly important in children, who have little fat and lack intrinsic contrast differences.

Scanning during peak contrast levels optimizes the evaluation of mediastinal and hilar lymph nodes and masses. Mediastinal vascular structures and masses are easily differentiated (Fig. 3.9). Helical CT is the procedure of choice for evaluating anterior or middle mediastinal masses. Posterior mediastinal masses can also be studied by helical CT, but MRI is the procedure of choice in these cases. Special attention should be given to intraspinal extension.

An important indication for helical CT is tumor staging and the follow-up evaluation of treatment. Compared with conventional CT, helical CT can facilitate identification of infiltration, vascular encasement, airway displacement and hilar lymph nodes. Multiplanar reconstructions can be very useful for identifying infiltration, encasement or compression of vital structures, and intraspinal extension. The resulting information can facilitate surgical planning or radiation therapy. Another advantage is that chest-abdominal studies can be performed in a single session with a single dose of IV contrast material. This is especially important in the evaluation of patients with lymphoma.

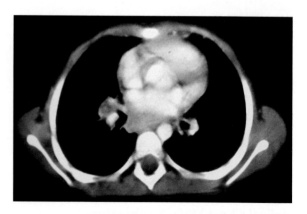

Fig. 3.9. Axial enhanced CT image in a 3-year-old boy with tuberculous lymph nodes. Right hilar and subcarinal lymph nodes well differentiated from vascular and mediastinal structures

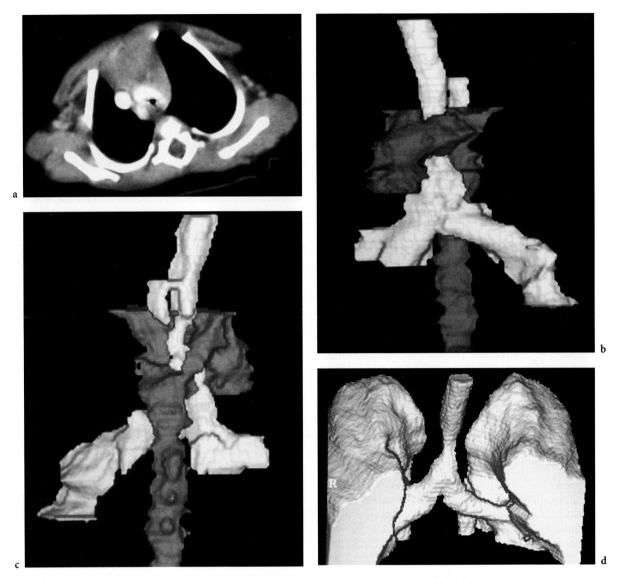

Fig. 3.10a–d. Double aortic arch in a 1-month-old boy with important respiratory distress. **a** Axial enhanced CT image. Double aortic arch surrounding the trachea, which appears very narrow. **b** Anteroposterior shaded surface display (SSD) image of the aorta and trachea. A double aortic arch encases the trachea. **c** Posteroanterior SSD image of the aorta and trachea. Both aortic arches join the descending aorta. **d** Anteroposterior SSD image of the trachea. The tracheal stenosis is due to compression by the double aortic arch

Other abnormalities that can benefit from helical CT studies at peak contrast enhancement include congenital large vessel abnormalities (Fig. 3.10), congenital chest masses (pulmonary sequestration, cystic adenomatoid malformation) (see Fig. 3.2), pulmonary and pleural infections (Fig. 3.11), chest trauma, the definition of surgical shunts and postoperative vascular anatomy, vascular masses (angiomas), and central pulmonary thromboemboli (REMY-JARDIN et al. 1992).

3.3.2
Evaluation of Vascular Anatomy: CT Angiography

CT angiography is a new and important application of helical CT. CT angiography can depict congenital and acquired vascular abnormalities of the chest in children because of its high-quality vascular imaging. Standardized CT angiography and arterial timing test (or bolus-tracking technique) protocols are rec-

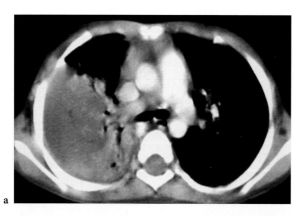
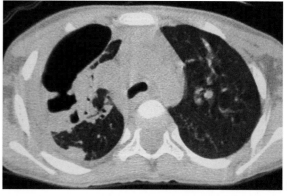

a   b

Fig. 3.11a,b. Right lung pleuropneumonia in a 3-year-old boy with persistence of clinical symptoms despite treatment. **a** Axial enhanced CT image. Intrapleural fluid and consolidation of the pulmonary parenchyma. The lack of pulmonary parenchyma enhancement has been described as a sign of a bad prognosis. **b** Follow-up low-dose high-resolution CT image 3 weeks later. The pulmonary parenchyma shows necrotic areas with a pleuropulmonary fistula and residual pleural thickening

ommended in such cases (see above). Optimal contrast enhancement is best achieved using a power injector. We never use manual injection. With CT angiography one can analyze vascular abnormalities of the pulmonary arteries, aortic arch and large vessels (double aortic arch, pulmonary sling, etc.) (KATZ et al. 1995) (Fig. 3.10b,c), as well as congenital chest masses (pulmonary sequestration, cystic adenomatoid malformation) (Fig. 3.12) in which depiction of the systemic vessel is important for the diagnosis.

<The improved contrast enhancement and the use of multiplanar and 3-D reconstructions afforded by helical CT are useful for characterizing normal and abnormal vascular anatomy. MRI is usually the technique of choice for evaluating congenital large vessel anomalies and other vascular anomalies, but helical CT could be an alternative in patients whose clinical condition requires a quick exam and where a lengthy MRI study would not be advisable. They can benefit from the high-speed scan acquisition and the low requirements of sedation.

There are several postprocessing techniques available to analyze the vascular anatomy. Curved multiplanar reconstructions are useful for displaying serpentine vascular structures, such as a systemic vessel in pulmonary sequestration, but they are highly operator-dependent and time-consuming (Fig. 3.2c,d). STS-MIP requires less computer time and can be used as an alternative to curved MPR to improve the depiction of vessels.

MIP, SSD and VR images, the most frequently used to provide information on vascular anatomy, are similar or comparable to angiograms. Since these images can be rotated in a movie-loop, they enable the visualization of lesions from innumerable viewing angles. This can facilitate the analysis of underlying pathologies and improve the display of the vessel's origin on superimposed images (Fig. 3.12b,c).

CT angiography can replace conventional angiography in selected applications. Helical CT angiocardiography with 3-D reconstructions is superior to echocardiography for the noninvasive assessment of pulmonary artery anatomy and is equal to angiography in patients with complex congenital heart disease (VESTRA et al. 1999). As compared to conventional arteriography, CT angiography has the advantages of lower patient morbidity, and reductions in cost and time.

3.3.3
Evaluation of Central Airways

Helical CT of the central airways is performed with thin collimation during one breath-hold or during quiet respiration (see Sect. 3.2.9.2). As a result of the volumetric scanning, more detailed anatomy can be obtained by reconstructions at 50% overlap increment. A comparison of standard CT at 8 mm contiguous increment and helical CT with thin collimation and reconstruction at 50% overlap showed that helical CT was the superior imaging technique (SHAFER et al. 1991).

Helical CT demonstrates 95% of the normal segmental bronchial anatomy. The inferior and superior lingular segmental bronchi, which are often difficult

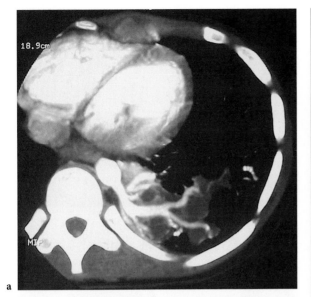

a

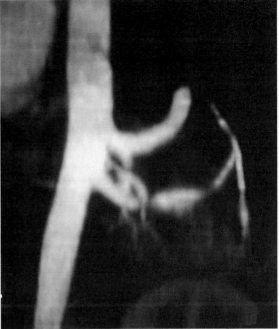

b

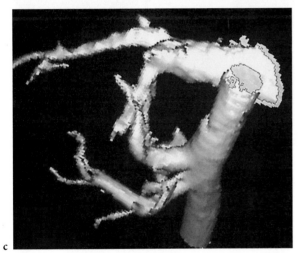

c

Fig. 3.12a–c. CT angiography of a pulmonary sequestration in a 6-year-old boy who was asymptomatic, but had a persistent dense image in the left pulmonary base. **a** Axial CT image. A large vessel is seen arising from the aorta, with multiple branches supplying a pulmonary mass. **b** Anteroposterior maximum intensity projection image. Three systemic vessels coming from the aorta are seen to feed the pulmonary sequestration. **c** Posteroanterior shaded surface display (SSD) image. The 3-D depth perception created by the SSD technique improves recognition of the spatial relationships of the three vessels arising from the aorta. Two veins are also shown in the upper area of the image. With a cine-loop rotating image, the origin and the course of vessels can be better depicted

to visualize on conventional CT scans, can be demonstrated in 85% of patients on helical scans (COSTELLO et al. 1992b). MPR, MIP, SSD and VR images beautifully depict the central airways and are of great clinical value in their assessment (KAUCZOR et al. 1996; NICOTRA et al. 1997).

Helical CT of the airways is mainly indicated in the study of congenital and acquired abnormalities of the tracheobronchial tree (Fig. 3.13), postpneumectomy complications (Fig. 3.14), complications after lung transplantation (Fig. 3.3), and endobronchial lesions (Fig. 3.15).

Postoperative patients are good candidates for assessment by helical CT. Following pneumectomy, a dehiscence or a bronchopleural fistula can occur at the anastomotic region (Fig. 3.14). Bronchopleural fistulae are best shown on coronal reformations. After lung transplantation, complications at the sites of tracheobronchial anastomosis such as dehiscences and stenosis are common. Helical CT may demonstrate a minor dehiscence at an anastomotic site even when conventional CT shows no abnormalities. Two- and 3-D images are better than axial ones to identify stenotic lesions, especially stenoses in obliquely oriented bronchi. Multiplanar reconstructions along the axis of the bronchus are also useful.

Endobronchial lesions and intrabronchial stent location are best shown on multiplanar reconstructions along the axis of the bronchus. Endobronchial lesions (endobronchial tumors, long-standing foreign

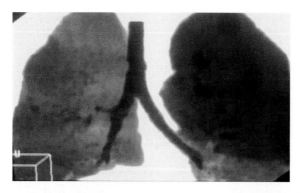

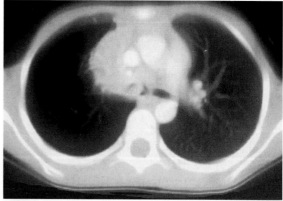

a

Fig. 3.13. Anteroposterior maximum intensity projection image. Bronchial atresia in a 4-year-old girl with cough and minor respiratory infections. Note the absence of the left upper lobe bronchus. There is a hyperlucency of the left upper lobe caused by pulmonary emphysema

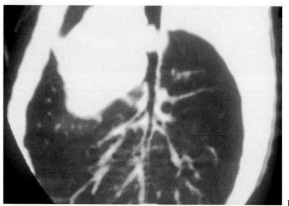

b

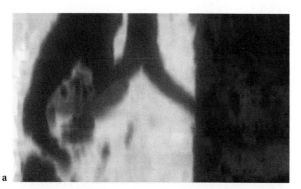

a

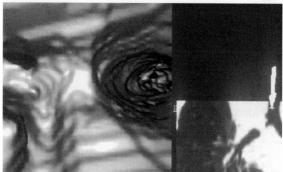

c

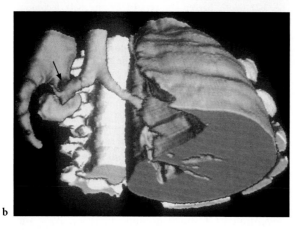

b

Fig. 3.15a–c. Intrabronchial carcinoid tumor in a 9-year-old boy with a persistent right upper lobe atelectasis. **a** Axial CT image. The right main bronchus seems to be occupied by a mass. **b** Oblique multiplanar reformation (MPR) image through the right main bronchus. An intrabronchial mass located in the right main bronchus is confirmed. **c** Virtual bronchoscopy (view from the carina). The coronal MPR image at the right indicates the viewpoint. The right main bronchus is occupied by a mass

Fig. 3.14a,b. Three-dimensional images of the tracheobronchial tree in a 7-year-old boy with a previous right pneumectomy for necrotizing pneumonia. **a** Anteroposterior maximum intensity projection image. There is a right pneumothorax and a bronchopleural fistula in the area of the bronchial suture line. **b** Tilted anteroposterior shaded surface display image viewed from below. Three-dimensional perception is better with this technique. The bronchopleural fistula is well depicted. The spine is shown posteriorly

bodies) can also be shown with virtual endoscopy images (Fig. 3.15c). Intrabronchial foreign bodies can be difficult to diagnose. There is often no history of foreign body aspiration. These patients are usually set for thoracic CT examination due to foreign body complications. CT scanning can help in detecting the intrabronchial lesion in these cases.

Helical CT can be very useful in evaluating the tracheobronchial tree when using bronchographic images depicted by the VR technique. Tracheobronchography is quite invasive and can carry a significant risk in pediatric patients. This risk is greatest in conditions that compromise the tracheal lumen. Moreover, airway lesions may not be isolated anomalies. It is important to emphasize the possibility offered by helical CT of simultaneously providing bronchographic images as well as angiographic reconstructions. This combination of data allows the evaluation of complex malformations in a single examination and can avoid unnecessary invasive diagnostic procedures.

Developing applications, such as virtual bronchoscopy (FERRETI et al. 1996) and real-time VR (REMY-JARDIN et al. 1998; JOHNSON et al. 1998a), are currently being explored.

3.3.4
Evaluation of Difficult Areas: Cervicothoracic Junction, Peridiaphragmatic Area and Chest Wall

Helical CT is useful for imaging lesions in areas that are difficult to evaluate on axial images and are better assessed on 2- or 3-D reformatted images. Multiplanar reconstructions, generated from helical CT data, are particularly helpful in lesions located in cervicothoracic and apical areas (HARTY and KRAMER 1998) (Fig. 3.16a,b), peridiaphragmatic and diaphragmatic areas (ISRAEL et al. 1996) (Fig. 3.16c,d) and the chest wall. The reformatted images better depict the extension of lesions and their relationship to adjacent anatomic structures.

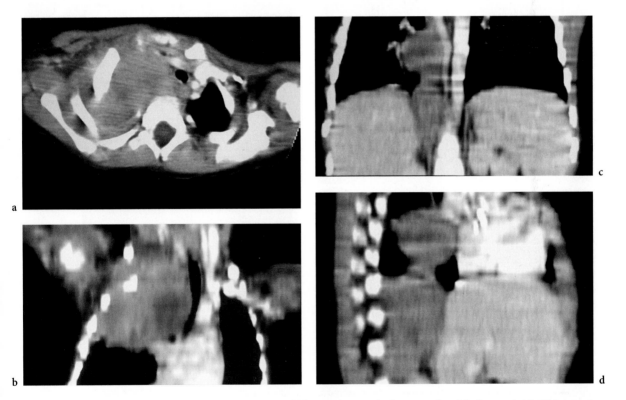

Fig. 3.16a–d. Cervicothoracic tumor (PNET) in a 3-year-old boy with a cervical mass and weight loss. **a** Axial CT image. A heterogeneous mass located in the thoracic apex is seen to displace the trachea. **b** Coronal multiplanar reformation (MPR) image. The extension of the apical mass into the neck and to the lateral chest wall is better shown. **c** Coronal MPR image from the same patient 1 year after the diagnosis demonstrates mediastinal metastasis progressing to the abdomen. MPR images better show the anatomical relationship between the abdominal mass and the diaphragm. The hourglass-shaped mass displaces the diaphragm laterally. **d** Sagittal MPR image. The mass extends to the abdomen and displaces the diaphragm anteriorly

Although uncommon in children, tumors of the chest wall are frequently malignant and may aggressively invade the pleural space, lung, spinal canal or mediastinum. The preoperative imaging evaluation should focus on assessment of the size and extent of the primary tumor and any possible bone invasion or involvement of the chest wall musculature. Both CT and MRI can identify bone and soft-tissue involvement by chest wall tumors (DONNELLY et al. 1997). CT is more sensitive in detecting cortical bone disruptions and calcifications, but MRI is better at depicting soft-tissue and marrow involvement. Three-D reconstructions also play a role in the depiction of bony structures of the chest wall and the spine. SSD images can be useful in depicting the chest wall deformity in pectus excavatum.

3.3.5
Evaluation of Critically Ill Patients

One of the greatest advantages of helical CT is its speed; examinations are shorter and the need for sedation is greatly reduced. This means that some patient groups (e.g. very ill patients and trauma cases), not previously considered to be good candidates, can now benefit from CT studies. In these patients the speed of helical CT allows an enormous amount of information to be obtained in a very short time, and enables both the chest and abdomen to be examined with only one data acquisition and a single dose of intravenous contrast material (Fig. 3.17). Helical CT studies in these cases should be done under the supervision of the intensive care physician, who also oversees the transport of the child to the

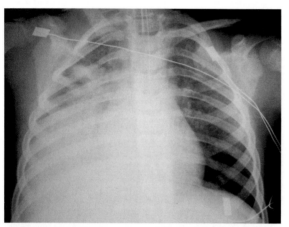
a

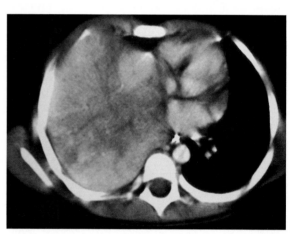
b

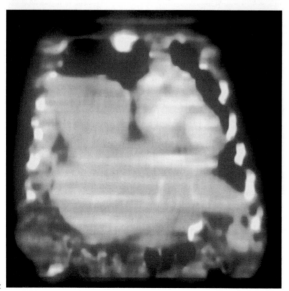
c

Fig. 3.17a–c. Traumatic diaphragmatic hernia due to a traffic accident in a 4-year-old boy. **a** Chest X-ray shows opacification of the right pulmonary base and no definition of the diaphragm. **b** Axial enhanced CT image. There is heterogeneous enhancement of the intrathoracic liver due to ischemia. **c** Coronal multiplanar reformation image shows an intrathoracic liver. Note the defect through which the liver migrated to the thorax (collar sign).

CT facilities. The images can be reconstructed and reformatted retrospectively after the patient has been returned to the intensive care unit.

3.3.6
Evaluation of Dubious Images on Chest Radiography

Helical CT and its technical capabilities of multiplanar and 3-D imaging are often useful for defining a "peculiar" image seen on chest X-rays (Fig. 3.18) and for establishing its exact anatomical location (Fig. 3.19).

3.4
Conclusions

Helical CT technology has several potential clinical benefits when used in pediatric patients. These include speed, improved image quality and reductions in the volume of contrast material required, in the use of sedation, and in radiation exposure (using extended pitch). Two- or 3-D reformatted images that are of great value in clinical diagnosis can be generated with the available post-processing methods. The technical aspects of this technique, the clinical indications and the suggested protocols to be used have been set out in this chapter.

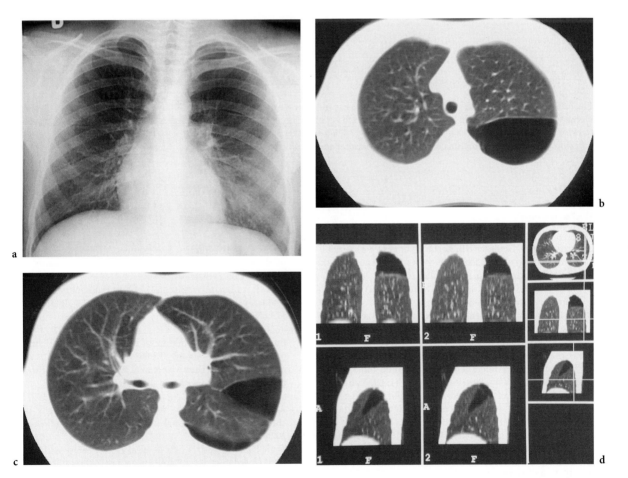

Fig. 3.18a–d. Pneumothorax located in the left major fissure in an 11-year-old boy with chest pain. A pneumothorax had been diagnosed 3 months earlier. **a** Anteroposterior chest X-ray. A hyperlucency and a small linear density of questionable etiology are noted at the left apex. **b** Axial CT image taken at the supracarinal level. There is a posterior left pneumothorax. **c** Axial CT image at the subcarinal level. The pneumothorax is located posteriorly and in the major fissure. **d** Coronal and sagittal multiplanar reformation images. The pneumothorax in the major fissure is shown best on these multiplanar images

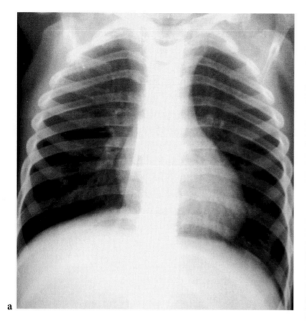
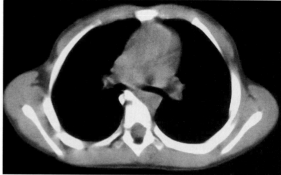
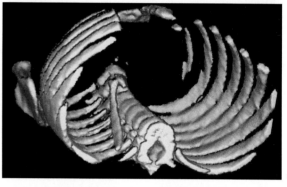

Fig. 3.19a–c. Intrathoracic rib in an asymptomatic 3-year-old boy. **a** Anteroposterior chest X-ray. There is an abnormal, dense, elongated structure in a right paravertebral position. **b** Axial CT image at the subcarinal level. The dense bony image is seen to arise from the anterior area of the vertebral body. **c** Shaded surface display image better shows the intrathoracic rib with its anterior vertebral origin and its course, running parallel and oblique to the spine

References

Ambrosino MM, Genieser NB, Roche KJ et al (1994) Feasibility of high-resolution low-dose chest CT in evaluating the pediatric chest. Pediatr Radiol 24:6–10

Brink JA (1995) Technical aspects of helical (spiral) CT. Radiol Clin North Am 33:825–841

Brink JA, Heiken JP, Semenkovich J et al (1994a) Abnormalities of the diaphragm and adjacent structures: findings on multiplanar spiral CT scan. AJR 163:307–310

Brink JA, Heiken JP, Wang G et al (1994b) Helical CT: principles and technical considerations. Radiographics 14:887–893

Buckley JA, Scott WWJ, Siegelman SS et al (1995) Pulmonary nodules: effect of increased data sampling on detection with spiral CT and confidence in diagnosis. Radiology 196:395–400

Coakley FV, Cohen MD, Waters DJ et al (1997a) The detection of pulmonary metastases with pathologic correlation in canine model: effect of breathing on the accuracy of helical CT. AJR 169:1615–1618

Coakley FV, Cohen MD, Waters DJ et al (1997 b) Detection of pulmonary metastases with pathologic correlation: effects of breathing on accuracy of spiral CT. Pediatr Radiol 27:576–579

Cook BA, Bass JW, Nomizu S, Alexander ME (1992) Sedation of children for technical procedures: current standards of practice. Clin Pediatr 31:137–142

Costello P, Anderson W, Blume D (1991) Pulmonary nodule: evaluation with spiral volumetric CT. Radiology 179:875–876

Costello P, Dupuy DE, Ecker CP et al (1992a) Spiral CT of the thorax with reduced volume of contrast material: a comparative study. Radiology 183:663–666

Costello P, Kruskal J, Dupuy D et al (1992b) Evaluation of tracheobronchial tree with spiral CT. Radiology 185:355

Donnelly LF, Taylor CNR, Emery KH et al (1997) Asymptomatic, palpable, anterior chest wall lesions in children: is cross-sectional imaging necessary? Radiology 202:829–831

Egelhoff JC, Ball WS Jr, Kock BL et al (1997) Safety and efficacy of sedation in children using a structured sedation program. AJR 168:1259–1262

Engeler CE, Tashjian JH, Engeler CM (1994) Volumetric high-resolution CT in the diagnosis of interstitial lung disease and bronchiectasis: diagnostic accuracy and radiation dose. AJR 163:31–35

Ferreti GR, Vining DJ, Knoplioch J et al (1996) Tracheobronchial tree: three-dimensional spiral CT with bronchoscopic perspective. J Comput Assist Tomogr 20:777–781

Frush DP, Donnelly LP (1998) Helical CT in children: technical considerations and body applications. Radiology 209:37–48

Frush DP, Bisett GS III, Hall SC (1996) Pediatric sedation in radiology: the practice of safe sleep. AJR 167:1381–1387

Frush DP, Siegel MJ, Bisset GS III (1997) Challenges of pediatric spiral CT. Radiographics 17:939–959

Garcia-Peña P, Lucaya J (1999) Chest CT-scan in children: main applications and advantages. Pediatr Pneumonol 18:56–59

Gartenschläger M, Schweden F, Gast K et al (1998) Pulmonary nodules: detection with low-dose vs conventional-dose spiral CT. Eur Radiol 8:609–614

Harty MP, Kramer SS (1998) Recent advances in pediatric pulmonary imaging. Curr Opin Pediatr 10:227–235

Hopper KD, Singapuri K, Finkel A (2000) Body CT and oncologic imaging. Radiology 215:27–40

Hu H, He HD, Foley WD et al (2000) Four multidetector-row helical CT: image quality and volume coverage speed. Radiology 215:55–62

Israel RS, Mayberry JC, Primack SL (1996) Diaphragmatic rupture. Use of helical CT scanning with multiplanar reformations. AJR 167:1201–1203

Johnson PT, Fishman EK, Duckwall JR et al (1998a) Interactive three-dimensional volume rendering of spiral CT data: current applications in the thorax. Radiographics 18:165–187

Johnson JL, Kramer SS, Mahboubi S (1998b) Air trapping in children: evaluation with dynamic lung densitometry with spiral CT. Radiology 206:95–101

Kaste SC, Young CW (1996) Safe use of power injectors with central patient motion and peripheral venous access devices for pediatric CT. Pediatr Radiol 26:449–501

Kaste SC, Young CW, Holmes TP et al (1997) Effect of helical CT on the frequency of sedation in pediatric patients. AJR 168:1001–1003

Katz M, Konen E, Rozenman J, Szeinberg A et al (1995) Spiral CT and 3d image reconstruction of vascular rings and associated tracheobronchial anomalies. J Comput Assist Tomogr 19:564–568

Kauczor HU, Wolcke B, Fisher B et al (1996) Three-dimensional helical CT of the tracheobronchial tree: evaluation of imaging protocols and assessment of suspected stenosis with bronchoscopic correlation. AJR 167:419–424

Lucaya J, Garcia-Peña P, Herrera L et al (2000a) Expiratory chest CT in children. AJR 174:1–7

Lucaya J, Piqueras J, Garcia-Peña P et al (2000b) Low-dose high-resolution CT of the chest in children and young adults: dose, cooperation, artifacts incidence, and image quality. AJR 175:985–992

Napel SA, Jeffrey RB Jr (1993) STS-MIP: a new reconstruction technique for CT of the chest. J Comput Assist Tomogr 17:832–838

Napel SA (1995) Basic principles of spiral CT. In: Fishman EK, Jeffrey RB Jr (eds) Spiral CT: principles, techniques, and clinical application. Raven, New York, pp 1–9

Nicotra JJ, Mahboubi S, Kramer SS (1997) Three-dimensional imaging of the pediatric airway. Int J Pediatr Otorhinolaryngol 41:299–305

Pappas JN, Donnelly LF, Frush DP (2000) Reduced frequency of sedation of young children with multisection helical CT. Radiology 215:897–899

Paterson A, Frush DP, Donnelly LF (2001) Helical CT of the body: are settings adjusted for pediatric patients? AJR 176:1–6

Remy-Jardin M, Remy J, Wattinne L et al (1992) Central pulmonary thromboembolim: diagnosis with spiral volumetric CT with the single-breath-hold tecnique comparison with pulmonary angiography. Radiology 185:381–387

Remy-Jardin M, Remi J, Giraud F et al (1993) Pulmonary nodules detection with thick-section spiral CT versus conventional CT. Radiology 187:513–520

Remy-Jardin M, Remy J, Artaud D et al (1998) Volume rendering of the tracheobronchial tree: clinical evaluation of bronchographic images. Radiology 208:761–770

Rogalla P, Stöver B, Scheer I et al (1999) Low-dose spiral CT: applicability to paediatric chest imaging. Pediatr Radiol 28:565–569

Rubin GD, Leung AN, Robertson VJ et al (1998) Thoracic spiral CT: influence of subsecond gantry rotation on image quality. Radiology 208:771–776

Shafer CM, Prokop M, Dohring W et al (1991) Spiral CT of the tracheobronchial system: optimized technique and clinical applications. Radiology 181:274

Siegel MJ, Luker GD (1995) Pediatric applications of helical (spiral) CT. Radiol Clin North Am 33:997–1022

Sillverman PM, Cooper CI, Welman DI et al (1995) Helical CT: practical considerations and potential pitfalls. Radiographics 15:25–36

Stokberger SM Jr, Hicklin JA, Liang Y et al (1998) Spiral CT with ionic and non-ionic contrast material: evaluation of patient motion and scan quality. Radiology 208:631–636

Takahashi M, Maguire WM, Ashtari M et al (1998) Low-dose spiral computer tomography of the thorax. Invest Radiol 33:68–73

Vestra SJ, Hill JA, Alejos JC et al (1999) Tree-dimentional helical CT of pulmonary arteries in infants and children with congenital heart disease. AJR 173:109–115

Wang G, Vannier MW (1994) Stair-step artifacts in three-dimensional helical CT: an experimental study. Radiology 191:79–83

White KS (1995) Reduced need for sedation in patients undergoing helical CT of the chest and abdomen. Pediatr Radiol 25:344–346

4 High-Resolution CT of the Lung in Children

Javier Lucaya and Hubert Ducou Le Pointe

CONTENTS

Javier Lucaya, MD
Department of Pediatric Radiology, Vall d'Hebron Hospitals, ps. Vall d'Hebron 119–129, Barcelona 08035, Spain
Hubert Ducou Le Pointe, MD
Service de Radiologie Pédiatrique, Hôpital d'Enfants Armand-Trousseau, 26, Av. du Docteur-Arnold-Netter, 75012 Paris, France

I.
Technique, Indications, Anatomy, Features of Lung Disease

Javier Lucaya

4.1
Introduction

High-resolution computed tomography (HRCT) of the chest is a technique capable of imaging the lung with excellent spatial resolution, offering precise anatomic detail. HRCT can demonstrate the morphologic characteristics of both the normal and abnormal lung parenchyma and its interstitium (Webb et al. 1996). In this regard, it provides more information than chest radiographs and conventional chest CT. This explains the increasing demand for this technique in the evaluation of most pediatric lung disorders.

4.2
Technique

To optimize spatial resolution it is necessary to use thin sections. In keeping with most authors, we use 1.0-mm collimation, but good images can be obtained with 3-mm collimation. It has been shown that there is no diagnostic difference with use of 1.5- or 3-mm thick sections (Murata et al. 1988). However, since radiation dose with 1.0-mm sections at 10-mm intervals is lower than with 3-mm scans at the same intervals (Rothenberg and Pentlow 1992), we recommend using the thinner sections. As a general rule we use 10-mm intervals and in premature infants we sometimes use 5-mm intervals.

Use of a high-spatial frequency algorithm (bone algorithm) is critical when performing HRCT of the lungs. The bone algorithm reduces image smoothing and increases spatial resolution, making the structures appear sharper (Mayo et al. 1987). In contrast to what occurs with the lungs, the quality of mediastinal images is poor with all HRCT techniques. This is because low-contrast structures, such as the mediastinum, are affected more by noise than high-contrast structures, such as the lung. The quality of mediastinal imaging improves somewhat with use of the low-spatial frequency (standard) algorithm; thus, we always use this filter to reconstruct mediastinal images.

Scanning should be performed with the smallest field of view (FOV) able to encompass the patient. Decreasing the FOV effectively reduces pixel size and improves spatial resolution (Mayo et al. 1987; Murata et al. 1989). The combination of a 512+512 matrix and a 40-cm FOV results in a pixel size of 0.78 mm. With targeted image reconstruction using a FOV of 25 cm, pixel size decreases to 0.49 mm and spatial resolution correspondingly increases. With an 18-cm FOV, pixel size is further reduced to 0.35 mm. We recommend use of a 15–18 cm FOV for neonates and small infants, 25 cm for larger infants and 35–45 cm for older children and adolescents. Generally the smallest structures visible on HRCT range from 0.3–0.5 mm in thickness. Thinner structures, measuring 0.1–0.2 mm are occasionally seen (Webb et al. 1996).

In addition to increasing image sharpness, HRCT techniques increase image noise. Much of this noise is quantum-related and it can be reduced by increasing the kilovolt peak or milliamperes used during scanning, thus improving scan quality. Noise is inversely proportional to the square root of the product of the milliamperage and scan time (Mayo et al. 1987; Webb et al. 1996). Although increasing kilovolt peak and milliamperage reduces image noise, the issue as to whether it is necessary to use high kilovolt peak and mAs settings for HRCT is somewhat subjective. Most authors recommend a 120–140 kVp and 100–200 mAs technique for HRCT in children (Lynch et al. 1999a; Moon et al. 1996; Siegel 1999). Nonetheless, reliable diagnostic scans can also be obtained using significantly lower milliamperages (Ambrosino et al. 1994; Zwirewich et al. 1991).

Since 1995 we routinely perform our HRCT scans using 50 mA and 0.6 s (34 mAs) for children able to follow breath-holding commands and 50 mA and 1 s (50 mAs) for non-cooperative children. We ran a study comparing visualization of the bronchi, vessels, and fissures, and sharpness of peripheral structures in scans performed with either 34 or 50 mAs and 180 mAs, keeping all the remaining technical parameters

constant. There were no differences in image quality between scans performed with 50 and 180 mAs. Small differences, consisting of slight blurring of fissures and peripheral structures, were apparent in the 34 mAs as compared to the 180 mAs images. In addition, when examining patients unable to follow breath-holding commands, there was an increased incidence of streak artifacts in the 34 mAs scans. The study demonstrated that HRCT performed with 180 or 50 mAs techniques produces images of similar quality in children regardless of their ability to cooperate. The 34 mAs technique offers good quality exams but its use should be reserved for cooperative children (Lucaya et al. 2000).

In the last six month we have reduced our mAs even further. Most cooperative children are studied with 25 mA and 1 second, and those who do not follow breath-holding commands with 50 mA and 1 second.

We also measured and compared radiation dose in scans performed with 180 mAs vs. 34 and 50 mAs. HRCT dose results were 5.4±1.6 mSv for 180 mAs, 1.5±0.5 mSv for 50 mAs and 1.1±0.3 mSv for 34 mAs. As compared to the 180 mAs technique, low-dose techniques resulted in dose reductions of 72% for 50 mAs and 80% for 34 mAs (Lucaya et al. 2000). Combining HRCT scans at 20-mm intervals with low-dose scans (40 mA) would result in an average skin dose comparable to that associated with chest radiography (Mayo et al. 1993). Moreover, with properly performed HRCT, one can manage to study the lung with less radiation to the female breast than with conventional radiography.

When examining children, the potential side effects of radiation exposure should always be kept in mind. With use of data obtained in A-bomb survivors it has been predicted that delivery of 1 Rad (0.01 Gy) of radiation to a woman's breast before the age of 35 fractionally increases her risk of breast cancer by 13.6% over the expected spontaneous rate for the general population (Land et al. 1993). This is one of the main reasons why we strongly support the use of low-dose techniques for children. When examining children with HRCT, we try to either skip the area around the nipple or protect the breasts with thin layers of radiation-absorbent material such as bismuth-coated latex shields. These measures provide girls with some breast radiation protection without affecting the diagnostic quality of the images (Hopper et al. 1998). In our experience over the last 6 months, the use of 2-mm thick bismuth-coated latex shielding in girls examined with low-dose (50 mA) HRCT saves an average of 40% of radiation dose to the breast without affecting the quality of the CT images (Fig. 4.1).

In children under 8 years of age the mean attenuation value of normal lung ranges from –500 HU to –700 HU and in those 8 years or older it is about –800 HU, which is similar to the attenuation value in healthy adults (between –700 HU and –800 HU). It should be emphasized that there are no "correct" or ideal window settings for demonstrating lung anatomy, to be used when photographing an HRCT study. Often the precise window width and levels chosen are a matter of personal preference. However, it is important that at least one lung window setting be used consistently in all patients. If this is not done, it is difficult to develop an understanding of what appearances are normal and abnormal, to compare cases and to compare sequential examinations in the same patient. Level and width settings of approximately –700/1000 HU are appropriate for routine lung windows. Window level/width settings of 50/350 are best for evaluating the mediastinum and hila (WEBB et al. 1996). The recommended scanning parameters for HRCT of the chest in children are shown in Table 4.1.

Since the diagnostic sensitivity and specificity of HRCT of the lung are superior those of conventional chest X-rays, the indications for HRCT in children will undoubtedly increase. We are convinced that in the future the study of several lung diseases in children

Table 4.1. Recommended scanning parameters for HRCT of the chest in children

Slice thickness	1 mm
Interval	10 mm (in premature infants we may use 5 m
kVp	120–140
mA	25–50
Seconds	1
FOV	15–40
Filter	High-spatial-frequency algorithm (bone). Use standard for mediastinum

will be routinely performed with HRCT. Therefore, we should ensure that the examination is as little aggressive as possible. For this purpose, scans should be tailored to the specific clinical problem, the number of sections and exposure parameters should be decreased as much as possible, low-dose techniques should be used routinely and scout views spared.

To tailor the examination to diagnostic needs, the radiologist should know the patient's clinical features and previous imaging findings. Furthermore, to obtain the greatest diagnostic information that HRCT can provide, the radiologist should directly supervise the study and decide whether additional or special slices (prone, lateral decubitus, expiratory, etc.) are required. This approach avoids unnecessary examinations and virtually eliminates incomplete studies.

Needless to say, the routine use of low-dose techniques is mandatory to minimize the potential side effects of ionizing radiation exposure. This is extremely important for extending the indications of HRCT in children so they can benefit from the excellent diagnostic information it provides.

4.3
Sedation

Another important measure aimed at reducing the aggressiveness of HRCT is to avoid anesthesia and use sedation as little as possible. In our practice we have never used general anesthesia for HRCT in children and we have reduced the use of sedation in children under 6 years old to a mere 2.4%. The introduction of modern, silent scanners has been very helpful in this regard. With the old scanners our incidence of sedated patients was approximately 15%. Since we could not know in advance which patients would require sedation and aspiration is a major clinical concern in sedated children, we used to keep all our

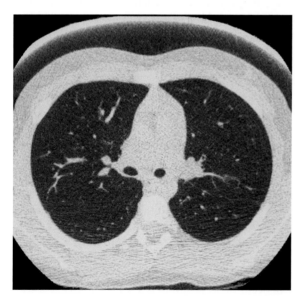

Fig. 4.1. A 10-year-old girl. HRCT of the lungs performed using a 2-mm-thick bismuth-coated latex shield over both nipples. Notice there are no significant artifacts

patients NPO (nothing by mouth) for 4 h before the exam in children under 1 year old and for 6 h in those 1 year or older. Considering the extremely low incidence of sedation currently required for HRCT, we have recently changed this policy. Nowadays none of our patients are kept NPO and those who, once in the gantry, behave poorly and require sedation, are rescheduled. Since well-fed infants behave better than hungry ones, this policy will undoubtedly further reduce the 2.4% of patients needing sedation.

We resort to all sorts of tricks to keep the non-sedated patients still. We make sure they are warm and allow the parents to hold their hands and talk to them. To attract a fidgety child's attention, we project some "teletubbies" or other t.v. characters onto the gantry. They usually become captivated at once and stop moving and crying. At that moment, we take a section. Occasionally, we ring a gantry bell to attract their attention. It is also helpful to offer them a bottle of glucose water.

When all our maneuvers fail, we reschedule the study, keep the patient NPO for 4–6 h and administer sedation before the exam. We use chloral hydrate p.o. at a dose of 50–75 mg/kg, with a maximum dosage of 2.000 mg. Children are given an initial dose of 50 mg/kg and are kept in the sedation area. If after 20–30 min the patient has not fallen asleep, a second dose of chloral hydrate, usually half the initial dose (25 mg/kg) is given. Exceptionally, we may go up to a total dose of 100 mg/kg. The onset of action is usually within 25–30 min and the duration of sedation is 30–40 min. Chloral hydrate has a bitter taste that children dislike. Attempts to conceal it with sweeteners like cherry syrup are not very helpful. Although the taste improves somewhat, it still remains unpleasant. Furthermore, the total volume of fluid to be administered increases and dose control becomes difficult. Consequently, we always use undiluted chloral hydrate administered directly by syringe or with a nipple connected to a syringe. With time and patience most children swallow it well. Although we use chloral hydrate mainly in children under 2 years of age, it can also be used in older patients.

Chloral hydrate is a successful sedative in 95%–99% of children (KARIAN et al. 1999; PEREIRA et al. 1993) and it has a very low rate of side effects. Transient respiratory depression (oxygen desaturation 10% below baseline for that patient for more than 15 s, despite repositioning of the head and neck to clear the airway) is the most common during or after sedation, yet it occurs in less than 1% of patients. Delayed complications such as vomiting, irritability and mild

respiratory difficulty are also rare (EGELHOFF et al. 1997). Certain patients are difficult to sedate, such as children with mental retardation, patients receiving chemotherapy or antiseizure medication and those habituated to sedation (HUBBARD et al. 1992).

All sedated patients are given oxygen by mask or nasal prong to increase pulmonary oxygen reserves and permit prolonged apnea or airway obstruction without hypoxia. Oxygen should be administered to all patients receiving sedative medications with the possible exception of neonates at risk for retinopathy of prematurity, in which case a neonatologist should be consulted. There are no rules about the amount of supplemental oxygen that a patient requires; rather, administration of any amount improves the margin of safety. Thus, there is no legitimate reason to not administer oxygen routinely when patients are sedated (FISHER 1990). Continuous monitoring of the vital signs (at least every 5 min) must be performed and recorded during each use of sedation.

The physiologic measurements we monitor include oxygenation (with pulse oximetry), heart rate, respiratory rate and temperature. The alarm on the pulse oximeter is usually set at 90% oxygen saturation, but any decrease below 95% is immediately investigated. The majority of apparent desaturations are due to patient motion and loss of sensor contact. A small number of patients, however, demonstrate significant decreases in pO_2. Most of these are transient and are quickly corrected by repositioning the head and extending the neck. Occasionally, a patient requires suctioning of the oral cavity. A suction device and size-appropriate recovery equipment must be on hand during each sedation procedure. Children who have medical conditions that compromise the airway require special attention with respect to cardiopulmonary monitoring and airway management. These children may not be appropriate candidates for sedation by personnel who do not routinely deal with pediatric airway management and cardiopulmonary resuscitation. Children who fall into this monitoring category include those with anatomic airway anomalies (craniofacial defects), those with airway diseases such as obstructive adenotonsillar hyperplasia, acute respiratory infection, and uncontrolled asthma, and those with significant cardiopulmonary, neurologic and hepatorenal disorders. Life-threatening airway obstruction or respiratory depression with hypoxia can occur in these children (VADE et al. 1995).

Once the examination is over, all sedated patients are discharged home or transported to the inpatient wards when they meet the postanesthesia care unit discharge criteria recommended by the American Academy of Pediatrics (AAP 1992): (1) Cardiovascular function and airway patency are satisfactory and stable; (2) the patient is easily arousable, and protective reflexes are intact; (3) the patient can talk (if age appropriate); (4) the patient can sit unaided (if age-appropriate); (5) the state of hydration is adequate; (6) for a very young or handicapped child, incapable of the expected responses, the presedation level of responsiveness or a level as close as possible to the normal level for that child should be achieved. Parents are instructed not to feed the children until their level of consciousness and motor function have returned to presedation ranges. They should also be instructed not to use the children's car seats on their way home after a procedure. Children may fall asleep with the rhythmic motion of the automobile and the head fall forward, thereby obstructing the upper airway (CoTé et al. 2000). When examining critically ill patients, we require the assistance of a pediatrician from the intensive care unit. After the examination is completed, these patients are returned to their wards immediately under the supervision of the specialist. Other sedation regimes (see Chap. 3) are practically never required for HRCT. There have been some reports in the literature on the use of oral pentobarbital sodium, claiming that its acceptance is better than that of choral hydrate (CHUNG et al. 2000). However, we have not used it.

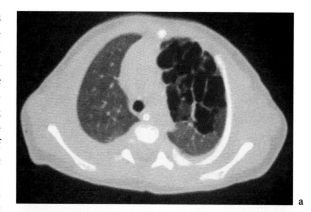

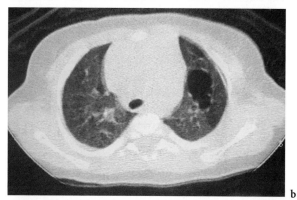

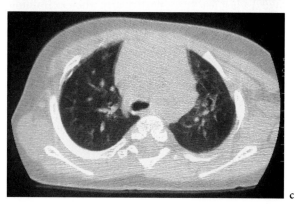

4.4
Special Techniques

4.4.1
"Focused" Chest CT

In patients with known "localized" lung disorders we recommend a "focused" technique, performing 1-mm slices at 10-mm intervals through the abnormal area of the lung. The rest of the lung is not scanned. We believe that study of the entire lung should not be performed in patients being controlled for known localized disease whose clinical symptoms and/or chest radiographs do not suggest progression to other lobes. The "focused" scan is used in the follow up of bronchiectasis, right middle lobe syndrome, cystic emphysema (Fig. 4.2), cavitated pneumonia and some pulmonary malformations not considered tributary of surgical treatment. In many of these cases, three

Fig. 4.2a–c. A 2-week-old premature baby with RDS treated with mechanical ventilation. Developed localized pulmonary emphysema in left upper lobe (**a**). Three months later (**b**) the lesions have decreased in size. At the age of 10 months (**c**) the CT is normal

or four low-dose HRCT slices will provide more information with less radiation dose to the female breast than PA and lateral chest radiographs. As always with HRCT, we try to skip the scout view to save on radiation exposure, though occasionally, and particularly when we want to reduce the exam to a mere two or three slices, we may use it. We center the exam with the light collimator. When we want to explore the right middle lobe, lingula and both lower lobes, we start the study midway between the sternal manubrium and the xiphoid. When examining the upper lobes, we start the study at the level of the clavicles and stop at the inferior border of the abnormal lobe.

4.4.2
"Limited Slice" Chest CT

The "limited slice" technique, consisting of 1-mm slices at 20-mm intervals, is a type of "sampling" technique that can be used for studying generalized lung disorders. Radiation dose is halved with this technique, making it particularly useful for follow up of patients with chronic lung disorders who require repeated examinations. The main indication for limited slice is in the control of patients with cystic fibrosis, bronchopulmonary dysplasia (Fig. 4.3), Langerhans' cell histiocytosis, alveolar proteinosis, and interstitial pneumonias.

In our experience use of both the "focused" and the "limited-slice" techniques has increased steadily over the last few years, particularly when examining female patients with chronic lung disorders. In addition to providing reliable diagnostic information, these techniques permit a reduction in radiation exposure to the breasts. If radiographs are still required in this group of patients we obtain the AP or PA views only. The lateral projection is not routinely performed.

4.4.3
Expiratory Slices. Lateral Decubitus
and Prone Views

Expiratory slices are extremely helpful when examining patients suspected of having airway abnormalities or patients with a history of repeated pulmonary infections who are found to have a normal or questionably normal inspiratory CT exam (Lucaya et al. 1999) (Fig. 4.4). They are also useful when the inspiratory sections demonstrate a mosaic pattern, characterized by visible differences in lung attenuation. Since children do not usually suffer pulmonary thromboembolic disorders, a mosaic pattern is almost always due to small airway disease with obstruction.

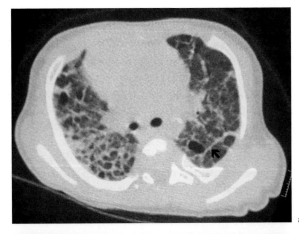

a

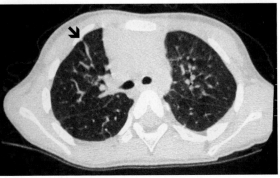

b

Fig. 4.3a,b. Bronchopulmonary dysplasia at the age of 2 months (**a**) shows marked septal thickening, parenchymal bands (*arrow*) and multifocal areas of hyperaeration. Repeated HRCT at the age of 2 years (**b**) shows a mosaic pattern and some residual parenchymal bands (*arrow*)

When the examined child presents clinical or radiological features commonly associated with small airway disease, we routinely complete the HRCT examination with three additional expiratory slices at three equally-spaced levels, one in the upper, one in the middle and one in the lower lobes. We use the table level information provided by the inspiratory exam to center these slices. Whereas the "level" of the upper lobes does not change significantly on expiration, the middle lobe, lingula and particularly the lower lobes will "move upwards" significantly, from 2–5 cm, depending on the size of the patient. To obtain good expiratory scans it is mandatory to spend some time teaching the child how to exhale well.

A useful method for obtaining expiratory scans in uncooperative children is to use the lateral decubitus technique (Capitanio and Kirkpatrick 1972; Lucaya et al. 1999). The patients are scanned in both

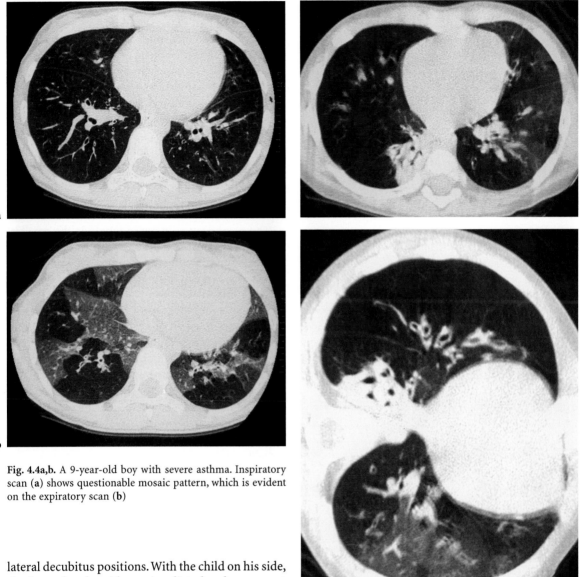

Fig. 4.4a,b. A 9-year-old boy with severe asthma. Inspiratory scan (a) shows questionable mosaic pattern, which is evident on the expiratory scan (b)

lateral decubitus positions. With the child on his side, the dependent hemithorax is splinted and movement of the thoracic cage is restricted on that side. When movement of the hemithorax is limited, the lung on the dependent side tends to be underaerated. Conversely, the hemithorax facing upwards is not restricted and the lung is well aerated. If air trapping is present, the affected lung, lobe or segment will remain hyperlucent when that side of the thorax is in the dependent position (Fig. 4.5).

This simple technique can also be used when trying to obtain good inspiratory examinations in noncooperative patients. As mentioned, the lung facing upwards is usually well aerated. Awareness of this fact is particularly helpful when examining noncooperative patients whose supine scans show a ground glass pattern consistent either with lung dis-

Fig. 4.5a,b. A 10-month-old baby with bilateral RSV pneumonia. Supine scan (a) demonstrates bilateral mosaic pattern. Air trapping confirmed on the left lateral decubitus view (b)

ease or with normal lung on expiration. When the lungs are normal the ground glass pattern will no longer persist in the lung facing upwards (Fig. 4.6). This same principle of gravity-dependent aeration is the rationale for using prone views to obtain good inspiratory scans of the lower lobes.

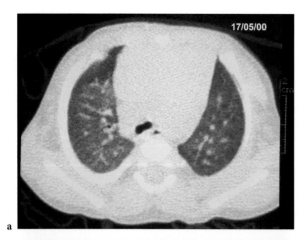

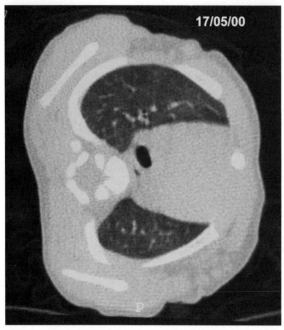

Fig. 4.6a,b. A 4-month-old infant with leukemia, fever and questionable pneumonia. Supine HRCT (**a**) shows ground glass in right upper lobe, which is no longer identified in left lateral decubitus view (**b**)

4.5
Normal Lung Anatomy

The lung is supported by a network of connective tissue fibers known as the lung interstitium (Fig. 4.7). For the purpose of interpreting HRCT images and identifying abnormal findings, the interstitium can be thought of as having several components. The peribronchovascular interstitium is a system of fibers

that invests the large bronchi and pulmonary arteries in the parahilar regions and forms a continuum with the centrilobular interstitium, surrounding the small centrilobular bronchi, arteries and some lymphatic vessels. The subpleural interstitium is located beneath the visceral pleura and envelops the lung in a fibrous sac from which connective tissue septa (interlobular septa) invaginate into the lung parenchyma. The pulmonary veins and lymphatic vessels travel in the interlobular septa. The last component is the intralobular interstitium, a network of thin fibers in the walls of the alveoli bridging the gap between the centrilobular interstitium and the interlobular septa or subpleural interstitium (WEIBEL 1979).

The secondary pulmonary lobule is the smallest lung unit delineated by the connective tissue septa and the smallest functional unit that can be discretely visualized by HRCT (Fig. 4.8). With a diameter of 1–2.5 mm, it can have a polyhedric or prismatic shape, but more frequently resembles a truncated pyramid. Each secondary lobule has a central supporting tissue (centrilobular interstitium) containing a small bronchiole, pulmonary artery and lymphatic vessel (bronchovascular bundle) and is marginated by interlobular septa that contain pulmonary veins and lymphatic branches. The substance of the secondary lobule, surrounding the lobular core and contained within the interlobular septa, consists of a variable number of lung acini (ranging from 3 to 24) and the associated capillary bed, supplied by small airways and branches of the pulmonary arteries and veins (GIOVAGNORIO and CAVALLO 1995). Secondary lobules are difficult to visualize in HRCT scans of children except in patients with abnormal septal thickening (see Figs. 4.9, 4.10, 4.22, 4.23, 4.33, 4.49, 4.51 and 4.53).

The terminal bronchiole and the artery supplying the lobule are located in its center and give off smaller branches at intervals along their courses. On HRCT scans the vessels can be seen as linear, branching or dot-like structures near the center of the secondary pulmonary lobule and extending to within 5–10 mm of the pleural surface; the smallest arteries resolved are as small as 0.2 mm. Normal intralobular bronchioles cannot be identified because their walls are less than 0.15 mm thick. In one in vitro study only bronchioles having a diameter of 2 mm or more were visible using HRCT (MURATA et al. 1986). This explains why normal bronchi within 2 cm of the pleural surface are not visible (Fig. 4.11) (TEEL et al. 1996). Bronchiolar abnormalities can be detected only when there is thickening of the bronchiolar wall, peribronchial inflammation,

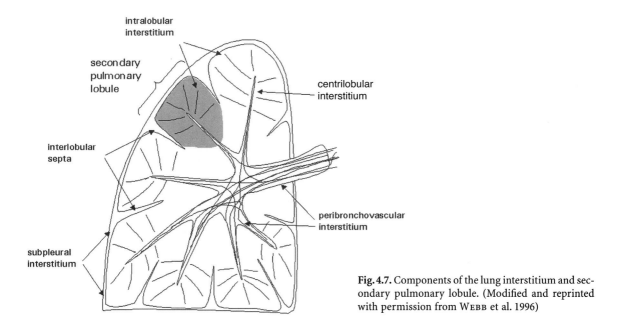

Fig. 4.7. Components of the lung interstitium and secondary pulmonary lobule. (Modified and reprinted with permission from Webb et al. 1996)

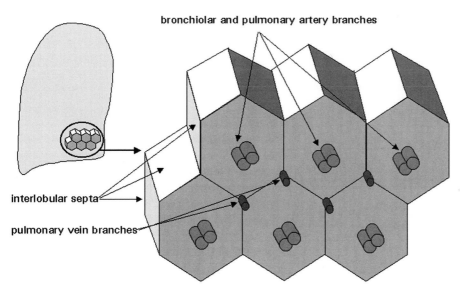

Fig. 4.8. The secondary pulmonary lobule, as defined by Miller. (Modified and reprinted with permission from Webb et al. 1996)

fibrosis or bronchiolectasis, with or without filling of the dilated bronchiole with secretions.

The attenuation of the normal air-containing lung varies with the phase of respiration and with the region of the lung being examined. With the child in a supine position, attenuation is usually higher posteriorly (lower lobes) than anteriorly (right middle lobe and lingula). This is due to physiologic hyperemia and the tendency of the dependent lobes to be incompletely expanded. This gravity-dependent density is accentuated at partial expiration, is reversible with full inspiration or with the patient in a prone position, and is most frequently observed in scans of children not following breath-holding commands whose studies are practically never performed on full inspiration. The opposite situation, i.e. anterior lobes denser than the dependent lobes, is always abnormal and indicates disease in the anterior lobes or air trapping in the dependent lobes (Fig. 4.12).

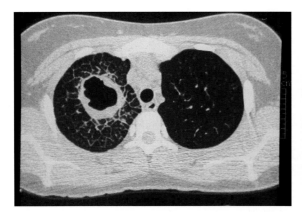

Fig. 4.9. A 15-year-old girl with fever and cough of 10 days' duration, treated with oral antibiotics. HRCT demonstrates a cavity with a thick, irregular wall in the right upper lobe. There is marked interlobular septal thickening around the lesion. Cultures were negative. The patient responded to intravenous antibiotic therapy

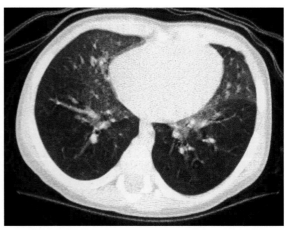

Fig. 4.12. Reversal of the normal aeration pattern in a 13-month-old girl with airway disease secondary to gastro-esophageal reflux with repeated episodes of aspiration. Air-trapping is present in both lower lobes. This finding was confirmed in the lateral decubitus views (not shown)

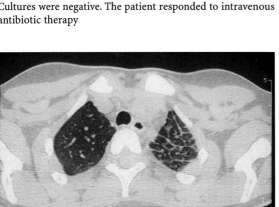

Fig. 4.10. Septal thickening delineating the secondary pulmonary lobule in a 2-year-old patient with congenital atresia of the pulmonary veins

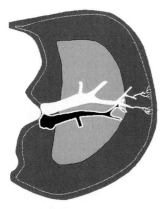

Fig. 4.11. Extent of visualization of airways (in *black*) and vessels (in *white*) at HRCT. (Modified and reprinted with permission from TEEL et al. 1996)

4.6
HRCT Features of Lung Disease

The most common HRCT features of lung disease in children are grouped in Fig. 4.13.

4.6.1
Ground-glass Opacity

Ground-glass opacity (GGO) refers to hazy increased attenuation of the lung with preservation of the bronchial and vascular margins, caused by partial filling of the air spaces, interstitial thickening, partial collapse of alveoli, normal expiration, or increased capillary blood volume. It is sometimes associated with air bronchograms and it can be patchy, resulting in a mosaic pattern of lung attenuation (AUSTIN et al. 1996; COLLINS and STERN 1997).

Lung attenuation normally increases with expiration. This increased attenuation can mask underlying GGO from infiltrative lung disease or create an appearance of diffuse lung disease if the expiratory nature of the examination is not recognized. The tracheal configuration changes from round on inspiration to flat

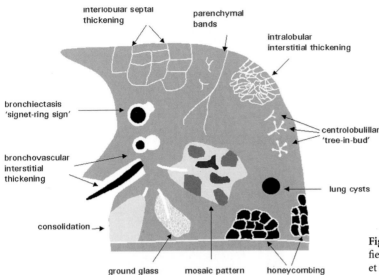

Fig. 4.13. HRCT features of lung disease. (Modified and reprinted with permission from WEBB et al. 1996)

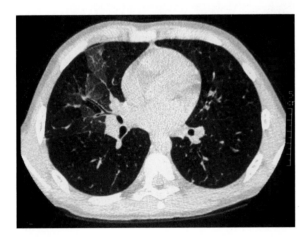

Fig. 4.14. Ground-glass pattern due to infectious right middle lobe pneumonia in a 9-year-old girl

or crescent-shaped on expiration and can be used to determine at what phase of respiration the HRCT scan was performed (COLLINS and STERN 1997).

Recognition of GGO is based on subjective assessment of the lung attenuation (see Fig. 4.6). When uniform GGO is observed in scans of children not following breath-holding commands, it probably corresponds to normal lung on expiration. Lateral decubitus views can help in this regard. When the GGO is patchy, it can cause a mosaic pattern of lung attenuation, which in children is usually due to small airway disease, with the GGO corresponding to areas of normal lung on expiration (see Fig. 4.4b). Again, lateral decubitus views will help to establish whether the mosaic pattern corresponds to patchy groundglass secondary to lung disease or to patchy air-trapping. Assessment of true GGO in the scans of children

following breath-holding commands is significantly easier. Its presence in these patients, whose scans are usually obtained in full inspiration, is always abnormal and is due to air-space or interstitial disease or both. The differential diagnosis of pathological GGO in the pediatric age group is extensive, being infectious pneumonia of any etiology its most common cause (Fig. 4.14). GGO can also be seen in pulmonary edema, hemorrhage (see Fig. 4.52), leukemic infiltration of the lung, lung contusion, acute lung transplant rejection, adult respiratory distress syndrome, collagen disease, extrinsic allergic alveolitis (see Fig. 4.43), drug toxicity, interstitial pneumonia, sarcoidosis (see Fig. 4.44), alveolar proteinosis (see Fig. 4.45), bronchiolitis obliterans organizing pneumonia, idiopathic pulmonary fibrosis (see Fig. 4.47) and following bronchoalveolar lavage.

4.6.2
Consolidation

A homogeneous increase in pulmonary parenchymal attenuation that obscures the margins of vessels and airway walls is referred to as consolidation (see Fig. 4.45). Air bronchograms may be present. By definition, diseases that produce consolidation are characterized by a replacement of alveolar air by fluid, cells, tissue or other material. The differential diagnosis of consolidation overlaps that of GGO and, in fact, it is common to find a mixture of both findings. Pneumonia of any etiology, pulmonary edema or hemorrhage and lung contusion are the most common causes of lung consolidation in children.

4.6.3
Pulmonary Nodule

Pulmonary nodules are focal, rounded opacities of varying size, which can be well- or ill-defined. They have been described as either air space or interstitial nodules, but it is more practical to classify them according to their size and distribution. Small nodules (<5 mm) can be centrilobular or distributed at random (Fig. 4.15). Centrilobular nodules are located in the region of the bronchioarteriolar core of secondary pulmonary lobules. On HRCT they are adjacent to, surround, or obscure the centrilobular arter-

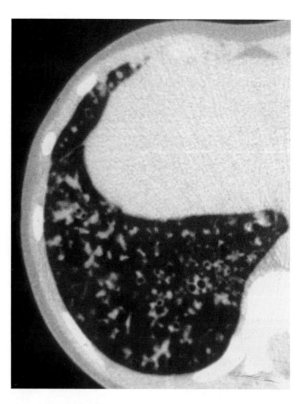

Fig. 4.16. Centrilobular nodules and tree-in-bud in a 12-year-old girl with postinfectious bronchiectasis

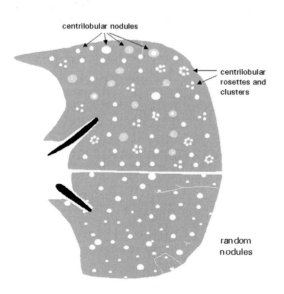

Fig. 4.15. Appearance of centrilobular and randomly distributed nodules. (Modified and reprinted with permission from WEBB et al. 1996)

ies, and are centered or clustered 5–10 mm from the periphery of the lobe, pleural surface or interlobar septa. Most centrilobular nodules in children are secondary to bronchiolar disease that also involves the peribronchiolar interstitium. They are common in cystic fibrosis, bronchiectasis (Fig. 4.16), infectious bronchitis and bronchogenic spread of tuberculosis. They may also be present in immotile cilia syndrome (Fig. 4.17), hypersensitivity pneumonia, asthma (especially when there is superimposed infection), Langerhans' cell histiocytosis, lymphocytic interstitial pneumonitis (LIP) in immunocompromised patients (see Fig. 4.48), congenital pulmonary lymphangiectasia, bronchiolitis obliterans, and pulmonary hemosiderosis (GRUDEN et al. 1994).

Small nodules that appear randomly distributed in relation to secondary lobule structures are often seen in patients with miliary tuberculosis (CHOI et al. 1999) fungal infections, hematogenous metastasis (Fig. 4.18) and Langerhans' cell histiocytosis (MOON et al. 1996). Contrary to what occurs with centrilobular nodules, these can be seen in close proximity to the interlobular septa and the pleural surfaces.

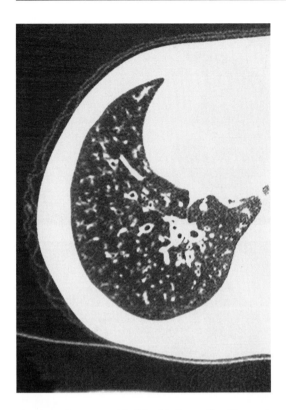

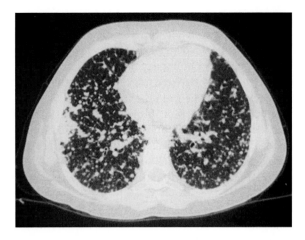

Fig. 4.18. Lung metastasis from thyroid carcinoma in a 6-year-old girl. Pulmonary nodules are distributed at random

Fig. 4.17. A 14-year-old girl with immotile cilia syndrome. HRCT shows centrilobular nodules, bronchiectasis and peribronchial thickening

The differential diagnosis of multiple, larger (>5 mm) nodules includes metastatic disease, tuberculosis, histoplasmosis, mycotic infections, lymphoproliferative disorders, pulmonary spread of laryngeal papillomatosis, septic emboli, vasculitis, Langerhans' cell histiocytosis (see Fig. 4.40), bleomycin lung, lipid granulomas in patients with total parenteral nutrition and bronchiolitis obliterans with organizing pneumonia (Fig. 4.19) (KUHN 1999; LANDRY and MELHEM 1989; RIMMER et al. 1985).

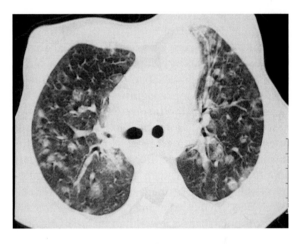

Fig. 4.19. Biopsy-proven bronchiolitis obliterans organizing pneumonia in a 15-year-old girl with hypogammaglobulinemia and respiratory difficulty. HRCT shows multiple nodules and some areas of ground glass. Lesions disappeared with steroid therapy

4.6.4
Bronchiolar Disease and Tree-in-Bud

The direct CT findings of bronchiolar disease include bronchiolar wall thickening, bronchiolar dilatation, and luminal impaction. Assessment of bronchial wall thickening on HRCT is quite subjective. Moreover, the apparent thickening of the bronchial wall represents not only the wall itself, but also the surrounding peribronchovascular interstitium. Peribronchovascular interstitial thickening, also known as peribronchial cuffing, can result in apparent bronchial wall thickening on HRCT. Bronchial wall/peribronchial thickening should be suspected when the bronchial "walls" are clearly seen in the distal third of the lung or when the walls of the more proximal aspects represent more than one third of the bronchial diameter (see Fig. 4.37) (AMBROSINO et al. 1994).

Small airways that are dilated and/or filled with mucus, pus or inflammatory material appear in some patients as small, well-defined, centrilobular, nodular, linear or branching structures of soft tissue opacity.

The "tree-in-bud" pattern represents severe bronchiolar impaction with "clubbing" of distal bronchioles. Seen in profile, the pattern resembles the "finger-in-glove" appearance of impacted bronchi. In cross section, tree-in-bud patterns may resemble childhood toy jacks. The tree-in-bud pattern is most commonly seen in infectious bronchiolitis of any etiology (see Fig. 4.16) endobronchial spread of tuberculosis, cystic fibrosis, allergic bronchopulmonary aspergillosis, immotile cilia syndrome (see Fig. 4.38), bronchiolitis obliterans and asthma (AQUINO et al. 1996).

4.6.5
Air-Trapping

The retention of excess air in all or part of the lung (especially during expiration), as a result of complete or partial airway obstruction or local abnormalities in pulmonary compliance, is known as air-trapping. Partial airway obstruction is particularly frequent in children. Recognition of a mosaic perfusion pattern on the inspiratory scans can suggest its presence. However, the expiratory scans often demonstrate marked air-trapping while the inspiratory scans show normal findings or only subtle abnormalities, such as decreased vascularity of the affected segment or lobe (Arakawa and Webb 1998). In our experience, the diagnostic yield of inspiratory scans is lower than that of expiratory scans in children with peripheral airway disease. The latter should always be included when performing HRCT of the lungs in cooperative children with clinical features suggesting airway disease (see Fig. 4.4).

Air trapping is particularly common in bronchiolitis obliterans (see Fig. 4.27), cystic fibrosis (see Fig. 4.37), bronchiectasis (see Fig. 4.21) and asthma (see Fig. 4.4), in which it can disappear following bronchodilator therapy (Fig. 4.20). It has also been reported in children with follicular hyperplasia of a bronchus (OH et al. 1999). Since bronchiolitis obliterans distal to bronchiectasis is a universal finding (SHEPARD 1995), air trapping is always found in the segments or lobes harboring bronchiectasis. This is a feature of significant diagnostic value, particularly when examining children whose studies show "questionable" bronchiectasis. In such cases the presence of associated air-trapping favors the diagnosis (HANSELL et al. 1994). It also helps in the

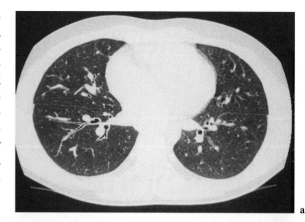

a

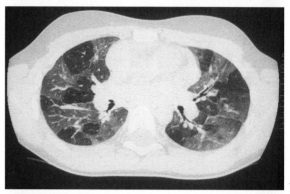

b

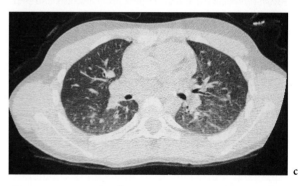

c

Fig. 4.20a–c. Example of air trapping in a 9-year-old patient with asthma. Inspiratory scan (**a**) is normal. Expiratory scan (**b**) shows severe air trapping. Repeated expiratory scan after bronchodilator therapy (**c**) is normal

follow up evaluation of children with known cylindrical bronchiectasis that have been treated and maintained infection-free. Occasionally the bronchiectasis becomes difficult to identify, yet the air trapping persists (Fig. 4.21).

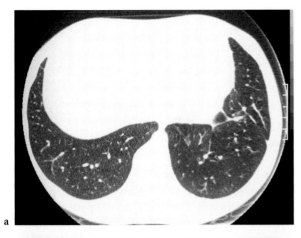

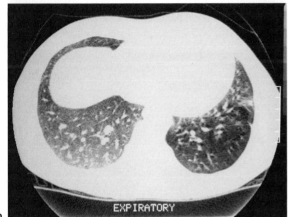

Fig. 4.21a,b. A 14-year-old girl with long-standing left lower lobe bronchiectasis treated with physiotherapy and antibiotics. Follow-up inspiratory HRCT (**a**) shows some architectural distortion and hypovascularity in the left lower lobe. Bronchiectases are no longer seen. Marked air trapping is evident on the expiratory scan (**b**)

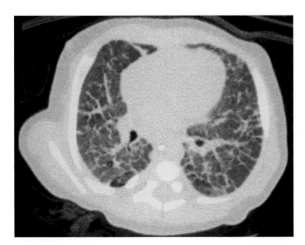

Fig. 4.22. Septal lines in a 2-month-old infant with bronchopulmonary dysplasia

4.6.6
Septal Thickening

Interlobular septal thickening, also known as septal lines, is defined as abnormal widening of an interlobular septum or septa. On HRCT it presents as short (1–2 cm in length), fine linear opacities perpendicular to and abutting the pleural surface (Fig. 4.22), or as a fine, polygonal pattern of lines in the more central lung (see Figs. 4.9, 4.10, 4.23, 4.51 and 4.53). Interlobular septal thickening is usually due to interstitial edema of any cause (see Fig. 4.10), but it is also seen in neoplasms (see Fig. 4.49), infectious processes (see Fig. 4.9), pulmonary fibrosis, bronchopulmonary dysplasia (Fig. 4.22), pulmonary lymphangiectasia (see Fig. 4.51), Niemann-Pick disease (Fig. 4.23) (FERETTI et al. 1996), Gaucher's disease (see Fig. 4.53) collagen vascular disorders, tuberous sclerosis, alveolar proteinosis (see Fig. 4.33) and sarcoidosis. Septal thickening is usually smooth. It can be irregular in cases of fibrosis and irregular or nodular in sarcoidosis or lymphangitic spread of tumor (Fig. 4.24) (LYNCH et al. 1999a; MOON et al. 1996).

Intralobular lines, rarely observed in children, correspond to thickening of the intralobular interstitium. When numerous, they may appear as a fine reticular pattern.

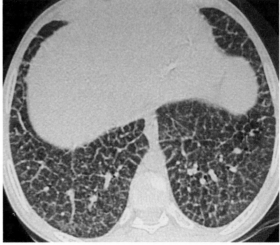

Fig. 4.23. A 16-year-old boy with Niemann-Pick disease and respiratory insufficiency. HRCT shows thickening of the interlobular septa. Areas of ground glass were seen in other slices (not shown). Interstitial thickening is due to infiltration of lymphatics and interlobular septa with lipid-laden macrophages. (Courtesy of Dr. Ucar, Argentina)

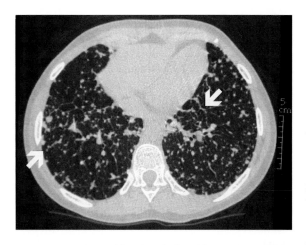

Fig. 4.24. A 14-year-old girl with thyroid carcinoma. HRCT demonstrates irregular nodular thickening of interlobular septa (*arrows*) corresponding to lymphangitic spread. Small nodules randomly distributed through both lungs, characteristic of hematogenous metastasis, are also seen

4.6.7
Parenchymal Bands

Visualized as elongated opacities, parenchymal bands are usually 2–5 cm in length and often represent several contiguous thickened septa. They can also correspond to areas of peribronchovascular fibrosis, coarse scars or atelectasis associated with lung or pleural fibrosis. Parenchymal bands can extend to the pleura, which may be thickened and retracted at the site of contact. The pleural retractions are visualized as pleural-based triangular opacities. These features are commonly seen in children with long-standing bronchopulmonary dysplasia (Figs. 4.3b, 4.25) (AQUINO et al. 1999; OPPENHEIM et al. 1994).

4.6.8
Honeycombing

A sign of destroyed, fibrotic and cystic lung, honeycombing represents complete loss of acinar and bronchiolar architecture at the end stage of fibrosing lung disease. On HRCT of the lung it presents as clustered cystic air spaces with clearly definable walls, measuring 1–3 mm in thickness and predominantly found in peripheral and subpleural lung regions, often in several contiguous layers. True honeycomb cysts do not change in size during exhalation (JOHKOH et al. 1999d). Honeycombing is not a common finding in children, but it can be seen in

chronic interstitial lung disorders, such as non-specific interstitial pneumonitis (see Fig. 4.47), desquamative interstitial pneumonitis (COPLEY et al. 2000), scleroderma (SEELY et al. 1998), lupus (see Fig. 4.50) and end-stage pulmonary fibrosis (Fig. 4.26).

4.6.9
Mosaic Perfusion

A patchwork of varied attenuation, mosaic perfusion has been interpreted as secondary to regional differences in perfusion. The HRCT mosaic pattern of lung attenuation is a nonspecific finding that can reflect the presence of airway abnormalities, ground-glass interstitial or air-space infiltrates or vascular dis-

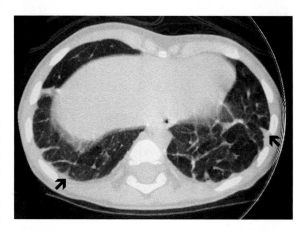

Fig. 4.25. Parenchymal bands in a 2-year-old infant with bronchopulmonary dysplasia. Peripheral wedge-shaped densities (*arrows*) are also present

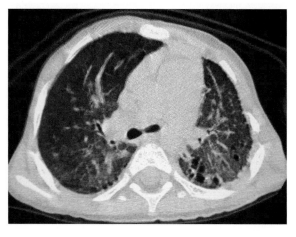

Fig. 4.26. Honeycombing secondary to pulmonary fibrosis in a 3-year-old girl with congenital pulmonary vein atresia

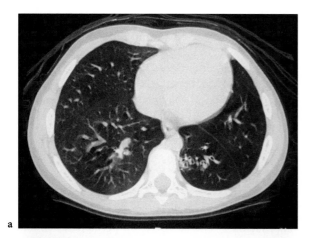

a

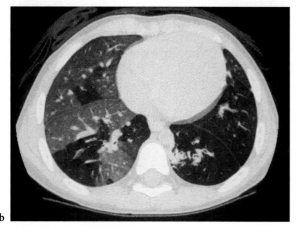

b

Fig. 4.27a,b. Inspiratory (**a**) and expiratory (**b**) HRCT scans in a 6-year-old boy with postinfectious bronchiolitis obliterans (Swyer-James syndrome). There is left lower lobe bronchiectasis and a bilateral mosaic perfusion pattern with air trapping

ease (STERN et al. 1995). In small airway disease and pulmonary vascular disease, the pulmonary vessels within the lucent regions of the lung are small relative to the vessels in the more opaque lung. In primary vascular diseases, such as thromboembolism or pulmonary hypertension, which are exceedingly rare in children, the reduced vascularity in the lucent lesions results from the primary vascular disease. In contrast, when mosaic perfusion is due to small airway disease, the commonest cause of this pattern in children, the reduced vascularity in the lucent areas results from abnormal ventilation, air-trapping and secondary hypoxic vasoconstriction. Recognition of a mosaic perfusion pattern secondary to airway disease is enhanced with the use of expiratory slices. Asthma (see Figs. 4.4 and 4.20), bronchiolitis obliterans (Figs. 4.27 and 4.39), cystic fibrosis and bronchopulmonary

dysplasia are the most common causes of a mosaic perfusion pattern in the pediatric age group.

The third cause of HRCT mosaic patterns of lung attenuation is infiltrative lung disease, producing areas of ground-glass attenuation in a lobular or multilobular distribution. The areas of ground-glass can be due to interstitial or air-space infiltrates, or both. In these cases the vessel caliber and number are similar in both the normal lower attenuation regions and the abnormal higher attenuation regions of lung. Furthermore, there is no air-trapping on expiration.

4.6.10
Architectural Distortion

A manifestation of lung disease in which bronchi, pulmonary vessels, fissures and/or septa are abnormally displaced. Usually there are fewer vessels and their branching pattern is anomalous. This finding can be observed in pulmonary hypoplasia (Fig. 4.28), but it is most common in lung diseases associated with small airway obstruction (see Fig. 4.21). In the latter, architectural distortion may be the only abnormality seen in the inspiratory slices; expiratory scans will demonstrate air- trapping (see Fig. 4.21).

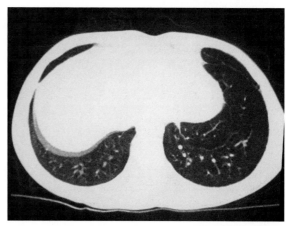

Fig. 4.28. Example of architectural distortion of the left lower lobe in a 5-year-old boy with unilateral pulmonary hypoplasia secondary to congenital left-sided diaphragmatic hernia operated in the neonatal period

4.6.11
Air-Filled Cystic Lung Lesions: Bullae, Pneumoceles and Cysts

Air-filled cystic lung lesions correspond to intrapulmonary air collections surrounded by a visible wall of varying thickness. In our experience, it is extremely difficult, if not impossible, to differentiate between air-filled cysts, bullae, pneumatoceles and even some cases of cystic bronchiectasis or localized emphysema on imaging findings alone. Clinical features and evolution are essential to establish the diagnosis.

The differential diagnosis of air-filled cystic lung lesions in children includes congenital cyst, inflammatory pneumatoceles secondary to hydrocarbon ingestion (Fig. 4.29) or infectious pneumonia (Fig. 4.30), traumatic pneumatoceles, pseudocysts due to barotrauma (see Fig. 4.2), Langerhans' cell Langerhans' cell histiocytosis (Figs. 4.31, 4.40 and 4.41), tuberous sclerosis, papillomatosis, septic pulmonary emboli, Wegener's granulomatosis, and Ehlers-Danlos, Marfan or Williams-Campbell syndromes (HARTMAN et al. 1994).

4.6.12
Dependent Increased Attenuation

Increased subpleural attenuation (sometimes appearing as a subpleural line) occurs in a region of the dependent lung and disappears when the lung is nondependent. Dependent increased attenuation is a normal finding. The opposite indicates airway disease (see Fig. 4.12).

4.6.13
Emphysema

Emphysema is characterized by permanent, abnormal enlargement of the air spaces distal to the terminal bronchioles, accompanied by destruction of their walls. It is visible on HRCT as a focal region or regions of low attenuation, usually without visible walls, resulting from actual or perceived enlarged air spaces and destroyed alveolar walls (AUSTIN et al. 1996). It can be associated with air-trapping. Emphysema is classified morphologically relative to the pulmonary lobule as centrilobular, panlobular or paraseptal.

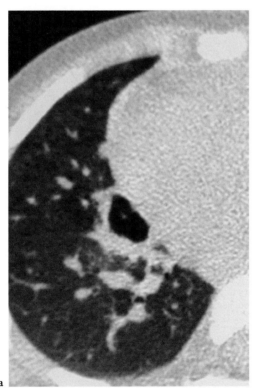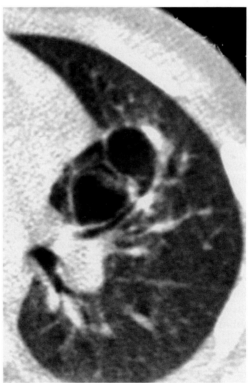

a   b

Fig. 4.29a,b. Bilateral pulmonary pneumatoceles, which appeared 6 days after hydrocarbon ingestion in an 18-month-old girl

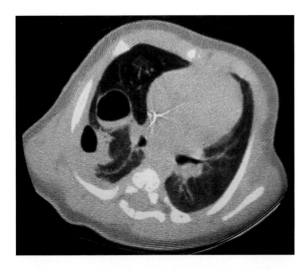

Fig. 4.30. Infectious pneumatocele in a 3-month-old infant

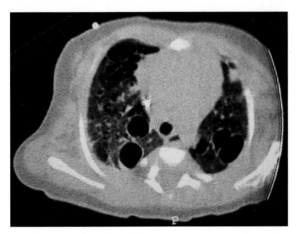

Fig. 4.31. Cystic pulmonary lesions in a 3-month-old infant with Langerhans' cell histiocytosis

4.6.14
Halo Sign

The halo sign is a GGO surrounding the circumference of a nodule or mass. It can be seen in patients with invasive pulmonary aspergillosis, tuberculosis, lymphoproliferative disorders, Wegener's, pulmonary hemorrhage and metastatic osteosarcoma (TOMIYAMA et al. 1994; KIM et al. 1999; PRIMACK et al. 1994).

4.6.15
Signet-Ring Sign

A ring of opacity (usually representing a dilated, thick-walled bronchus) associated with a smaller,

round, soft-tissue opacity (the adjacent pulmonary artery) is known as signet-ring sign. In children this finding indicates bronchiectasis (Fig. 4.32) (OUELLETE 1999).

4.6.16
Crazy Paving Pattern

Crazy paving pattern is a combination of areas of ground glass attenuation and smoothly thickened interlobular septa, within the areas of air space disease (Fig. 4.33). This finding has been considered to be strongly suggestive of alveolar proteinosis. However, it can occur in other diseases such as lipoid pneumonia, adult respiratory distress syndrome, acute interstitial pneumonia and drug-induced pneumonitis (FRANQUET et al. 1998; JOHKOH et al. 1999b).

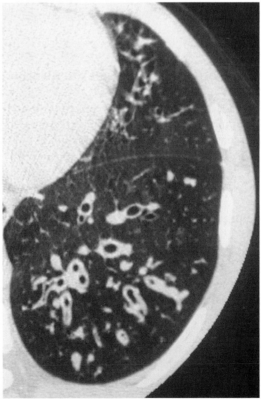

Fig. 4.32. Signet-ring sign in an 8-year-old patient with cystic fibrosis and left lower lobe bronchiectasis

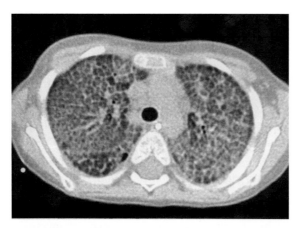

Fig. 4.33. A 3-year-old girl with alveolar proteinosis. HRCT shows thickened interlobular septa in background of ground-glass opacification (crazy-paving pattern). (Reprinted with permission, from COPLEY et al. 2000)

II.
Clinical Applications

HUBERT DUCOU LE POINTE

4.7
HRCT Features in Diseases of the Airways

HRCT is the imaging technique of choice for the evaluation of most lesions of the bronchial tree: bronchiectasis, constrictive bronchiolitis, bronchiolitis obliterans organizing pneumonia (BOOP), and asthma.

4.7.1
Bronchiectasis

Bronchiectasis is defined pathologically as the irreversible dilatation of the bronchial tree. Numerous disorders are associated with bronchiectasis (postinfective bronchial damage, bronchial obstruction, immune deficiency, mucociliary clearance defect, fibrosis, etc.).

HRCT has proven to be a reliable, noninvasive technique for assessing the presence, severity and extension of bronchiectasis and has largely eliminated the need for bronchography in children (HERMAN et al. 1993). In our institution, bronchography is not even performed prior to surgery.

The HRCT criteria for diagnosing bronchiectasis have been well described (HANSELL 1998): internal diameter of the bronchus larger than the diameter of the adjacent pulmonary artery branch, absence of normal tapering of bronchi, bronchial wall thickening, and visualization of a bronchus in the lung periphery. This last criterion is not clearly defined in the literature. Several authors (GRENIER et al. 1986; WEBB 1994; McGUINNESS and NAIDICH 1995) consider all bronchi visible within 2–3 cm from the pleural surface to be abnormal. J.S. KIM et al. (1997) defined the visualization of bronchi within 1 cm of costal or paravertebral pleura or visualization of

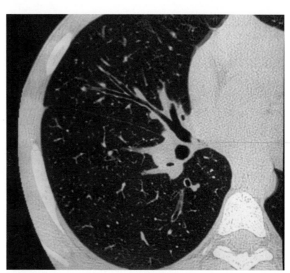

Fig. 4.34. A 14-year-old boy with cylindrical bronchiectasis in the middle lobe. Bronchi are dilated and slightly irregular

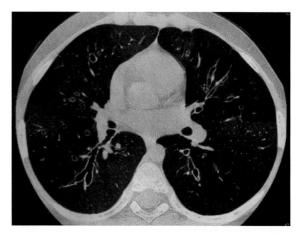

Fig. 4.35. An 11-year-old boy with varicose bronchiectasis in the right lower lobe. Bronchi have an irregular and beaded appearance

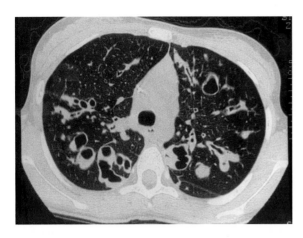

Fig. 4.36. A 14-year-old girl with cystic bronchiectasis. Saccular bronchiectasis with retained secretions are seen in both upper lobes

bronchi abutting the mediastinal pleura as abnormal. These differences in criteria could be related to improvements in CT technology. We consider abnormal the visualization of bronchi in the peripheral 1 cm of the lung.

Bronchiectasis has been classified into three types – cylindrical, varicose and cystic – based on the morphology of the abnormal bronchi. Cylindrical bronchiectasis is diagnosed when there is a lack of bronchial tapering and bronchial walls are smooth or slightly irregular (Fig. 4.34). Varicose bronchiectasis is easily recognized when bronchi are parallel to the scan plane, as the dilated bronchi have a beaded appearance (Fig. 4.35). Cystic bronchiectasis has a cystic or saccular appearance (Fig. 4.36). Air-fluid levels caused by retained secretions are sometimes seen in the dilated bronchi. Cystic and varicose bronchiectasis imply more bronchial destruction than cylindrical bronchiectasis.

Retained bronchial secretions, atelectasis, and/or mosaic perfusion, can also be seen in HRCT scans of patients with bronchiectasis. When the bronchus is perpendicular to the scan plane, retained bronchial secretions in the central lung appear as nodular or oval shaped opacities. When the bronchus is parallel to the scan plane, they are recognized as lobulated linear or branching structures. In the peripheral bronchi, retained mucus is visualized as centrilobular nodules or tree-in-bud appearance (GRENIER et al. 1990). Mosaic perfusion, secondary to air-trapping and reflecting the presence of small airway disease distal to the bronchiectasis, is extremely common.

The pattern and distribution of abnormalities revealed by HRCT in patients with bronchiectasis

are influenced by the underlying cause, and distinctive HRCT appearances have been well-described in a few conditions: cystic fibrosis, immotile cilia, allergic asthma, bronchopulmonary aspergillosis, tuberculosis and hypogammaglobulinemia (CARTIER et al. 1999).

4.7.1.1
Cystic Fibrosis

Cystic fibrosis is the most common cause of pulmonary insufficiency in childhood (RUZAL-SHAPIRO 1998). Bronchiectasis in cystic fibrosis is usually widespread, with upper lobe involvement being almost universal and both central and peripheral bronchiectasis being present in approximately two-thirds of patients. Although cystic and varicose types are not uncommon, cylindrical bronchiectasis usually predominates, particularly in young children. Peribronchial thickening, mucoid impaction and a mosaic perfusion pattern secondary to air-trapping

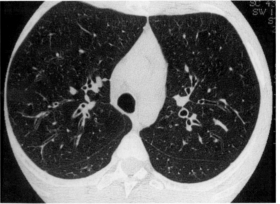

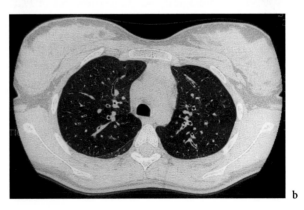

Fig. 4.37a,b. A 15-year-old girl with cystic fibrosis. HRCT detects cylindrical bronchiectasis with bronchial wall thickening (**a**). Expiratory air-trapping reflects the presence of small airway disease (**b**)

are very common in cystic fibrosis (Fig. 4.37). Mosaic perfusion may be the only HRCT abnormality early in the course of the disease. Mucoid impaction can present as large nodules in the central lung or as centrilobular or tree-in-bud pattern in the lung periphery. Mucus plugging may lead to lobar and segmental atelectasis. Partial or total resolution of mucus plugging is a finding that can reflect therapeutic efficacy and is useful for monitoring

Several authors have devised scoring systems based on chest X-ray findings to assess the severity of the disease (NATHANSON et al. 1991; SOCKRIDER et al. 1994; CLEVELAND et al. 1998). The Brasfield method is one of the most commonly used (BRASFIELD et al. 1980). New scoring systems based on HRCT have been proposed (SHAH et al. 1997; BRODY et al. 1999; HELBICH et al. 1999). The most popular is the Bhalla method (BHALLA et al. 1991), which attempts to provide an objective assessment of the severity and extension of lung disease. However, the clinical relevance of HRCT scoring systems has not yet been demonstrated.

4.7.1.2
Immotile Cilia

Immotile cilia or primary ciliary dyskinesia (PCD) is a term including diseases that occur as a direct result of congenital defects in the airway cilia (MEEKS and BUSH 2000). The main features of PCD are recurrent sinopulmonary infections, situs inversus and subfertility. The association between chronic respiratory disease and PCD is well recognized. Kartagener's syndrome, characterized by situs inversus totalis, bronchiectasis and paranasal sinusitis accounts for 50% of all patients with PCD (HIDDEMA and ENGELSHOVE 1999). The radiological and clinical features of PCD are similar to those of cystic fibrosis but are less severe and progressive. Hyperinflation and bronchial thickening are the most common abnormalities. Bronchiectasis (particularly in the right middle lobe), mucus plugging (Figs. 4.17, 4.38), atelectasis and consolidation are also frequent (NADEL et al. 1985; FAURÉ et al. 1986; REYES DE LA ROCHA et al. 1987).

4.7.2
Asthma.
Allergic Bronchopulmonary Aspergillosis

Asthma is a disorder of the tracheobronchial tree characterized by inflammation, reversible airway obstruction and tracheobronchial mucosal hyperre-

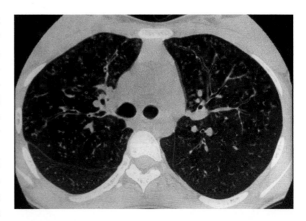

Fig. 4.38. A 16-year-old girl with primary ciliary dyskinesia. Cylindrical bronchiectasis with mucus plugging (tree-in-bud pattern) is seen in both lungs

activity to numerous stimuli. Asthma often coexists with other allergic disorders (e.g. allergic rhinitis and atopic dermatitis). Radiography is indicated to exclude other causes of wheezing and to detect complications. Air-trapping due to small airway disease is the most common HRCT feature in children with asthma (see Fig. 4.4) and can disappear after therapy with bronchodilators (see Fig. 4.20) (LUCAYA et al. 2000). Atelectasis, particularly in the right middle lobe, is also common (ALTAMIRANO et al. 1991).

Other reported HRCT features include bronchial wall thickening, bronchiectasis and mucoid impaction (McLEAN et al. 1998; PAGANIN et al. 1992; GRENIER et al. 1996). The pathogenesis of bronchial wall thickening in asthmatic patients is not clear. LYNCH (1998) has suggested that it is due to inflammation, muscle hypertrophy and peribronchial fibrosis. The prevalence of bronchiectasis seems to be associated with disease severity (PAGANIN et al. 1992; GRENIER et al. 1996). In our experience bronchiectasis is infrequent in asthmatic children.

Central bronchiectasis associated with asthma is considered to be highly suggestive of allergic bronchopulmonary aspergillosis (ABPA) (SHAH et al. 1992). ABPA is an immunological disorder characterized by immediate hypersensitivity due to endobronchial growth of *Aspergillus fumigatus*. In patients with IgE-mediated asthma, *A. fumigatus* may trigger an asthmatic reaction. The diagnosis of ABPA is based on a clinical history of asthma, skin test reactivity, elevated IgE and measurement of serum precipitins. WARD et al. (1999) suggested that the presence of randomly distributed, predominantly central, moderate to severe bronchiectasis affecting three or more lobes, bronchial wall thickening and centrilobular nodules in an asthmatic patient is highly suggestive of ABPA.

4.7.3
Constrictive Bronchiolitis

Constrictive bronchiolitis (bronchiolitis obliterans) is a rare disease characterized by thickening of the bronchiole walls due to submucosal collagenization, with few changes in the distal parenchyma (COLBY 1998). Progressive bronchiole narrowing is associated with distortion of the lumen, mucostasis and chronic inflammation. Bronchiolectasis and bronchiolar smooth-muscle hypertrophy may also be seen.

Constrictive bronchiolitis can be idiopathic or secondary to various insults, such as viral, bacterial or mycoplasma infections, bone marrow or lung transplantation, collagen vascular diseases or toxic fume inhalation (CHANG et al. 1998; LAU et al. 1998; SARGENT et al. 1995; SIEGEL 1999). It has also been reported to occur in association with Stevens-Johnson syndrome (KIM and LEE 1996). Chest X-rays are usually normal, although hyperaeration and vascular attenuation are sometimes seen. HRCT demonstrates a mosaic perfusion pattern due to oligemia and air-trapping, which is better detected on expiratory scans. Central or peripheral bronchiectasis, bronchial thickening and mucus plugging of the centrilobular bronchioles may also be noted.

Swyer-James or Macleod's syndrome is a variant of postinfectious constrictive bronchiolitis (MARTI-BONMATI et al. 1989), and is characterized by unilateral small or normal-sized hyperlucent lung with air-trapping (STERN and SAMPLES 1992; MOORE et al. 1992). It is usually the result of a viral or mycoplasma respiratory infection in early childhood. HRCT reveals unilateral hyperlucency and decreased pulmonary vascularity in all patients. Other common findings are a mosaic perfusion pattern and bronchiectasis, each of which are seen in approximately 70% of patients. Expiratory HRCT scans show air-trapping in the hyperlucent lung in all cases. Contralateral lung involvement, characterized by patchy areas of air-trapping, is present in half the patients (see Fig. 4.27). Bronchiectasis can be cylindrical or varicose and may be associated with collapse. Children without bronchiectasis or with cylindrical bronchiectasis had a lower incidence of pneumonia

episodes than those with varicose bronchiectasis (LUCAYA et al. 1998).

Constrictive bronchiolitis may occur after heart-lung transplantation (50% of patients) or bone-marrow transplantation (10% of patients). It is thought to be the consequence of repeated episodes of rejection. Clinically, the patients may present with cough and dyspnea. The triad of mosaic perfusion pattern, bronchial dilatation and bronchial wall thickening after lung transplantation is indicative of bronchiolitis obliterans syndrome, a term referring to lung graft deterioration due to progressive airway disease for which no other cause has been identified (Fig. 4.39). A mosaic perfusion pattern without the associated bronchial changes has been observed in a large percentage of transplant patients with normal pulmonary function tests (LAU et al. 1998).

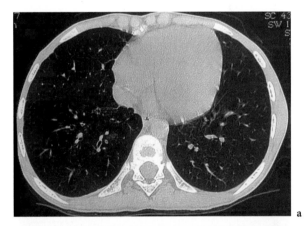

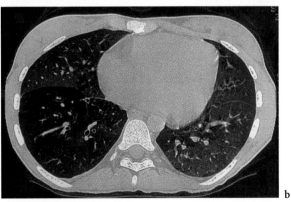

Fig. 4.39a,b. A 17-year-old girl with constrictive bronchiolitis after heart-lung transplantation. Bronchial dilatation in the right lower lobe with bronchial wall thickening are seen on inspiratory HRCT (**a**). Mosaic perfusion is better seen on expiratory HRCT (**b**)

4.7.4
Bronchiolitis Obliterans Organizing Pneumonia

Bronchiolitis obliterans organizing pneumonia (BOOP) is characterized pathologically by the presence of granulation tissue within the lumen of bronchioles and alveolar ducts and associated patchy areas of organizing pneumonia. BOOP rarely occurs in children. It may be idiopathic but is more commonly seen in children after chemotherapy. It can also occur after bone marrow transplantation or as a response to toxic inhalants, drugs, or viral, mycoplasmal or bacterial infection (INOUE et al. 1996; MATHEW et al. 1994; KLEINAU et al. 1997). The main symptoms are cough, dyspnea, fever and weight loss. Physical examination is unremarkable except for crackles on auscultation of the lungs. Pulmonary function tests show a restrictive ventilatory defect with impaired gas transfer.

The HRCT findings in BOOP most commonly consist of patchy consolidation or ground glass opacities, often with a subpleural and/or peribronchial distribution (MÜLLER et al. 1990; FLOWERS et al. 1992; AKIRA et al. 1998). Peripheral nodular opacities (see Fig. 4.19), irregular linear opacities, bronchial wall thickening and dilatation, and small pleural effusions may also be present (WEBB et al. 1996; LEE et al. 1994a). Although nonspecific, the HRCT findings can suggest the diagnosis and help to select the site for biopsy.

4.8
HRCT Features in Specific Lung Diseases

4.8.1
Chronic Diffuse Infiltrative Lung Disease

A specific diagnosis of chronic diffuse infiltrative lung disease (CDILD) is essential to prescribe treatment. The diagnosis is based on clinical information, pulmonary function tests, bronchoalveolar lavage and chest imaging. Studies in adults have demonstrated the superiority of HRCT over radiography for obtaining the correct diagnosis of CDILD because many of these patients have distinguishing features (characteristic appearances and distributions) when evaluated with this technique (GRENIER et al. 1994; LEE et al. 1994b; BONELLI et al. 1998; SWENSEN et

al. 1997). According to recent publications the same results were obtained in children (LYNCH et al. 1999a; COPLEY et al. 2000; KOH and HANSELL 2000). In some cases, lung biopsy can be avoided. HRCT can also be useful to determine the optimal site for biopsy and to assess the extent of the disease. Because CDILD is uncommon in children, the applications of HRCT are less developed. Our experience suggests that HRCT contributes to the diagnosis and monitoring of pediatric CDILD.

4.8.1.1
Langerhans' Cell Histiocytosis

Infiltration and accumulation of monocytes and large histiocytes in various tissues and organs characterize the histological appearance of Langerhans' Cell Histiocytosis (LCH). Pulmonary involvement is present in 23%–50% of children with the multisystemic form (SMETS et al. 1997). Localized LCH is the mildest and most common form (70% of all cases) and involves either bone or lung. The lung is the second most common site of LCH (SMINIOTOPOULOS et al. 1999). The lesions are more often diffuse with a topographic predominance in the upper or middle lung zones and tend to spare the costophrenic angles (MOORE et al. 1989). HRCT detects peribronchial or peribronchiolar granulomas, usually 1–10 mm in diameter; larger nodules are less common. These nodules can disappear or cavitate (BRAUNER et al. 1989b) and become thick-walled cysts that can progress to thin-walled cysts (BRAUNER et al. 1997) (Fig. 4.40).

Thick or thin-walled pulmonary cysts are the main feature of LCH. They may be round or irregularly shaped, probably due to the fusion of several cysts (Fig. 4.41). Rupture of subpleural cysts may cause pneumothorax (Fig. 4.42). Pneumothorax is a potentially fatal complication of LCH and relapsing cases may even require bilateral total pleurectomy (YULE et al. 1997). In children, LCH lesions may remain stable over long periods or progress rapidly, leading to destruction of the pulmonary parenchyma within a few weeks or months after diagnosis (SEELY et al. 1997). Thymic involvement associated with parenchymal lesions has been also reported (DONNELLY 2000). In the multisystemic form of LCH pulmonary involvement does not mean that the disease is more severe or suggest a poorer prognosis (SMETS et al. 1997), yet it may influence the choice of treatment.

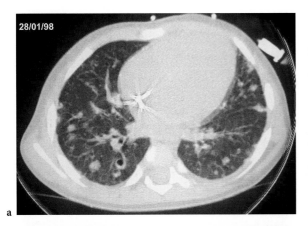

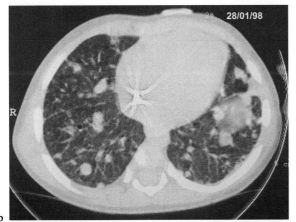

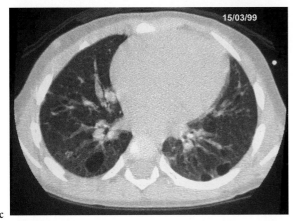

Fig. 4.40a–c. A 14-month-old girl with Langerhans' cell histiocytosis. Initial HRCT (**a,b**) shows nodules and small cystic lesions. Follow-up HRCT (**c**) at the age of 30 months shows larger cystic lesions

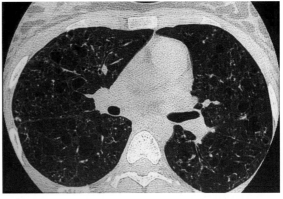

Fig. 4.41. A 16-year-old girl with Langerhans' cell histiocytosis. HRCT shows thick- and thin-walled cysts; a few micronodules are also seen

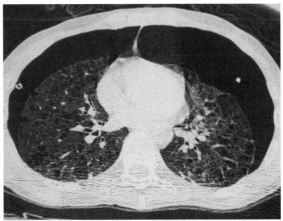

Fig. 4.42. A 15-year-old boy with Langerhans' cell histiocytosis, with multiple skin lesions, diabetes insipida and recurrent bilateral pneumothoraces. Chest CT shows multiple pulmonary cystic lesions, some located subpleurally, and bilateral pneumothorax

4.8.1.2
Extrinsic Allergic Alveolitis

Extrinsic allergic alveolitis (EAA) is caused by the repeated inhalation of particulate organic antigens. Farmer's lung is the best-known EAA syndrome. The development of EEA requires massive acute or prolonged low-grade exposure. Many inhaled responsible antigens have been described, including animal and plant proteins and fungal microorganisms (thermophilic actinomycetes). Extrinsic allergic alveolitis is divided into acute, subacute and chronic forms (VINCENT et al. 1992). The diagnosis of EAA in its earliest stages is controversial and remains primarily clinical. Symptoms occur 4–8 h after exposure, and include shortness of breath, dry cough, malaise and fever. Subacute and chronic forms have an insidious onset with progressive shortness of breath and cough.

HRCT abnormalities depend on the stage of the disease. HRCT is rarely performed in the early stage. In the acute and subacute stages EAA presents as airway disease characterized by small poorly defined centrilobular nodules (<5 mm in diameter) and areas of ground glass (HANSELL and MOSKOVIC 1991) (Fig. 4.43). GGOs are slightly more marked in the middle and lower lung zones. Areas of decreased attenuation and air-trapping, consistent with small airway disease, are also common findings (SMALL et al. 1996).

Chronic EAA is characterized by fibrosis that seems to spare the lung bases.

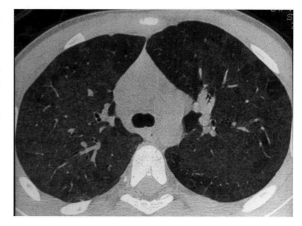

Fig. 4.43. A 12-year-old boy with extrinsic allergic alveolitis. HRCT shows small, ill-defined rounded opacities with patchy ground-glass opacities

4.8.1.3
Sarcoidosis

Sarcoidosis is a chronic granulomatous disorder of unknown etiology. It is uncommon in children and occurs most often in young adults (PATTISHALL and KENDIG 1996). The majority of pediatric patients are 9–18 years of age (GROSSMAN et al. 1985). Respiratory symptoms include cough, dyspnea and, sometimes, chest pain. Mediastinal and/or bilateral hilar adenopathy, often isolated, is the most common intrathoracic finding in sarcoidosis. The characteristic HRCT finding consists in small 2–10 mm nodules with irregular margins distributed along the lymphatics in the bronchovascular sheath and in the interlobar septa and pleura. This distribution can produce a beaded appearance of the bronchovascular bundles and interlobular septa and fissural nodularity (BRAUNER et al. 1989a; DAWSON and MÜLLER 1990; TRAILL et al. 1997) (Fig. 4.44).

Confluence of granulomas may result in large opacities with poorly defined contours, or areas of frank consolidation. Air-bronchograms may be seen within these opacities. Large nodules can cavitate, but this is uncommon. Patchy areas of ground-glass opacity may also be present and may be due to the presence of numerous sarcoid granulomas below the resolution of HRCT (NISHIMURA et al. 1995). Architectural distortion, displacement of interlobar fissures, traction bronchiectasis, cystic air spaces and

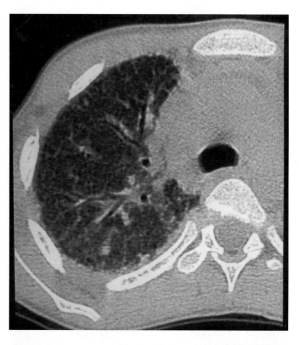

Fig. 4.44. An 11-year-old boy with sarcoidosis. HRCT detects small nodules in a perilymphatic distribution (note the beaded appearance of the bronchovascular bundles and subpleural nodularity) and ground-glass opacities

honeycombing are signs of advanced disease with fibrosis (ABEHSERA et al. 2000). Posterior displacement of the main or upper lobe bronchus is a classical finding, which indicates loss of volume in the posterior segment of the upper lobes.

4.8.1.4
Pulmonary Alveolar Proteinosis

Pulmonary alveolar proteinosis (PAP) is a rare intrinsic lung disease of unknown etiology characterized by alveolar filling with amorphous lipoproteinaceous material (SCHUMACHER et al. 1989). Plain films show alveolar infiltrates, a reticulonodular pattern or both. Pleural effusion and adenopathy are absent (McCOOK et al. 1981). HRCT shows areas of consolidation or ground glass, often with a geographic distribution, and/or widespread miliary nodules (GODWIN et al. 1988; MURCH and CARR 1989; ALBA-FOUILLE et al. 1999) (Fig. 4.45). Smooth thickening of the interlobular septa within the areas of air space disease resulting in a crazy paving appearance (see Fig. 4.33) suggests, but is not specific to, alveolar proteinosis (FRANQUET et al. 1999; COULIER et al. 1999; JOHKOH et al. 1999b).

4.8.1.5
Pulmonary Fibrosis and Chronic Interstitial Pneumonias

Pulmonary fibrosis is a chronic inflammatory interstitial lung disorder, characterized by an initial accumulation of inflammatory and immunoregulatory cells in the pulmonary interstitium and the alveolar space. Inflammation leads to modification of the alveolar structures with progression to interstitial fibrosis and thickening of alveolar walls. In children, pulmonary fibrosis is the result of a heterogeneous group of disorders that share common histological features

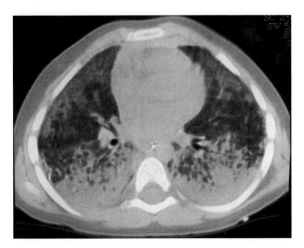

Fig. 4.45. A 3-year-old boy with biopsy-proven pulmonary alveolar proteinosis. Despite the 5-mm slice thickness alveolar consolidation and alveolar infiltrates are clearly visualized

(OSIKA et al. 1997). The known causes include infectious disorders, reactions to environmental exposures, drugs, collagen-vascular disorders or gastroesophageal reflux with chronic aspiration. For idiopathic pulmonary fibrosis (IPF), classification by histological features into usual interstitial pneumonitis (UIP) and desquamative interstitial pneumonitis (DIP) has been proposed. The distinction between these two forms of fibrosing alveolitis is now questioned (UIP and DIP can be seen simultaneously). These entities may represent different stages of a lung injury (WEBB et al. 1996) with associated thickening of alveolar walls and many mononuclear cells in the alveolar space.

Because of the rarity of these entities in children, most HRCT findings have been reported in adults. On HRCT, the main sign in DIP is the presence of bilateral and symmetric areas of GGO (the predominant lesion in DIP is alveolar spaces filled with macrophages) (HARTMAN et al. 1993). The ground-glass areas of attenuation are seen mainly in lower lung zones. Other findings in DIP are those of UIP: reticular opacities, which correspond to areas of irregular fibrosis, honeycombing and traction bronchiectasis (NISHIMURA et al. 1992). Less common HRCT findings include discrete nodules and interlobular septal thickening. Mild enlargement of mediastinal lymph nodes is commonly seen, whereas large lymph nodes are uncommon.

The main HRCT findings of IPF in children are areas of ground-glass attenuation involving mostly the subpleural regions (SEELY et al. 1997). Large subpleural air cysts in the upper lobes adjacent to areas of GGOs seem to be unique to childhood IPF. These cysts are interpreted as paraseptal or irregular emphysema (Fig. 4.46). Irregular interlobular septal thickening and honeycombing seem to be less common findings and, thus, less contributory to diagnosis.

Recently, two new forms of idiopathic interstitial pneumonia have been described: acute interstitial pneumonia (AIP) (KATZENSTEIN et al. 1986) and nonspecific interstitial pneumonia and fibrosis (NIPF) (KATZENSTEIN and FIORELLI 1994).

AIP is a fulminant disease of unknown etiology that is histologically characterized as diffuse alveolar damage. The latter manifests as injury to the alveolar lining and endothelial cells, pulmonary edema, hyaline membrane formation and, later, proliferative changes involving alveolar and bronchiolar lining cells, and interstitial cells. The histologic appearance of AIP can be separated into acute exudative, sub-

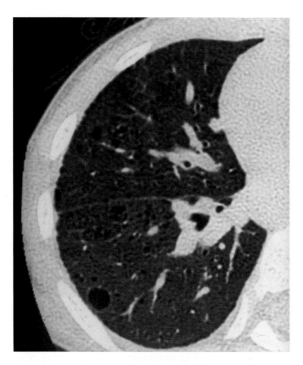

Fig. 4.46. A 7-year-old boy with biopsy-proven idiopathic pulmonary fibrosis. HRCT shows ground-glass attenuation and air cysts, involving mostly the subpleural regions

acute proliferative and chronic fibrotic phases. The radiological finding on chest radiographs is progressive parenchymal consolidation. HRCT images include diffuse air-space consolidation and patchy or diffuse GGOs, traction bronchiectasis and, occasionally, focal honeycombing (PRIMACK et al. 1993; ICHIKADO et al. 1997). These findings are usually bilateral, symmetrical, and basilar in distribution. GGOs are seen in all three histological phases and reflect different histological findings. During the acute exudative phase, they reflect the presence of alveolar septal edema and hyaline membranes along the alveolar walls. During the subacute proliferative phase, ground-glass opacities are due to intraalveolar and interstitial organization. During the fibrotic phase, ground-glass attenuation results from alveolar septal fibrosis (JOHKOH et al. 1999a,c).

NIPF describes the group of interstitial pneumonias that cannot be classified as UIP, DIP, AIP or BOOP. NIPF is essentially a diagnosis of exclusion. It is characterized by varying degrees of interstitial inflammation and fibrosis that persist (MÜLLER and COLBY 1997). COPLEY et al. (2000) reported six cases of NIPF in children. In three of them, HRCT showed a predominantly upper-zone honeycomb pattern with parenchymal distortion superimposed on a back-ground of widespread ground-glass opacification (Fig. 4.47). For the other three patients with NIPF, one had widespread ground-glass opacification, honeycombing with mid- and lower-zone predominance, and traction bronchiectasis; another had widespread ground-glass opacification; and the last one had widespread ground-glass opacification with peripheral consolidation. None of the patients had interlobular septal thickening.

4.8.1.6
Lymphocytic Interstitial Pneumonia (LIP)

LIP is a benign lymphoproliferative disorder described by LIEBOW and CARRINGTON (1973) and characterized by pulmonary infiltration of lymphocytes and plasma cells. LIP occurs in patients who have systemic disorders, such as Sjögren's syndrome, multicentric Castleman's disease or acquired immunodeficiency syndrome (AIDS). In children, LIP has been reported to be frequently associated with AIDS. In a series of 77 human immunodeficiency virus positive (HIV+) children evaluated by AMOROSA et al. (1992), 32 were diagnosed as having LIP. The appearance of LIP on chest radiography is nonspecific and includes a fine reticular pattern and nodular opacities or a diffuse confluent pattern. HRCT findings include extensive bilateral ground-glass attenuation, focal air-space consolidation, ill-defined, centrilobular and subpleural nodules, septal thickening and thin-walled cystic lesions (CARIGNAN et al. 1995; McGUINNESS and NAIDICH 1995) (Fig. 4.48). Associated bronchiectasis and hilar or mediastinal lymph-

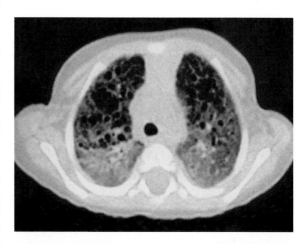

Fig. 4.47. A 10-month-old female infant with biopsy-proven non-specific interstitial pneumonitis. HRCT shows ground glass and honeycombing. (Reprinted with permission from COPLEY et al. 2000)

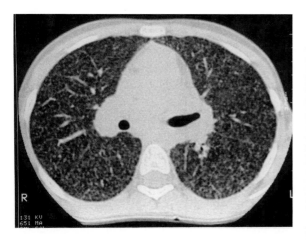

Fig. 4.48. A 13-year-old girl with biopsy-proven lymphocytic interstitial pneumonia. The patient was immunocompromised because of postviral neutropenia. HRCT shows profuse nodules. (Reprinted with permission from COPLEY et al. 2000)

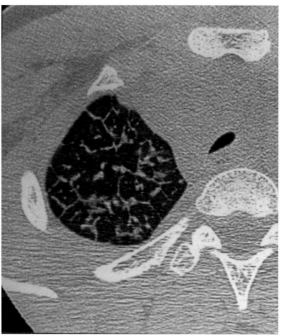

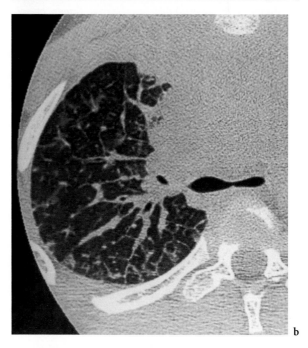

Fig. 4.49a,b. A 14-year-old boy with Hodgkin's disease. HRCT shows thickening of the interlobular septa (a), smooth peribronchovascular interstitial thickening (b), and ground-glass attenuation

adenopathy may be present (JOHKOH et al. 1999e). Pleural effusion is not seen in LIP.

4.8.1.7
Pulmonary Lymphangitic Carcinomatosis

Pulmonary lymphangitic carcinomatosis (PLC) refers to tumor growth in the lymphatics of the lung. The histological findings are characterized by thickening of the interlobular septa and the peribronchovascular interstitium. In most cases, the primary tumor disseminates hematogenously to the lungs and secondarily penetrates vessel walls and invades the surrounding interstitium and lymphatics. In children PLC is uncommon but can occur in lymphoma, thyroid carcinoma, sarcoma and neuroblastoma (KUHN 1999). In our experience, PLC has been most common in lymphoma.

Chest X-ray findings are normal or show nonspecific findings in many patients with PLC (MUNK et al. 1988). HRCT findings (JOHKOH et al. 1992) correlate well with the two types of lymphatic drainage systems described by pathologists. Axial drainage is seen on HRCT as smooth or nodular peribronchovascular interstitial thickening in the parahilar lung and enhanced visibility of the branching arteries in the pulmonary lobule. Peripheral drainage (interlobular and subpleural) is seen as interlobular septal thickening or as thickening of fissures, which may be smooth or nodular (Figs. 4.24 and 4.49). HRCT abnormalities can be focal, unilateral or diffuse.

Despite axial and peripheral interstitial abnormalities, lung architecture remains normal, a finding that is useful to differentiate between PLC and sarcoidosis.

4.8.1.8
Collagen-Vascular Disease and Pulmonary Vasculitis

Pulmonary vasculitis can be due to primary systemic vasculitides, such as Wegener's granulomatosis, Churg-Strauss angiitis or microscopic polyangiitis. In addition, pulmonary vasculitis may accompany systemic connective tissue disease, including systemic lupus erythematosus, dermatomyositis or systemic sclerosis. Connolly et al. (1996) identified a pattern on HRCT of perivascular, centrilobular, ill-defined densities in eight children with vasculitis. In the appropriate clinical setting this pattern indicates pulmonary involvement and may obviate the need for lung biopsy.

Collagen-vascular disease, especially progressive systemic sclerosis (PSS), is commonly associated with pulmonary fibrosis in children. SEELY et al. (1998) described a series of 11 patients with PSS who had interstitial lung disease. HRCT revealed abnormality in 91% of the patients. The main features were GGOs, subpleural micronodules, non-septal linear opacities, honeycombing and subpleural cysts. HRCT was able to demonstrate interstitial lung disease in 33% of patients with lupus erythematosus, mostly adults (FENLON et al. 1996) (Fig. 4.50). Juvenile rheumatoid arthritis, on the other hand, seldom leads to pulmonary fibrosis in children (SEELY et al. 1998). The HRCT pattern of fibrosis associated with collagen-vascular disease is similar to that of idiopathic pulmonary fibrosis and consists predominantly of areas of ground-glass involving mostly the subpleural lung regions, large and thin-walled cysts or bullae in the affected upper-lung zones, and smooth or irregular intralobular septal thickening.

4.8.1.9
Pulmonary Lymphangiectasia

According to NOONAN et al. (1970), pulmonary lymphangiectasia can be divided into three groups. In the first, pulmonary lymphangiectasia is part of a generalized disease, the major clinical manifestations being related to the intestinal involvement. The pulmonary involvement is less severe and is associated with a much better prognosis than for the following two groups. In the second group with associated heart disease, dilatation of the lung lymphatics occurs secondary to obstruction of pulmonary venous flow. The third group, termed congenital pulmonary lymphangiectasia (CPL), includes patients with a primary developmental defect of lung lymphatics, which are dilated. Histological examination is characterized by subpleural, interlobar, perivascular and peribronchial lymphatic dilatation. Radiological findings include bilateral pulmonary hyperinflation and a reticulonodular pattern throughout the lung fields. Occasional small cystic areas, representing aerated distal bronchial and alveolar ducts, may also be present. Pleural effusion and pneumothorax may be associated. Unilateral or lobar involvement has been reported (VERLAAT et al. 1994; LI et al. 1985; RETTWITZ-VOLK et al. 1999).

Prolonged survival of patients with CPL is rare. The chest radiograph and HRCT findings in survivors have recently been reviewed by CHUNG et al. (1999). Chest radiograph findings include increased interstitial markings, hyperinflation that generally increases with age, pleural effusion and pectus excavatum. The presence of patchy subpleural or perihilar ground glass opacities that are fixed in location and tend to decrease with time was the most characteristic HRCT feature. Hyperinflation and interstitial thickening were often seen.

4.8.1.10
Lymphangiomatosis and Gorham's Disease

Lymphangiomatosis, a malformation of the lymphatic system, is a very rare entity that occurs mainly in children and adolescents. It is believed to be caused by either a developmental defect or obstruction of the lymphatic channels. The main abnormalities seen on HRCT are smooth thickening of the interlobular septa and bronchovascular bundles, and areas of

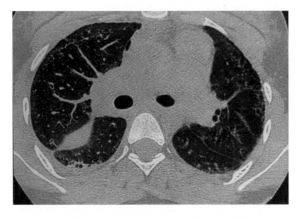

Fig. 4.50. A 16-year-old girl with systemic lupus erythematous. HRCT shows honeycombing, predominantly in the periphery, and pleural effusion. Note the right pneumomediastinum

ground glass opacification (SWENSEN et al. 1995). Bilateral pleural effusions or smooth thickening of the pleura and increased attenuation of the mediastinal fat are also seen in most patients (MITCHELL et al. 1993). Chest involvement in Gorham's or "vanishing bone" disease, in which there is replacement of a single or several contiguous bones by lymphangiomatous tissue, may present with severe and progressive osteolysis associated with septal thickening (Fig. 4.51) and chylothorax (DUTHEIL-DOCO et al. 1997; KONEZ et al. 2000).

4.8.1.11
Pulmonary Hemorrhage

Pulmonary hemorrhage is frequently found in children with idiopathic hemosiderosis (KIPER et al. 1999; KOH and HANSELL 2000) and may also be seen in systemic lupus erythematosus, Wegener's granulomatosis and Goodpasture's syndrome (RAMIREZ et al. 1984; VON VIGIER et al. 2000). Pulmonary hemorrhage appears on HRCT as patchy, frequently bilateral areas of ground-glass attenuation or consolidation (Fig. 4.52. Idiopathic hemosiderosis is characterized by recurrent pulmonary hemorrhages. The etiology remains unknown and prognosis is poor since pulmonary fibrosis develops rapidly (PRIMACK et al. 1995).

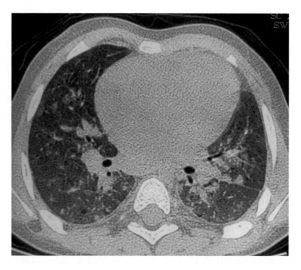

Fig. 4.52. A 3-year-old girl with hemosiderosis. HRCT shows ground-glass attenuation due to pulmonary hemorrhage

4.8.1.12
Pulmonary Alveolar Microlithiasis

Pulmonary alveolar microlithiasis (PAM) is characterized by calcium deposits within the alveoli of both lungs with a predominantly symmetrical middle- and lower-lung zone distribution. The etiology is unknown, but evidence supporting an autosomal recessively inherited defect is accumulating (WALLIS et al. 1996). HRCT findings are GGOs and tiny calcifications along the bronchovascular bundles, pleura and interlobular septa (CLUZEL et al. 1991). Parenchymal calcifications are described as nodular in adults and as micronodular in children. Parenchymal and subpleural cysts have also been reported as signs of fibrosis in PAM. However, in the two pediatric cases studied by HELBICH et al. (1997), no intraparenchymal cysts were seen.

4.8.1.13
Pulmonary Gaucher's Disease
and Niemann-Pick Disease

Gaucher's disease is a genetic disorder characterized by b-glucocerebrosidase deficiency with secondary accumulation of glucocerebrosides in the reticuloendothelial system. The liver, spleen, bone marrow, brain and lungs may be involved. Three clinical forms have been described. In the adult form (type I), the central nervous system is intact and pulmonary involvement is rare. The infantile form (type II) is

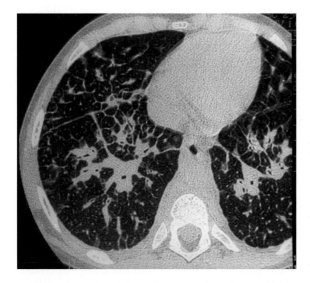

Fig. 4.51. A 6-year-old girl with Gorham's disease. Note the prominent diffuse smooth septal thickening, bronchovascular bundles and ground-glass attenuation

characterized by early CNS involvement and death within 2 years. The juvenile form (type III) is a sub-acute variant of the disease that comprises cases with combined involvement of the CNS and other organs. Pulmonary involvement is not unusual in the infantile form but is particularly rare in the adult form. However, HRCT pulmonary findings have only been reported in the adult type (TUNACI et al. 1995; AYDIN et al. 1997; YASSA and WILCOX 1998). These include interlobular and intralobular septal thickening, GGOs, and small nodules within the secondary lobules. Thickening of the septa reflects infiltration of the pulmonary interstitium by Gaucher cells (Fig. 4.53). GGOs may indicate interstitial or intra-alveolar involvement and micronodules are probably due to accumulation of Gaucher cells within air-spaces. Similar HRCT features have been reported in patients with Niemann-Pick disease (see Fig. 4.23) (FERETTI et al. 1996).

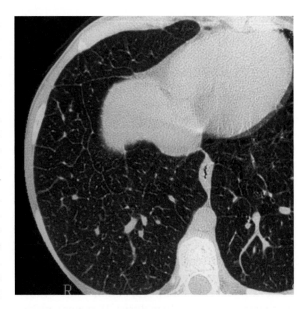

Fig. 4.53. A 13-year-old girl with Gaucher's disease. Interlobular septal and intralobular interstitial thickening are seen on HRCT

4.8.1.14
Bronchopulmonary Dysplasia

Bronchopulmonary dysplasia (BPD) occurs in premature infants and as the chronic sequela of lung disease (mostly surfactant deficiency) and its treatment. In the early phase HRCT shows thickening of the peribronchial and interlobular interstitium, sub-pleural parenchymal bands and hyperexpanded cyst-like areas, corresponding to hyperaerated lung and atelectasis, that give the lung a "cobblestone" appearance (see Fig. 4.3). In most survivors of BPD respiratory symptoms and radiologic abnormalities show a slow but continuous improvement. After the age of 2 years HRCT scans in children who have had BPD will be abnormal and characterized by the presence of a mosaic attenuation pattern due to air-trapping, parenchymal bands, thickened interlobular septa, peripheral wedge-shaped subpleural opacities, and architectural distortion (see Figs. 4.3 and 4.25) (OPPENHEIM et al. 1994; AQUINO et al. 1999). In the experience of AQUINO, the correlation between these findings and physiologic evidence of air-trapping and obstructive lung disease was statistically significant. The HRCT features of BPD in older children may resemble those seen in constrictive bronchiolitis. Whereas parenchymal bands and architectural distortion are more common in BPD, bronchiectasis is significantly more frequent in constrictive bronchiolitis.

4.8.2
Air-Space Disease

4.8.2.1
Bacterial, Mycoplasma and Tuberculous Pneumonia

Pneumonia due to bacterial or mycoplasma infection, the most frequent cause of parenchymal lung disease in immunocompetent children, is rarely studied with HRCT. Tuberculous pneumonia is extensively covered in other chapters.

4.8.2.2
Invasive Pulmonary Aspergillosis

Invasive pulmonary aspergillosis is a common complication in immunocompromised patients (acute leukemia with neutropenia, organ transplantation, use of immunosuppressive drugs) (BOMELBURG et al. 1992; TACCONE et al. 1993). The invasive form is characterized by occlusion of large or medium caliber arteries by plugs of hyphae. Lesions caused by Aspergillus microorganisms are endobronchial at the beginning followed by transbronchial vascular invasion.

Radiographic findings are initially nonspecific: patchy nodular opacities or lobar-type air-space disease. The two most common HRCT findings of invasive pulmonary aspergillosis are segmental consolidation with surrounding ground-glass attenuation and nodules surrounded by a halo corresponding to pulmonary hemorrhage (LOGAN et al. 1994; THOMPSON et al. 1995). These two signs are not specific and have been reported in many other entities (WON et al. 1998).

Cavitation occurs in half of the cases as a consequence of pulmonary infarction and increased granulocytic response associated with bone-marrow recovery. The cavitation process is characterized on HRCT by the air-crescent sign (Fig. 4.54), which represents air between retracted infarcted lung and the adjacent parenchyma. In the appropriate clinical setting though this sign is suggestive, but not diagnostic, of the disease. It may be seen in other diseases, such as tuberculosis, actinomycosis, bacterial abscess or septic emboli.

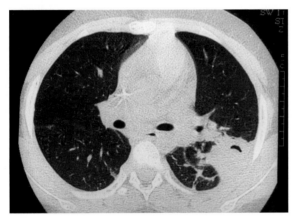

Fig. 4.54. A 7-year-old girl with acute leukemia and invasive pulmonary aspergillosis. HRCT shows pulmonary consolidation with an air crescent sign

4.8.2.3
Pneumocystis carinii Pneumonia

Pneumocystis carinii pneumonia (PCP) is the most common pulmonary opportunistic infection in immunosuppressed children, occurring in up to 90% of HIV+ patients during the course of their illness (SIVIT et al. 1995).

Radiographically, PCP presents as diffuse bilateral, progressively coalescing pulmonary infiltrates. In about 10%–20% of microbiologically documented cases, the chest radiograph remains normal.

HRCT is considered to be more sensitive than chest radiography for the detection of early parenchymal disease. HRCT findings include patchy airspace disease with a geometric or mosaic pattern and diffuse homogeneous GGOs (Fig. 4.55). Interlobular septal thickening and reticular densities have also been reported. Cysts are frequently observed and are highly suggestive of the diagnosis. Lymphadenopathy, pleural effusion and pulmonary nodules are uncommon.

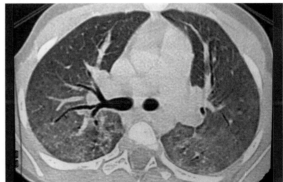

Fig. 4.55. A 6-year-old HIV+ girl with *Pneumocystis carinii* pneumonia. Diffuse homogeneous ground-glass opacities are seen on the HRCT scan

4.10
Conclusion

High resolution CT of the lung is an excellent technique for the study of lung disorders in the pediatric age group. In most cases it can be performed without the need for sedation and with techniques that deliver very little radiation to the patient. Careful technique is extremely important. In some cases, particularly in the study of chronic pediatric lung disorders, HRCT provides more information than conventional chest films with comparable radiation exposure; thus it could be an alternative for routine use in these patients. HRCT has replaced bronchography as the gold-standard for diagnosing bronchiectasis in children. We have described the normal anatomy of the lung and the HRCT features of pediatric lung disorders. Most HRCT features are non-specific, but when related to the clinical findings, they can suggest the proper diagnosis and obviate biopsy.

References

Abehsera M, Valeyre D, Grenier P et al (2000) Sarcoidosis with pulmonary fibrosis: CT patterns and correlation with pulmonary function. AJR 174:1751–1757

American Academy of Pediatrics Committee on Drugs (1992) Guidelines for monitoring and management of pediatric patients during and after sedation for diagnostic and therapeutic procedures. Pediatrics 89:1110–1115

Akira M, Yamamoto S, Sakatani M (1998) Bronchiolitis obliterans organizing pneumonia manifesting as multiple large nodules or masses. AJR 170:291–295

Albafouille V, Sayegh N, De Coudenhove S et al (1999) CT scan patterns of pulmonary alveolar proteinosis in children. Pediatr Radiol 29:147–152

Altamirano HG, McGeady SJ, Mansmann HC (1991) Right middle lobe syndrome in asthmatic children. Pediatr Asthma Allergy Immunol 5:33–37

Ambrosino NM, Genieser NB, Roche KJ et al (1994) Feasibility of high-resolution, low-dose chest CT in evaluation of the pediatric chest. Pediatr Radiol 24:6–10

Amorosa JK, Miller RW, Laraya-Cuasay L et al (1992) Bronchiectasis in children with lymphocytic interstitial pneumonia and acquired immune deficiency syndrome. Pediatr Radiol 22:603–607

Aquino SL, Gamsu G, Webb WR et al (1996) Tree-in-bud pattern: frequency and significance on thin section CT. J Comput Assist Tomogr 20:594–599

Aquino SL, Schechter MS, Chiles C et al (1999) High-resolution inspiratory and expiratory CT in older children and adults with bronchopulmonary dysplasia. AJR 173:963–967

Arakawa H, Webb WR (1998) Air-trapping on expiratory high-resolution CT scans in the absence of inspiratory scan abnormalities. AJR 170:1349–1353

Austin JHM, Müller NL, Friedman PJ et al (1996) Glossary of terms for CT of the lungs: Recommendations of the nomenclature committee of the Fleischner Society. Radiology 200:327–331

Aydin K, Karabulut N, Demirkazik F et al (1997) Pulmonary involvement in adult Gaucher's disease: high-resolution CT appearance. Br J Radiol 70:93–95

Bhalla M, Turcios N, Aponte V et al (1991) Cystic fibrosis: scoring system with thin-section CT. Radiology 179:783–788

Bomelburg T, Roos N, von Lengerke HJ et al (1992) Invasive aspergillosis complicating induction chemotherapy of childhood leukaemia. Eur J Pediatr 151:485–487

Bonelli FS, Hartman TE, Swensen SJ et al (1998) Accuracy of high-resolution CT in diagnosing lung diseases. AJR 170:1507–1512

Brasfield D, Hicks G, Soong SJ et al (1980) Evaluation of scoring system of the chest radiograph in cystic fibrosis: a collaborative study. AJR 134:1195–1198

Brauner MW, Grenier P, Mompoint D et al (1989a) Pulmonary sarcoidosis: evaluation with high-resolution CT. Radiology 172:467–471

Brauner MW, Grenier P, Mouelhi MM et al (1989b) Pulmonary histiocytosis X: evaluation with high-resolution CT. Radiology 172:255–258

Brauner MW, Grenier P, Tijani K et al (1997) Pulmonary Langerhans cell histiocytosis: evolution of lesions on CT scans. Radiology 204:497–502

Brody AS, Molina PL, Klein JS et al (1999) High-resolution computed tomography of the chest in children with cystic fibrosis: support for use as an outcome surrogate. Pediatr Radiol 29:731–735

Capitanio MA, Kirkpatrick JA (1972) Lateral decubitus film: an aid in determining air-trapping in children. Radiology 103:460–462

Carignan S, Staples CA, Müller NL (1995) Intrathoracic lymphoproliferative disorders in the immunocompromised patient: CT findings. Radiology 197:53–58

Cartier Y, Kavanagh PV, Johkoh T et al (1999) Bronchiectasis: accuracy of high-resolution CT in the differentiation of specific diseases. AJR 173:47–52

Chang AB, Masel JP, Masters B (1998) Post-infectious bronchiolitis obliterans: clinical, radiological and pulmonary function sequelae. Pediatr Radiol 28:25–29

Choi D, Lee KS, Suh GY et al (1999) Pulmonary tuberculosis presenting as acute respiratory failure: Radiol Find J Comput Assist Tomogr 23:107–113

Chung CJ, Fordham LA, Barker P et al (1999) Children with congenital pulmonary lymphangiectasia: after infancy. AJR 173:1583–1588

<Chung T, Hoffer FA, Connor L et al (2000) The use of oral pentobarbital sodium (Nembutal) versus oral chloral hydrate in infants undergoing CT and MRI imaging – a pilot study. Pediatr Radiol 30:332–335

Cleveland RH, Staub Neish A, Zurakowski D et al (1998) Cystic fibrosis: a system for assessing and predicting progression. AJR 170:1067–1072

Cluzel P, Grenier P, Bernadac P et al (1991) Pulmonary alveolar microlithiasis: CT findings. J Comput Assist Tomogr 15:938–942

Colby TV (1998) Bronchiolitis. Pathologic considerations. Am J Clin Pathol 109:101–109

Collins J, Stern EJ (1997) Ground-glass opacity at CT: the ABCs. AJR 169:355–367

Connolly B, Manson D, Eberhard A et al (1996) CT appearance of pulmonary vasculitis in children. AJR 167:901–904

Copley SJ, Coren M, Nicholson AG et al (2000) Diagnostic accuracy of thin-section CT and chest radiography of pediatric interstitial lung disease. AJR 174:549–554

Coté CJ, Karl HW, Notterman DA et al (2000) Adverse sedation events in pediatrics: analysis of medications used for sedation. Pediatrics 106:633–644

Coulier B, Mailleux P, Mairesse M et al (1999) Pulmonary alveolar proteinosis, high-resolution CT findings and evolution in 5 patients. JBR-BTR 82:277–281

Dawson WB, Müller NL (1990) High-resolution computed tomography in pulmonary sarcoidosis. Semin Ultrasound CT MR 11:423–429

Donnelly LF (2000) Langerhan's cell histiocytosis showing low-attenuation mediastinal mass and cystic lung disease. AJR 174:877–878

Dutheil-Doco A, Ducou le Pointe H, Larroquet M et al (1997) Maladie de Gorham à manifestation pleuro-pulmonaire prédominante. J Radiol 78:665–667

Egelhoff JC, Ball WS Jr, Koch BL et al (1997) Safety and efficacy of sedation in children using a structured sedation program. AJR 168:1259–1262

Fauré C, Verderi D, Schmit P et al (1986) The chest film in immotile cilia syndrome in children. Ann Radiol 29:301–311

Fenlon HM, Doran M, Sant SM et al (1996) High-resolution chest CT in systemic lupus erythematosus. AJR 166:301–307

Feretti GR, Lantuejoul S, Brambilla E et al (1996) Pulmonary involvement in Niemann-Pick disease subtype B: CT findings. J Comput Assist Tomogr 20:990–992

Fisher DM (1990) Sedation of pediatric patients: an anesthesiologist's perspective. Radiology 175:613–615

Flowers JR, Clunie G, Burke M et al (1992) Bronchiolitis obliterans organizing pneumonia: the clinical and radiological features of seven cases and a review of the literature. Clin Radiol 45:371–377

Franquet T, Gimenez A, Bordes R et al (1998) The crazy paving pattern in exogenous lipoid pneumonia. CT-Pathologic correlation. AJR 170:315–317

Giovagnorio F, Cavallo V (1995) HRCT evaluation of secondary lobules and acini of the lung. J Thorac Imaging 10:129–133

Godwin JD, Müller NL, Takasugi JE (1988) Pulmonary alveolar proteinosis: CT findings. Radiology 169:609–613

Grenier P, Maurice F, Musset D et al (1986) Bronchiectasis: assessment by thin-section CT. Radiology 161:95–99

Grenier P, Lenoir S, Brauner M (1990) Computed tomographic assessment of bronchiectasis. Semin Ultrasound CT MR 11:430–441

Grenier P, Chevret S, Beigelman C et al (1994) Chronic diffuse infiltrative lung disease: determination of the diagnostic value of clinical data, chest radiography, and CT with Bayesian analysis. Radiology 191:383–390

Grenier P, Mourey-Gerosa I, Benali K et al (1996) Abnormalities of the lung and lung parenchyma in asthmatics: CT observations in 50 patients and inter- and intraobsever variability. Eur Radiol 6:199–206

Grossman H, Merten DF, Spock A et al (1985) Radiographic features of sarcoidosis in pediatric patients. Semin Roentgenol 20:393–399

Gruden JF, Webb WR, Warnock M et al (1994) Centrilobular opacities in the lung on high-resolution CT: diagnostic considerations and pathologic correlation. AJR 162:569–574

Hansell DM (1998) Bronchiectasis. Radiol Clin North Am 36:107–128

Hansell DM, Moskovic E (1991) High-resolution computed tomography in extrinsic allergic alveolitis. Clin Radiol 43:8–12

Hansell DM, Wells AU, Rubens MB et al (1994) Bronchiectasis: functional significance of areas of decreased attenuation at expiratory CT. Radiology 193:369–374

Hartman TE, Primack SL, Swenson SJ et al (1993) Desquamative interstitial pneumonia: thin-section CT findings in 22 patients. Radiology 187:787–790

Hartman TE, Primack SL, Lee KS et al (1994) CT of bronchial and bronchiolar diseases. Radiographics 14:991–1003

Helbich TH, Wojnarovsky C; Wunderbaldinger P et al (1997) Pulmonary alveolar microlithiasis in children: radiographic and high-resolution CT findings. AJR 168:63–65

Helbich TH, Heinz-Peer G, Fleischmann D et al (1999) Evolution of CT findings in patients with cystic fibrosis. AJR 173:81–88

Herman M, Michalkova K, Kopriva F (1993) High-resolution CT in the assessment of bronchiectasis in children. Pediatr Radiol 23:376–379

Hiddema A, Engelshove HA (1999) Kartagener's syndrome. JBR-BTR 82:112

Hopper KD, King SH, Lobell ME et al (1998) The breast: in-plane x-ray protection during diagnostic thoracic CT-shielding with bismuth radioprotective garments. Radiology 205:853–858

Hubbard AM, Markowitz RI, Kimmel B et al (1992) Sedation for pediatric patients undergoing CT and MRI. J Comput Assist Tomogr 16:3–6

Ichikado K, Johkoh T, Ikezoe J et al (1997) Acute interstitial pneumonia: high-resolution CT findings correlated with pathology. AJR 168:333–338

Inoue T, Toyoichiro K, Kikui M (1996) Idiopathic bronchiolitis obliterans organizing pneumonia (idiopathic BOOP) in childhood. Pediatr Pulmonol 22:67–72

Johkoh T, Ikezoe J, Tomiyama N et al (1992) CT findings in lymphangitic carcinomatosis of the lung: correlation with histologic findings and pulmonary function tests. AJR 158:1217–1222

Johkoh T, Müller NL, Cartier Y et al (1999a) Idiopathic interstitial pneumonias: diagnostic accuracy of thin-section CT in 129 patients. Radiology 211:555–560

Johkoh T, Itoh H, Müller NL et al (1999b) Crazy-paving appearance at thin-section CT: spectrum of disease and pathologic findings. Radiology 211:155–160

Johkoh T, Müller NL, Taniguchi H et al (1999c) Acute interstitial pneumonia: thin section CT findings in 36 patients. Radiology 211:859–863

Johkoh T, Müller NL, Ichikado K et al (1999d) Respiratory change in size of honeycombing: Inspiratory and expiratory spiral volumetric CT analysis of 97 cases. J Comput Assist Tomogr 23:174–180

Johkoh T, Müller NL, Pickford HA et al (1999e) Lymphocytic interstitial pneumonia: thin-section CT findings in 22 patients. Radiology 212:567–572

Karian VE, Burrows PE, Zurakowski D et al (1999) Sedation for pediatric radiological procedures: analysis of potential causes of sedation failure and paradoxical reactions. Pediatr Radiol 29:869–873

Katzenstein AL, Fiorelli RF (1994) Nonspecific interstitial pneumonia/fibrosis. Histologic features and clinical significance. Am J Surg Pathol 18:136–147

Katzenstein AL, Myers JL, Mazur MT (1986) Acute interstitial pneumonia. A clinicopathologic, ultrastructural, and cell kinetic study. Am J Surg Pathol 10:256–267

Kim JS, Müller NL, Park CS et al (1997) Cylindrical bronchiectasis: diagnostic findings on thin-section CT. AJR 168:751–754

Kim MJ, Lee KY (1996) Bronchiolitis obliterans in children with Stevens-Johnson syndrome: follow-up with high-resolution CT. Pediatr Radiol 26:22–25

Kim Y, Lee KS, Jung KJ et al (1999) Halo sign on HRCT: findings in spectrum of pulmonary diseases with pathologic correlation. J Comput Assist Tomogr 23:622–626

Kiper N, Gocmen A, Ozcelik U et al (1999) Long-term clinical course of patients with idiopathic pulmonary hemosiderosis (1979–1994): prolonged survival with low-dose corticosteroid therapy. Pediatr Pulmonol 27:180–184

Kleinau I, Perez-Canto A, Schmid HJ et al (1997) Bronchiolitis obliterans organizing pneumonia and chronic graft-versus-host disease in a child after allogenic bone marrow transplantation. Bone Marrow Transplant 19:841–844

Koh DM, Hansell DM (2000) Computed tomography of diffuse interstitial lung disease in children. Clin Radiol 55:659–667

Konez O, Vyas PK, Goyal M (2000) Disseminated lymphangiomatosis presenting with massive chylothorax. Pediatr Radiol 30:35–37

Kuhn JP (1999) High-resolution CT of diffuse parenchymal disorders. In: Siegel MJ (ed) Special course in pediatric radiology: current concepts in body imaging at the millennium. RSNA 1999 syllabus_, Radiological Society of America, Oak Brook, Ill., USA, pp 57–67

Land CE, Tokunaga M, Tokuaka AS et al (1993) Early-onset breast cancer in A bomb survivors. Lancet 342:237

Landry BA, Melhem RE (1989) Pulmonary nodules secondary to total parenteral alimentation. Pediatr Radiol 19:456–457

Lau DM, Siegel MJ, Hildebolt CF et al (1998) Bronchiolitis obliterans syndrome: thin-section CT diagnosis of obstructive changes in infants and young children after lung transplantation. Radiology 208:783–788

Lee KS, Kullnig P, Hartman TE et al (1994a) Cryptogenic organizing pneumonia: CT findings in 43 patients. AJR 162:543–546

Lee KS, Primack SL, Staples CA et al (1994b) Chronic infiltrative lung disease: comparison of diagnostic accuracies of radiography and low- and conventional-dose thin-section CT. Radiology 191:669–673

Li YW, Snow J, Smith W et al (1985) Localized pulmonary lymphangiectasia. AJR 145:269–270

Liebow AA, Carrington CB (1973) Diffuse pulmonary lymphoreticular infiltrations associated with dysproteinemia. Med Clin North Am 57:809–843

Logan PM, Primack SL, Miller RR et al (1994) Invasive aspergillosis of the airways: radiographic, CT and pathologic findings. Radiology 193:383–388

Lucaya J, Gartner S, Garcia-Pena P et al (1998) Spectrum of manifestations of Swyer-James-MacLeod syndrome. J Comput Assist Tomogr 22:592–597

Lucaya J, Garcia-Peña P, Herrera L et al (1999) Expiratory chest CT in children. AJR 174:235–241

Lucaya J, Piqueras J, Garcia-Peña P et al (2000) Low-dose high-resolution CT of the chest in children and young adults: dose, cooperation, artifact incidence, and image quality. AJR 175:985–992

Lynch DA, Hay T, Newell JD Jr et al (1999a) Pediatric diffuse lung disease. AJR 173:713–718

Lynch DA (1998) Imaging of asthma and allergic bronchopulmonary mycosis. Radiol Clin North Am 36:129–142

Marti-Bonmati L, Ruiz Perales F, Catala F et al (1989) CT findings in Swyer-James syndrome. Radiology 172:477–480

Mathew P, Bozeman P, Krance RA et al (1994) Bronchiolitis obliterans organizing pneumonia (BOOP) in children after allogeneic bone marrow transplantation. Bone Marrow Transplant 13:221–223

Mayo JR, Webb WR, Gould R et al (1987) High resolution CT of the lungs: an optimal approach. Radiology 163:507–510

Mayo JR, Jackson SA, Müller NL (1993) High resolution CT of the chest: radiation dose. AJR 160:479–481

McCook TA, Kirks DR, Merten DF et al (1981) Pulmonary alveolar proteinosis in children. AJR 137:1023–1027

McGuinness G, Naidich DP (1995) Bronchiectasis: CT/clinical correlations. Semin Ultrasound CT MR 16:395–419

McLean AN, Sproule MW, Cowan MD et al (1998) High-resolution computed tomography in asthma. Thorax 53:308–314

Meeks M, Bush A (2000) Primary ciliary dyskinesia (PCD). Pediatr Pulmonol 29:307–316

Mitchell CS, Parisi MT, Osborn RE (1993) Gorham's disease involving the thoracic skeleton. Pediatr Radiol 23:543–544

Moon WK, Kim WS, Kim IO et al (1996) Diffuse pulmonary disease in children. High-resolution CT findings. AJR 167:1405–1408

Moore AD, Godwin JD, Müller NL et al (1989) Pulmonary histiocytosis X: comparison of radiographic and CT findings. Radiology 172:249–254

Moore AD, Godwin JD, Dietrich PA (1992) Swyer-James syndrome: CT findings in eight patients. AJR 158:1211–1215

Müller NL, Colby TV (1997) Idiopathic interstitial pneumonias: high-resolution CT and histologic findings. Radiographics 17:1016–1022

Müller NL, Staples CA, Miller RR (1990) Bronchiolitis obliterans organizing pneumonia: CT features in 14 patients. AJR 154:983–987

Munk PL, Müller NL, Miller RR et al (1988) Pulmonary lymphangitic carcinomatosis: CT and pathologic findings. Radiology 166:705–709

Murata K, Itoh H, Todo G et al (1986) Centrilobular lesions of the lung: demonstration by high-resolution CT and pathologic correlation. Radiology 161:641–645

Murata K, Khan A, Rojas KA et al (1988) Optimization of computed tomography technique to demonstrate the fine structure of the lung. Invest Radiol 23:170–175

Murata K, Khan A, Herman PG (1989) Pulmonary parenchymal diseases: evaluation with high resolution CT. Radiology 170:629–635

Murch CR, Carr DH (1989) Computed tomography appearances of pulmonary alveolar proteinosis. Clin Radiol 40:240–243

Nadel HR, Stringer DA, Levison H et al (1985) The immotile cilia syndrome: radiological manifestations. Radiology 154:651–655

Nathanson I, Conboy K, Murphy S et al (1991) Ultrafast computerized tomography of the chest in cystic fibrosis: a new scoring system. Pediatr Pulmonol 11:81–86

Nishimura K, Kitaichi M, Izumi T et al (1992) Usual interstitial pneumonia: histologic correlation with high-resolution CT. Radiology 182:337–342

Nishimura K, Itoh H, Kitaichi M et al (1995) CT and pathological correlation of pulmonary sarcoidosis. Semin Ultrasound CT MR 16:361–370

Noonan JA, Walters LR, Reeves JT (1970) Pulmonary lymphangiectasis. Am R Dis Child 120:314–319

Oh YW, Effmann EL, Redding GJ et al (1999) Follicular hyperplasia of bronchus-associated lymphoid tissue causing severe air-trapping. AJR 172:745–747

Oppenheim C, Mamou-Mani T, Sayegh N et al (1994) Bronchopulmonary dysplasia: value of CT in identifying pulmonary sequelae. AJR 163:169–172

Ouellette H (1999) The signet ring sign. Radiology 212:67–68

Osika E, Muller MH, Boccon-Gibod L (1997) Idiopathic pulmonary fibrosis in infants. Pediatr Pulmonol 23:49–54

Paganin F, Trussard V, Seneterre E et al (1992) Chest radiography and high-resolution computed tomography of the lungs in asthma. Am Rev Respir Dis 146:1084–1087

Pattishall EN, Kendig EL (1996) Sarcoidosis in children. Pediatr Pulmonol 22:195–203

Pereira JK, Burrows PE, Richards HM et al (1993) Comparison of sedation regimens for pediatric outpatient CT. Pediatr Radiol 23:341–344

Primack SL, Hartman TE, Ikezoe J et al (1993) Acute interstitial pneumonia: radiographic and CT findings in nine patients. Radiology 188:817–820

Primack SL, Hartman TE, Lee KS et al (1994) Pulmonary nodules and the CT halo sign. Radiology 190:513–515

Primack SL, Miller RR, Müller NL (1995) Diffuse pulmonary hemorrhage: clinical, pathologic, and imaging features. AJR 164:295–300

Ramirez RE, Glasier C, Kirks D et al (1984) Pulmonary hemorrhage associated with systemic lupus erythematosus in children. Radiology 152:409–412

Rettwitz-Volk W, Schlober R, Ahrens P et al (1999) Congenital unilobar pulmonary lymphangiectasis. Pediatr Pulmonol 27:290–292

Reyes de la Rocha S, Pysher TJ, Leonard JC (1987) Dyskinetic cilia syndrome: clinical, radiographic and scintigraphic findings. Pediatr Radiol 17:97–103

Rimmer MJ, Dixon AK, Flower DR et al (1985) Bleomycin lung: computed tomographic observations. Br J Radiol 58:1041–1045

Rothenberg LN, Pentlow KS (1992) Radiation dose in CT. Radiographics 12:1225–1243

Ruzal-Shapiro C (1998) Cystic fibrosis. An overview. Radiol Clin North Am 36:143–161

Sargent MA, Cairns RA, Murdoch MJ et al (1995) Obstructive lung disease in children after allogenic bone marrow transplantation: evaluation with high-resolution CT. AJR 164:693–696

Schumacher RE, Marrogi AJ, Heidelberger KP (1989) Pulmonary alveolar proteinosis in a newborn. Pediatr Pulmonol 7:178–182

Seely JM, Effmann EL, Müller NL (1997) High-resolution CT of pediatric lung disease: imaging findings. AJR 168:1269–1275

Seely JM, Jones LT, Wallace C et al (1998) Systemic sclerosis: using high-resolution CT to detect lung disease in children. AJR 170:691–697

Shah A, Pant CS, Bhagat R et al (1992) CT in childhood allergic bronchopulmonary aspergillosis. Pediatr Radiol 22:227–228

Shah RM, Sexauer W, Ostrum BJ et al (1997) High-resolution CT in the acute exacerbation of cystic fibrosis: evaluation of acute findings, reversibility of those findings, and clinical correlation. AJR 168:375–380

Shepard JO (1995) The bronchi: an imaging perspective. J Thorac Imaging 10:236–254

Siegel M (1999) Pediatric body CT. Lippincott, Philadelphia / Williams and Wilkins, Baltimore, pp 101–140

Sivit CJ, Miller CR, Rakusan TA et al (1995) Spectrum of chest radiographic abnormalities in children with AIDS and *Pneumocystis carinii* pneumonia. Pediatr Radiol 25:389–392

Small JH, Flower CD, Traill ZC et al (1996) Air-trapping in extrinsic allergic alveolitis on computed tomography. Clin Radiol 51:684–688

Smets A, Mortelé K, De Praeter G et al (1997) Pulmonary and mediastinal lesions in children with Langerhans cell histiocytosis. Pediatr Radiol 27:873–876

Sminiotopoulos JG, Lonergan GJ, Abbott RM et al (1999) Image interpretation session: 1998. Radiographics 19:205–233

Sockrider MM, Swank PR, Seilheimer DK et al (1994) Measuring clinical status in cystic fibrosis: internal validity and reliability of the modified NIH score. Pediatr Pulmonol 17:86–96

Stern EJ, Samples TL (1992) Dynamic ultrafast high-resolution CT findings in a case of Swyer-James syndrome. Pediatr Radiol 22:350–352

Stern EJ, Müller NL, Swensen SJ et al (1995) CT mosaic pattern of lung attenuation: etiologies and terminology. J Thorac Imaging 10:294–297

Swensen SJ, Hartman TE, Mayo JR et al (1995) Diffuse pulmonary lymphangiectasis: CT findings. J Comput Assist Tomogr 19:348–352

Swensen SJ, Aughenbaugh GL, Myers JL (1997) Diffuse lung disease: diagnostic accuracy of CT in patients undergoing surgical biopsy of the lung. Radiology 205:229–234

Taccone A, Occhi M, Garaventa A et al (1993) CT of invasive pulmonary aspergillosis in children with cancer. Pediatr Radiol 23:177–180

Teel GS, Engeler CE, Tashijian JH et al (1996) Imaging of small airway disease. Radiographics 16:27–41

Thompson BH, Stanford W, Galvin JR et al (1995) Varied radiologic appearances of pulmonary aspergillosis. Radiographics 15:1273–1284

Tomiyama N, Miyamoto M, Nakahara K (1994) CT halo sign in metastatic osteosarcoma. AJR 162:468

Traill ZC, Maskell GF, Gleeson FV (1997) High-resolution CT findings of pulmonary sarcoidosis. AJR 168:1557–1560

Tunaci A, Berkmen YM, Gokmen E (1995) Pulmonary Gaucher's disease: high-resolution computed tomographic features. Pediatr Radiol 25:237–238

Vade A, Sukhani R, Dolenga M et al (1995) Chloral hydrate sedation of children undergoing CT and MR imaging: safety as judged by American Academy of Pediatrics guidelines. AJR 165:905–909

Verlaat CW, Peters HM, Semmekrot BA et al (1994) Congenital pulmonary lymphangiectasis presenting as a unilateral hyperlucent lung. Eur J Pediatr 153:202–205

Vincent JM, Armstrong P, Wilson AG (1992) Extrinsic allergic alveolitis and eosinophilic pneumonia. Imaging 4:5–13

von Vigier RO, Trummler SA, Laux-End R et al (2000) Pulmonary renal syndrome in childhood: a report of twenty-one cases and a review of the literature. Pediatr Pulmonol 29:382–388

Wallis C, Whitehead B, Malone M et al (1996) Pulmonary alveolar microlithiasis in childhood: diagnosis by transbronchial biopsy. Pediatr Pulmonol 21:62–64

Ward S, Heyneman L, Lee MJ et al (1999) Accuracy of CT in the diagnosis of allergic bronchopulmonary aspergillosis in asthmatic patients. AJR 173:937–942

Webb WR (1994) High-resolution computed tomography of obstructive lung disease. Radiol Clin North Am 32:745–757

Webb WR, Müller NL, Naidich DP (1996) High-resolution CT of the lung, 2nd edn. Lippincott, Philadelphia / Raven, New York

Weibel ER (1979) Looking into the lung: what can it tell us? AJR 133:1021–1031

Won HJ, Lee KS, Cheon JE et al (1998) Invasive pulmonary aspergillosis: prediction at thin-section CT in patients with neutropenia – a prospective study. Radiology 208:777–782

Yassa NA, Wilcox AG (1998) High-resolution CT pulmonary findings in adults with Gaucher's disease. Clin Imaging 22:339–342

Yule SM, Hamilton JRL, Windebank KP (1997) Recurrent pneumomediastinum and pneumothorax in Langerhans cell histiocytosis. Med Pediatr Oncol 29:139–142

Zwirewich CV, Mayo JR, Müller NL (1991) Low-dose high-resolution CT of lung parenchyma. Radiology 180:413–417

5 Pulmonary Malformations Beyond the Neonatal Period

Josep M. Mata and Amparo Castellote

CONTENTS

5.1 Introduction

Congenital lung malformations include a heterogeneous group of anomalies affecting the lung parenchyma, the arterial supply to the lung and its venous drainage (Heitzman 1984). From the morphological-radiological viewpoint, these malformations can be divided into two groups: focal malformations (bronchial atresia, single congenital thoracic cyst, congenital adenomatoid malformation, pulmonary sequestration and isolated systemic supply to normal lung) and dysmorphic lung (lung agenesis-hypoplasia complex and lobar agenesis-aplasia complex).

Josep M. Mata, MD
UDIAT, Servei de Diagnòstic per la Imatge, Corporació Parc Tauli, Parc Tauli s/n, Sabadell 08208, Spain
Amparo Castellote, MD
Servei de Radiologia Pediàtrica, Hospital Vall d'Hebron, Ps. Vall d'Hebron 119–129, Barcelona 08035, Spain

5.2 Focal Malformations

Focal congenital malformations usually involve only a part of the lung. They are a heterogeneous group, whose boundaries are not well defined and whose radiologic and pathologic manifestations vary and can be difficult to classify, especially if infection is present. They may cause symptoms in early life or be discovered incidentally.

Focal congenital malformations can be separated according to their radiologic and pathologic manifestations, with the understanding that significant degrees of overlap may occur. They can be considered a spectrum: at one extreme we find isolated bronchopulmonary anomaly (bronchial atresia, single congenital thoracic cyst, congenital adenomatoid malformation); next, associated systemic vascularization in the diseased lung (pulmonary sequestration); and at the other extreme isolated systemic arterial anomalies (isolated systemic supply to normal lung).

5.2.1 Bronchial Atresia

Bronchial atresia is an anomaly characterized by obliteration of the proximal lumen of a segmental bronchus, with preservation of the distal structures. Its pathogenesis is unknown, although it may be due to a vascular insult. Air enters the affected segment via collateral channels, producing overinflation and air-trapping. The mucus secretions generated in the bronchi accumulate at the point of obstruction, originating mucus impaction (Lemire et al. 1970; Felson 1979). The mucocele can be linear, branched, ovoid or spherical. Bronchial atresia almost always affects just one segment, and rarely affects a lobar bronchus. Involvement of multiple segments has been reported in a few cases (Ward and Morcos 1999). Bronchial atresia is characteristically located in the left upper lobe (apico-posterior segment), but can involve any lobe (Remy-Jardin et al. 1989; MEDELLI et al. 1979) and can be associated with other congenital anomalies. It is usually asymptomatic and is an incidental finding on radiological study. Infection of the unconnected lung is rare.

The chest plain film usually demonstrates pulmonary insufflation with trapped air during expiration, accompanied by a tubular, branched or spherical image in a central position, which corresponds to the mucocele (JERDERLINIC et al. 1986). CT shows the segmental overinflation and mucous impaction with great precision. When bronchial atresia does not involve the left upper lobe or when it does not present characteristic radiological findings in the plain film, CT is diagnostic, demonstrating the combination of emphysema and bronchial impaction that is the hallmark of this condition (PUGATCH and GALE 1983; FINCK and MILNE 1988) (Fig. 5.1). In some cases, a cystic lesion containing gas and fluid corresponding to a severely dilated bronchus just distal to segmental bronchial atresia can also be seen (GRISCOM 1993) (Fig. 5.2).

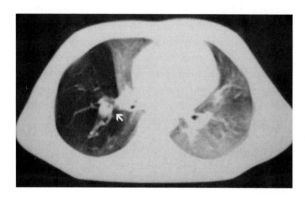

Fig. 5.1. Bronchial atresia in a 7-year-old girl. Expiratory CT scan imaged with lung window shows the bronchocele (*arrow*) and hyperinflation of the right upper lobe

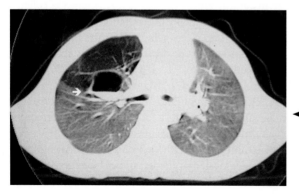

5.2.2
Single Congenital Thoracic Cyst

We include under the term single congenital thoracic cyst (SCTC) all congenital cysts located in the mediastinum (bronchogenic cysts, duplication cysts and pleuropericardial cysts) and lung parenchyma. Treatment of SCTC depends on the symptoms. The best approach in asymptomatic patients with mediastinal cysts is periodic control, avoiding surgery. For practical purposes of clinical management, all cysts located within the lung parenchyma can be considered bronchogenic cysts requiring surgery. The definitive diagnosis of SCTC should be established on the basis of the study of the cyst wall. When there is associated inflammation and in some cases of mediastinal cysts, diagnosis can be difficult.

The most frequent location of bronchogenic cyst varies according to the published series (DUMONTIER et al. 1985; BAKER 1989; PATCHER and LATTES 1963; ROGERS and OSMER 1964). In the most recent series including 68 bronchogenic cysts (MCADAMS et al. 2000), 58 (85%) were mediastinal and seven were intrapulmonary (10%), demonstrating a clear predominance of mediastinal cysts. Mediastinal cysts are most often found in a subcarinal location, whereas intrapulmonary bronchogenic cysts are most frequently located in the lower lobes. Bronchogenic cysts can be found in the diaphragm, below the diaphragm (BRAFFMAN et al. 1988) and even in the liver (KIMURA et al. 1990) or neck and can be associated with pericardial agenesis (KWAK et al. 1971). They are usually solitary and spherical in shape with thin walls of bronchial epithelium, and have a viscous gelatinous, mucoid, hemorrhagic or watery, translucent fluid content. They occasionally contain calcium, have calcified walls, or are completely calcified and they can be air-filled when they communicate with the bronchial tree (ROGERS and OSMER 1964; REED and SOBONYA 1975).

Fig. 5.2. Bronchial atresia in a 4-year-old boy. CT scan imaged with lung window shows a cystic lesion containing gas and fluid at the right hilum (*arrow*) corresponding to the dilated right upper lobe bronchus and hyperinflated right upper lobe

In infants mediastinal SCTC tend to compress or distort the esophagus, the trachea and bronchi, resulting in clinical respiratory compromise. Compression of a main bronchus may result in obstructive pulmonary hyperinflation of the ipsilateral lung (Fig. 5.3). These cysts can also compress the pulmonary artery or superior vena cava (BANKOFF et al. 1985). Mediastinal and intrapulmonary SCTC can disappear spontaneously (MARTIN et al. 1988), change form due to decreases in their internal pressure, or diminish in size, making themselves invisible to the chest plain film (Fig. 5.4).

The basic radiological study used to detect SCTC is the chest plain film. In the majority of cases, this technique detects the lesion and some of the complications (e.g. compression on neighboring structures). Ultrasound and CT allow a better evaluation of SCTC and its anatomic relationship with adjacent structures. Currently CT is the examination of choice for assessing SCTC (FITCH et al. 1986). CT reveals a round or ovoid mass with water or soft-tissue attenuation. Almost 50% of SCTC appear iso- or even hyperdense at CT due to intracystic hemorrhage, protein content, or milk of calcium. In these latter cases, MRI can contribute confirmatory information. On MRI, SCTC are homogeneously and markedly hyperintense on T2-weighted images. The intracystic signal intensity on T1-weighted images is more variable, and, depending upon the cyst content, low, intermediate, and high signal intensity cases have been reported (NAIDICH et al. 1998; NAKATA et al. 1993). Relatively high signal intensity on T1 is due to a high protein content and or the presence of methemoglobin. Fluid–fluid levels have also been reported (LYON and MCADAMS 1993). When air–fluid levels are seen within the cyst, it is usually infected, although we have seen cysts with air–fluid levels in asymptomatic patients (Fig. 5.5). Minimal wall enhancement is expected with gadolinium enhancement. The multiplanar imaging possibilities are an advantage of MRI in studying this entity.

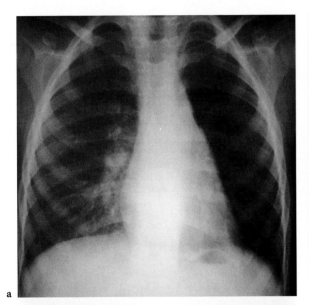

a

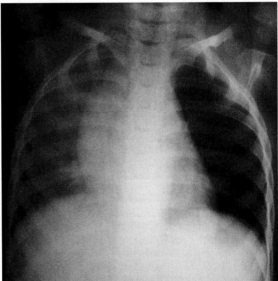

b

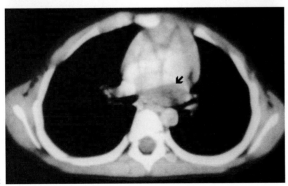

c

Fig. 5.3a–c. Bronchogenic cyst in a 3-year-old boy. **a** Inspiratory chest radiograph shows hyperlucency and decreased vascular perfusion in the left lung. **b** Expiratory chest radiograph demonstrates air-trapping in the left lung. **c** A subcarinal cyst compressing the left main bronchus is seen in the CT scan (*arrow*)

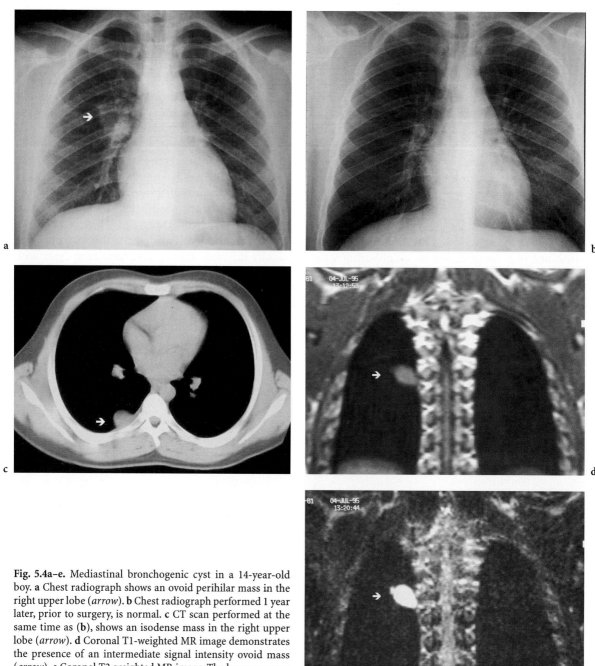

Fig. 5.4a–e. Mediastinal bronchogenic cyst in a 14-year-old boy. **a** Chest radiograph shows an ovoid perihilar mass in the right upper lobe (*arrow*). **b** Chest radiograph performed 1 year later, prior to surgery, is normal. **c** CT scan performed at the same time as (**b**), shows an isodense mass in the right upper lobe (*arrow*). **d** Coronal T1-weighted MR image demonstrates the presence of an intermediate signal intensity ovoid mass (*arrow*). **e** Coronal T2-weighted MR image. The homogeneous high signal intensity of the mass indicates a fluid content (*arrow*)

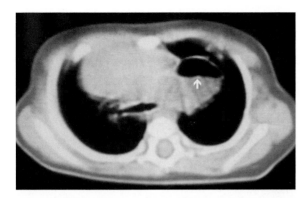

Fig. 5.5. Bronchogenic cyst in an asymptomatic 6-month-old boy. CT scan shows an air–fluid level within the cyst (*arrow*)

5.2.3
Congenital Adenomatoid Malformation–Pulmonary Sequestration Complex

5.2.3.1
Congenital Adenomatoid Malformation

Congenital adenomatoid malformation (CAM) consists of an intrapulmonary mass of disorganized pulmonary tissue that may or may not be accompanied by macroscopic cysts. When present, the cysts communicate with the airways and their vascular supply comes from pulmonary circulation. However, there are numerous examples of CAM fed by systemic blood vessels and in these cases it is extremely difficult to differentiate CAM from pulmonary sequestration, as they correspond to overlapping malformations (Winters et al. 1997). From the radiological viewpoint the differentiation between CAM with systemic supply and pulmonary sequestration is impossible. These malformations correspond to the same clinical and radiological entity, although they have a different anatomo-pathological expression.

Ch'in and Tang applied the name "congenital adenomatoid malformation" to a congenital cystic pulmonary anomaly for the first time in 1949. The essential discovery is an adenomatoid proliferation of the terminal bronchioles that produces cysts of varying sizes coated with bronchial epithelium. In 1977 Stocker et al. divided CAM into three groups, depending on whether the cysts were larger than 2 cm (type I), smaller than 2 cm (type II) or the malformation was solid without cysts (type III). Stocker's type I is the most frequent (50%), type II appears in 40% and the remaining 10% corresponds to type

III; in our experience type III is extremely infrequent (Stocker et al.1997). CAM can be associated with congenital bronchial atresia in the same lobe (Cachia and Sobonya 1981), can involve more than one lobe or be bilateral. It occurs with the same frequency in all lobes except the middle, where it is uncommon. CAM can cause severe respiratory distress in the neonatal period. Beyond this time it is usually discovered when it becomes infected or as an incidental radiological finding (Pulpeiro et al. 1987).

Chest X-rays play a fundamental role in detecting the anomaly. CAM can appear as single or multiple air-filled cavities that may have air-fluid levels, and occasionally, as a homogeneous mass. Spontaneous pneumothorax has been reported as a presenting finding, but is rare. CT better characterizes the malformed lung and its extension. The diverse features on CT scan result from variable content, number and size of the cysts. At CT study CAM appears as areas with small (<2 cm in diameter) or large (>2 cm in diameter) cysts with or without associated areas of consolidation, usually showing heterogeneous attenuation on enhanced scans. There can be areas of low attenuation around cystic pulmonary lesions. Cysts can have thick or thin walls and be filled with air, fluid or both. Fluid accumulation may transform air-filled cysts into fluid-filled cysts and this changing pattern can be seen on both chest X-rays and CT scans (Rosado-De-Christenson and Stocker 1991; Kim et al. 1997). Helical CT can facilitate the display of systemic aberrant arteries.

CAM may mimic some types of pleuropulmonary blastoma, a dysontogenetic neoplasm that occurs in children. Pleuropulmonary blastoma appears as a pulmonary and/or pleural-based aggressive neoplasm and can be cystic, cystic and solid, or solid. Pleuropulmonary blastoma is probably the same tumor that several authors have reported as mesenchymal sarcoma or rhabdomyosarcoma arising in congenital lung cysts (Ueda et al. 1977). It has also been stated that pleuropulmonary blastoma can arise from preexisting cystic lung disease, but is reasonable to assume that the cystic changes are a component of the pleuropulmonary blastoma, itself (Murphy et al. 1992). As the initial manifestation, pneumothorax is more frequently seen in pleuropulmonary blastoma than in adenomatoid congenital malformation (Fig.5.6) (Senac et al. 1991). However, pneumothorax can be found associated with both entities and the available information does not support the use of this finding as a differentiating diagnostic criteria (Lejeune et al. 1999).

Cases of CAM/pulmonary sequestration that dramatically decreased in size or disappear completely during pregnancy and infancy have been reported (Fig. 5.7). However, the clinical management of an asymptomatic child with a congenital mass of the lung remains controversial. Some authors advocate close clinical observation and radiological surveillance (MacGillivray et al. 1993), whereas others, considering the possibility that cystic pulmonary lesions may harbor or develop pleuropulmonary blastoma, favor elective surgical resection (Samuel and Burge 1999).

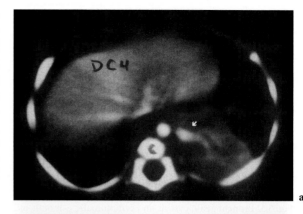

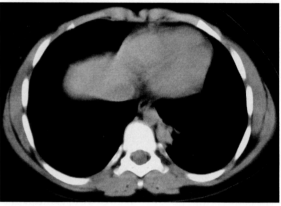

Fig. 5.7a,b. Spontaneous involution of a pulmonary sequestration. a Contrast-enhanced chest CT at the age of 3 months shows a soft tissue density mass with a large feeding vessel originating from the aorta (*arrow*). b Significant shrinkage of the mass is seen in the scan at the age of 10 years

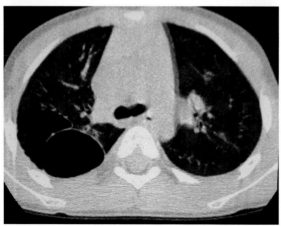

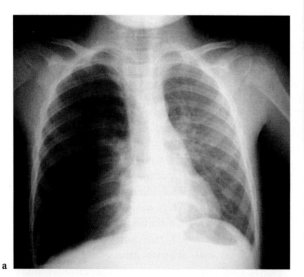

Fig. 5.6a,b. Congenital cystic adenomatoid malformation type I in a 6-year-old girl with chest pain and dyspnea. a Chest radiograph shows right-sided pneumothorax. A chest tube was inserted and the lung was re-expanded. b Chest CT performed 1 week later reveals multiple cysts at the right upper lobe

5.2.3.2
Pulmonary Sequestration

Pulmonary sequestration consists of a mass of pulmonary tissue disconnected from the bronchial tree that receives its blood supply from the systemic circulation (Heitzman 1984). Pulmonary sequestration is divided into two groups: intralobar sequestration, in which the tissue is surrounded by normal lung and found in the interior of the visceral pleura, and extralobar sequestration, in which the tissue is disconnected from the bronchial tree and has its own pleural coating. In 1946 Pryce identified intralobar sequestration as a clinical-pathological entity. He was the first to apply the term "sequestration" and further classified the lesion as intralobar or extralobar on the basis of the morphologic patterns of the malformation. There are also mixed cases with characteristics of both intralobar and extralobar sequestration.

Pulmonary sequestration is an uncommon anomaly; the intralobar form is more frequent than the extralobar. Intralobar sequestration constitutes 75% of all pulmonary sequestrations and is located en the left lower lobe in 60% of the cases. Only 2% occur in the upper lobes and 0.25% in the middle lobe. The affected lung can maintain the normal lung architecture, behave like a mass, or present internal cysts. Vascularization in the majority of cases is through the thoracic aorta (SAVIC et al. 1979), or less commonly, through systemic vessels originating from the abdominal aorta or one of its branches (PEDERSEN et al. 1988). The systemic supply can be formed by multiple, small-caliber blood vessels or by a single vessel, which are histologically similar to the pulmonary artery. This favors the early appearance of atherosclerosis (IKEZOE et al. 1990). Intralobar sequestration does not receive blood from the pulmonary arteries and it drains through pulmonary veins. In exceptional cases it communicates with the digestive tract (bronchopulmonary foregut malformation) (HRUBAN et al. 1989). It can be bilateral, or associated with other congenital malformations.

Since Pryce's description of pulmonary sequestration, there has been considerable controversy about its origin. Some authors contend that intralobar sequestration is, in fact, acquired (GEBAUER and MASON 1959; HOLDER and LANGSTON 1986), resulting from endobronchial obstruction leading to chronic pulmonary infection and hypertrophy of the systemic arteries in and around the area of the pulmonary ligament. This explains why, in the past, when infections were poorly controlled, intralobar sequestration was overdiagnosed. However, congenital intralobar sequestration does occur, since this anomaly has been detected in newborns (WEST et al. 1989; LAURIN and HÄGERTRAND 1999).

Intralobar sequestration is usually discovered because the patient has developed a pulmonary infection, although some patients are asymptomatic when the lesion is found. In a small number of cases intralobar sequestration debuts as a pleural effusion (KIM et al. 1997; LUCAYA et al. 1984), or pleural bleeding secondary to infarction of the sequestrated lung (ZUMBRO et al. 1974). On plain films, intralobar sequestration appears as a homogenous opacity mostly in the lower lobes. This opacity can simulate a mass with a well-defined border, or show internal air–fluid levels and a poorly defined border. In rare cases calcifications are present within the seques-

tration or in the systemic blood vessel. An unusual presentation of intralobar sequestration is localized emphysema without an associated opacity or mass (Ko et al. 2000).

Extralobar sequestration is usually located between the lower lobe and the diaphragm, more frequently at the left thoracic base, in 77% of cases (SAVIC et al. 1979). To a much lesser degree it has also been found in the mediastinum, pericardium (STOCKER and KAGAN-HALLET 1979), diaphragm or retroperitoneum (BAKER et al. 1982). Extralobar sequestration can connect with the digestive tract. Vascular supply occurs through a systemic artery and venous drainage through the azygos or portal system (REES 1981). Extralobar sequestration is associated with other congenital malformations in 65% of cases (SAVIC et al. 1979), and these are much more frequent and severe than those associated with the intralobar form. Extralobar sequestration is usually detected fortuitously and can also be associated with pleural effusion. It may be seen as a homogeneous mass or a small bump on the posterior hemidiaphragm that may be subtle and occasionally inapparent on the chest radiograph.

Ultrasound, CT and MRI are useful in the study of sequestrations, since they enable characterization of the lesion and identification of the anomalous arterial blood supply (Fig. 5.8). CT not only recapitulates the radiographic findings but also shows the complexity of the sequestration. Intralobar sequestration typically manifests as a homogeneous or inhomogeneous solid mass, with or without definable cystic changes. It can also appear as an aggregate of multiple small cystic lesions with air or fluid content (Fig. 5.9), a well-defined cystic mass, or a large cavitary lesion with air–fluid level. The lesion may enhance with contrast material (FRAZIER et al. 1997; ROSADO-DE-CHRISTENSON et al. 1993). An appearance simulating emphysema, possibly resulting from collateral ventilation and air-trapping, can sometimes be seen in sequestration. Expiratory CT scans are helpful for delineating the extent of the malformation (Fig. 5.10) (STERN et al. 2000; LUCAYA et al. 2000). Extralobar sequestration is seen on chest CT as a homogeneous, well-delimited mass, sometimes with internal cystic areas (ROSADO-DE-CHRISTENSON et al. 1993).

MR imaging is well suited for the diagnosis of bronchopulmonary sequestration (NAIDICH et al. 1988) This anomaly is seen as a well-defined, irregular or branch-like mass. MR can also reveal the presence of cystic areas, as well as the variable solid, fluid, hemorrhagic and mucus-containing compo-

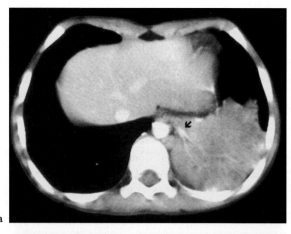

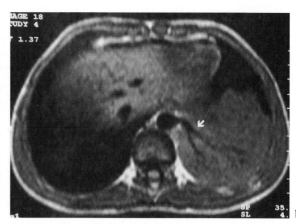

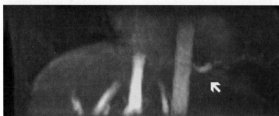

Fig. 5.8a–c. Intralobar pulmonary sequestration of the left lower lobe in a 2-year-old boy. **a** Contrast-enhanced chest CT shows the sequestration and a systemic branching vessel originating from the aorta (*arrow*). **b** Axial SE T1-weighted and **c** coronal 2D TOF MIP reconstruction images demonstrate a branching feeding vessel originating from the descending aorta and supplying the pulmonary sequestration (*arrows*)

nents. However, MR imaging cannot delineate focal thin-walled cysts or the emphysematous changes of sequestration as clearly as CT. The size, origin and course of the aberrant systemic artery and the venous drainage can be demonstrated by MR imaging. Two-dimensional time-of-flight MR angiography can reveal the aberrant artery, but this method is limited by low spatial resolution and turbulent flow. According to some reports and in our experience, breath-hold (if possible) or non breath-hold three-dimensional contrast-enhanced MR angiography offer excellent display of the aberrant vessel without flow artifacts (Ko et al. 2000).

As helical CT provides better evaluation of lung parenchyma, some authors consider it to be the technique of choice to study children with bronchopulmonary sequestration. In our experience of five cases of sequestration studied by helical CT and MRI, the feeding vessel was identified by both techniques, but in one case the origin and course of the aberrant vessel was better illustrated by MR. To our knowledge no study has objectively compared the various imaging techniques for depiction and definition of pulmonary sequestrations (FRUSH and DONELLY 1997).

Bronchopulmonary sequestration can decrease and even spontaneously disappear; therefore some authors recommend nonsurgical management in asymptomatic patients (see Fig. 5.7) (GARCIA-PEÑA et al. 1998).

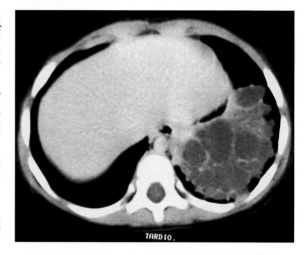

Fig. 5.9. Intralobar pulmonary sequestration in a 2-year-old boy. CT scan shows a mass with multiple fluid-filled cysts in the left lower lobe

5.2.4
Isolated Systemic Supply to Normal Lung

Isolated systemic supply to normal lung is a variant of pulmonary sequestration. This malformation corresponds to type I of Pryce's classification (PRYCE et al. 1947). The artery is typically large and supplies

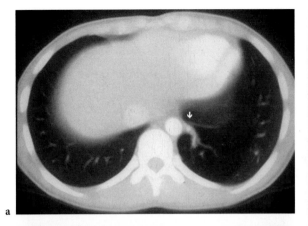

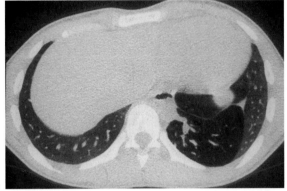

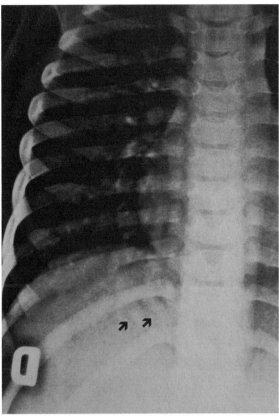

Fig. 5.10a,b. Intralobar pulmonary sequestration in left lower lobe in a 15-year-old boy. **a** Enhanced CT scan shows hyperlucency in left lower lobe. A systemic vessel (*arrow*) originating from the aorta and feeding the sequestration is well defined. **b** In an expiratory high-resolution CT scan at same level as (**a**), air-trapping can be seen within the sequestered lung. (Reprinted with permission)

Fig. 5.11. Isolated systemic supply to normal lung in a 14-year-old boy. Chest radiograph shows tubular images produced by anomalous vessels in the right lower lobe in an otherwise normal lung (*arrows*). Angiography (not shown) demonstrated two systemic arteries arising from the aorta. (Reprinted with permission)

the normal lung connected to the bronchial tree; the lung bases are affected more often (MÄKINEN et al. 1981). Patients are usually asymptomatic, although there may be a continuous murmur on the thoracic wall or heart failure secondary to left-to-left shunt. Associated hemoptysis occurs occasionally.

Chest radiographs show increased opacity due to the systemic artery. Sometimes well-defined tubular or rounded images produced by the anomalous vessels can be recognized (Fig. 5.11). The pulmonary parenchyma does not present any other changes, unless there is associated hemorrhage. Definitive diagnosis can be established with CT identification of a systemic artery originating in the thoracic or abdominal aorta and absence of pathology of the underlying lung (MATA et al. 1991).

5.3
Dysmorphic Lung

Dysmorphic lung (DL) is characterized by arrested development of either a whole lung (lung agenesis–hypoplasia complex) or a lobe (lobar agenesis–aplasia complex). Absence of a lobe may be associated with other abnormalities, some of them common and others highly unusual. Dysmorphic lung can be recognized on chest radiographs when we are aware of its existence and it is sometimes possible to reach a diagnosis based solely on plain film evidence. In doubtful cases it is advisable to use CT (MATA et al. 1990; WOODRING et al. 1994), or MRI (BAXTER et al. 1990) to confirm the diagnosis.

5.3.1
Lung Agenesis-Hypoplasia Complex

Arrested development of a whole lung (lung agenesis–hypoplasia complex) is uncommon and occurs equally often in either hemithorax. Although the terms agenesis (absence of bronchus and lung), aplasia (absence of lung with bronchus present), and hypoplasia (bronchus and rudimentary lung present) describe different anomalies (BOYDEN 1955), we group all three under the term "agenesis–hypoplasia complex" because all have a similar radiologic appearance on the chest radiograph. In pediatric patients the prognosis for right-sided agenesis is worse than for left-sided lesions, due to a greater shift of the heart and mediastinum, resulting in a greater distortion of the airway and great vessels. Respiratory distress and recurrent infections are common in children with right-lung agenesis. Airway compression by vascular structures, such as the aortic arch, pulmonary artery and patent ductus arteriosus, as well as intrinsic tracheobronchial anomalies and tracheobronchomalacia have been described in patients with right-lung agenesis (NEWMAN and GONDOR 1997) (Fig. 5.12). A similar appearance has been reported in patients with the so-called right postpneumectomy syndrome.

Lung agenesis–hypoplasia complex can be associated with malformations in other systems, including the skeletal, digestive, cardiac and urinary systems, and even in the contralateral lung (BRÜNNER and NISSEN 1963). The incidence of lung agenesis–hypoplasia with malformations in the skeleton or other organs is very high in some series (OSBORNE et al. 1989). A common origin, such as insult to the neural crest in the embryo has been postulated to explain these phenomena, giving rise to the VACTERL syndrome of anomalies (KNOWLES et al. 1988).

Characteristically, lung agenesis–hypoplasia complex appears on the posteroanterior view as a diffuse opacity of one hemithorax with mediastinal shift, reminiscent of the appearance of whole lung atelectasis. Occasionally it presents an atypical appearance that is more difficult to recognize on plain film. The small hemithorax, aerated lung and apparent pleural thickening, simulate chronic pleural disease (CALENOFF and FRIEDERICI 1964). This appearance results from the marked herniation of the contralateral lung. Typical and atypical cases show the same radiological appearance on the lateral chest view: retrosternal hyperclarity with the heart and large mediastinal vessels displaced backwards (MATA and CÁCERES 1996).

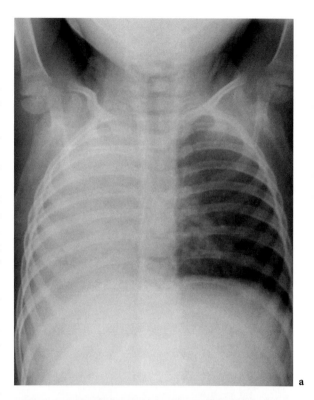

a

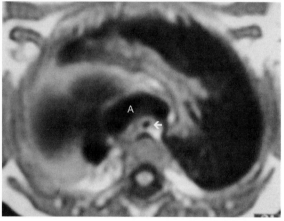

b

Fig. 5.12a,b. Right lung aplasia in a 2-year-old boy with respiratory symptoms. **a** Chest radiograph shows opaque right hemithorax with cardiomediastinal displacement and left lung hyperinflation. **b** Axial MR image at the level of the aortic arch demonstrates severe narrowing and posterior displacement of the distal trachea (*arrow*) by the crossing arch (*A*)

CT demonstrates the reasons for the two distinct radiological presentations. Pulmonary herniation takes place behind the sternum in both groups and accounts for the retrosternal hyperclarity. Mediastinal rotation explains the posterior displacement of the heart and mediastinum. If the herniation of the contralateral lung is not severe, the plain film shows the typical appearance of a small opaque hemithorax. In atypical cases, the extensive herniation of the contralateral lung crosses the midline to penetrate deep into the malformed hemithorax, giving the appearance of aerated lung on plain films. The pseudo-thickening of the pleura is produced by accumulation of subpleural fatty tissue, filling the space left by the absent or underdeveloped lung (MATA et al. 1990). Lung agenesis, aplasia and hypoplasia can be differentiated with use of CT, although the distinction is of little clinical significance. CT reveals the presence or absence of bronchi and pulmonary tissue, and allows measurement of the ipsilateral pulmonary artery (MATA and CÁCERES 1996). Although lung agenesis–hypoplasia complex is said to go together with a small ipsilateral pulmonary artery, on CT or MRI studies a small number of patients show a near normal-sized pulmonary artery with substantial blood flow.

Absence (atresia or interruption) of the main right or left pulmonary artery (APA) is an isolated vascular malformation that goes together with small homolateral lung, but should not be considered a part of lung agenesis–hypoplasia complex. It usually occurs in association with cardiac anomalies; isolated APA is rare (KLEINMAN 1979). During childhood APA produces substantial bronchial and transpleural (intercostal arteries) collateral circulation. The enlarged bronchial and intercostal arteries that feed the lung sometimes produce hemoptysis. At radiologic study, APA is seen as a small lung with mediastinal shift and no identifiable pulmonary artery. Collateral systemic supply produces peripheral linear opacities and pleural thickening. CT and MRI show absence of the pulmonary artery and can identify the enlarged systemic arteries (Fig. 5.13).

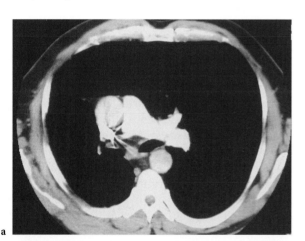

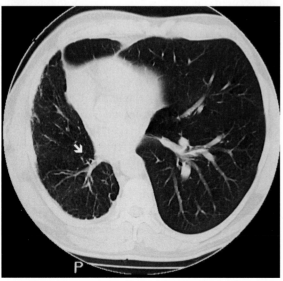

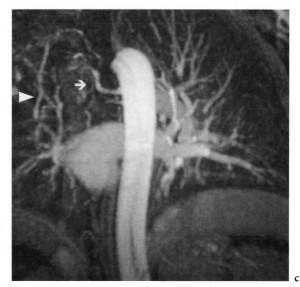

Fig. 5.13a–c. Absence of proximal right pulmonary artery. **a** Contrast-enhanced CT scan reveals absence of the right pulmonary artery. **b** Axial CT image at lung window shows volume loss on right side with shift of heart and mediastinum and a tiny pulmonary vein (*arrow*). **c** Breath-hold coronal 3D GRE MIP reconstruction after dynamic gadolinium injection shows the presence of intercostal vessels (*arrowhead*) and bronchial arteries (*arrow*) arising from the aorta supplying the right lung

a

b

c

5.3.2
Lobar Agenesis–Aplasia Complex

Lobar agenesis–aplasia complex is a group of pulmonary malformations affecting, almost exclusively, the right hemithorax. All of these malformations present pulmonary anomalies in the form of one or more absent or underdeveloped pulmonary lobe. Depending upon the associated venous malformation, we can look at this group as a continuum. At one extreme, the pulmonary malformation is isolated and the veins are normal (hypogenetic lung syndrome). The second step in the continuum includes the anomalous unilateral single pulmonary vein, which drains all the lung parenchyma into the left atrium (Hasuo et al. 1981). Next in line is the levo-atriocardinal vein; in this malformation there is an anomalous vein that drains the entire lung and connects the left atrium with a systemic vein (Edwards and DuShane 1950). Last in the continuum is an anomalous vein draining into the systemic venous system (venolobar syndrome). Accessory diaphragm (part of the right lung trapped by a membranomuscular duplication of the diaphragm) (Nazarian et al. 1971) and horseshoe lung (tissue from the malformed lung crossing the mediastinum to meet or fuse with the left lower lobe) (Dische et al. 1974) can accompany any of these malformations (Fig. 5.14). Systemic supply from the thoracic aorta is almost always present, although it is hardly ever seen on plain film or CT scans. Sometimes the systemic artery is thick, mimicking a scimitar vein (Partridge et al. 1988).

5.3.2.1
Hypogenetic Lung Syndrome

In hypogenetic lung syndrome there is agenesis or aplasia of one or two pulmonary lobes. Patients are usually asymptomatic. This entity almost always occurs in the right hemithorax; left hemithorax involvement is exceptional.

The chest radiograph shows a small right hemithorax with mediastinal shift to the right and haziness of the right cardiac border. In some cases, the right hilum is hidden by mediastinal rotation and cannot be seen, and in others the shape of the hilum is reminiscent of the left hilum. In most cases, lateral chest films show a retrosternal band caused by the interface between the shifted mediastinum and the anterior border of the underdeveloped lung (Ang and Proto 1984).

CT provides a wealth of information (Godwin and Tarver 1986; Mata and Cáceres 1996) by demonstrating the size of the pulmonary artery, the branching of the bronchi, and accompanying anomalies of the diaphragm (diaphragmatic hernias). If underdevelopment is very pronounced, one can observe extrapleural fat deposits along the thoracic wall simulating pleural thickening similar to, though not as striking as, those seen in the lung agenesis-hypoplasia complex (Mata et al. 1990). The right upper lobe is the most often affected. This gives a bronchial pattern of the right lung similar to that observed in the left lung in normal conditions (hypoarterial bronchus) (Fig. 5.15). CT demonstrates the pulmonary veins draining into their normal location, ruling out venous anomalies.

5.3.2.2
Lobar Agenesis–Aplasia with Anomalous Unilateral Single Pulmonary Vein

The second step in the continuum is a symptom-free malformation, first described by Benfield et al. in 1971. It has received several names since its description: pulmonary varix, meandering right pulmonary vein or scimitar sign with normal pulmonary venous drainage. In our experience, in most cases this malformation consists of a hypogenetic lung with a single anomalous vein draining the entire lung parenchyma into the left atrium. The vein follows an unusual pathway before it meets the left atrium.

In the chest radiograph anomalous unilateral single pulmonary vein usually has the same appearance as hypogenetic lung syndrome, plus a tubular and serpiginous shadow due to the anomalous vein. In rare cases the anomalous vein mimics a scimitar vein (Herer et al. 1988). CT and MRI provide the right diagnosis, showing a serpiginous shadow running through the lung and ending in the left atrium (Mata and Cáceres 1996) (Fig. 5.16). In some cases of anomalous unilateral single pulmonary vein, the vein drains into an extracardiac chamber located behind the left atrium (cor triatriatum).

Exceptionally we can see atypical cases with anomalous pulmonary veins affecting both lungs. This has been described as idiopathic prominence of pulmonary veins or "meandering pulmonary veins" (Kriss et al. 1995; Mata et al. 2000). The veins of both lungs follow an unusual pathway and drain into the left atrium (see Chap. 3, Fig. 3.5). Meandering pulmonary veins is occasionally associated with hypogenetic lung.

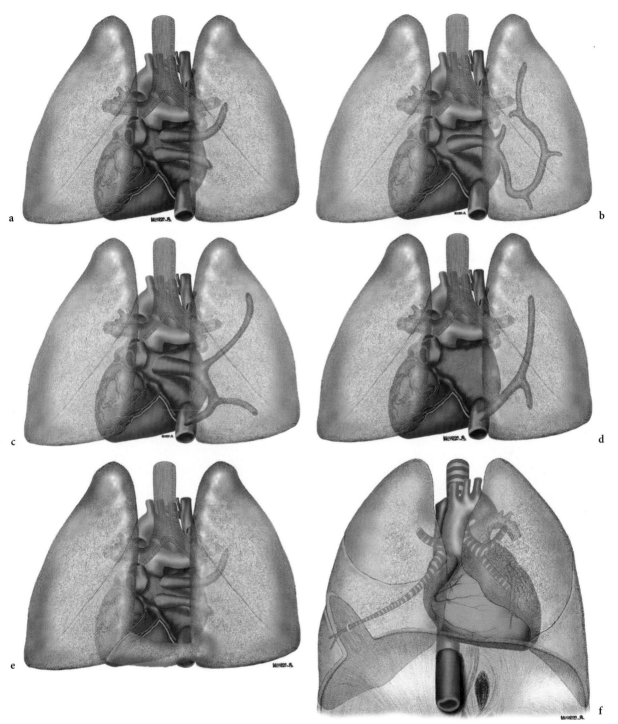

Fig. 5.14a–f. The term lobar agenesis–aplasia comprises a complex group of pulmonary malformations with one or more absent or underdeveloped pulmonary lobes. Depending on the associated venous malformation, this group can be viewed as a continuum. At one extreme, the pulmonary malformation is isolated, and the veins are normal and drain into the left atrium (**a**). The second step of the continuum includes the anomalous unilateral single pulmonary vein, which drains the entire lung parenchyma into the left atrium (**b**). Next in line is the levo-atriocardinal vein, in which there is an anomalous vein that drains the entire lung and connects the left atrium with a systemic vein (inferior vena cava in the drawing) (**c**). Last in the continuum is an anomalous vein draining into the systemic venous system (venolobar syndrome) (**d**). Horseshoe lung (tissue from the malformed lung crossing the mediastinum to meet or fuse with the left lower lobe) (**e**) and accessory diaphragm (part of the right lung trapped by a membranomuscular duplication of the diaphragm) (**f**) can accompany any of these malformations

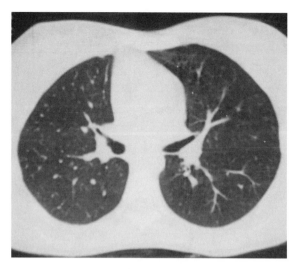

Fig. 5.15. Hypogenetic lung syndrome. CT scan shows left bronchial pattern in both lungs. The right lung is smaller than the left lung. (Reprinted with permission)

5.3.2.3
Lobar Agenesis-Aplasia with Levo-atriocardinal Vein

Levo-atriocardinal vein is defined as an anomalous vein that connects the left atrium and one vein of the systemic venous system. The systemic venous system derives from the embryological system known as cardinal veins. The malformation consists of a hypogenetic lung with the anomalous vein connecting the left atrium and one of the main systemic veins. Levo-atriocardinal vein would be the mid-point in the continuum between anomalous unilateral single pulmonary vein and venolobar syndrome. It is a very uncommon malformation.

On chest radiography the levo-atriocardinal vein looks very similar to the anomalous unilateral single pulmonary vein. CT demonstrates the usual findings of hypogenetic lung syndrome and the vein joining

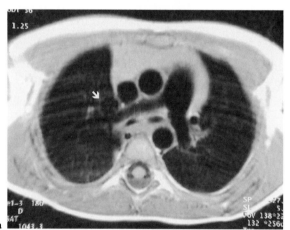

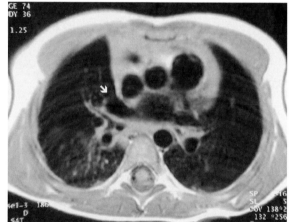

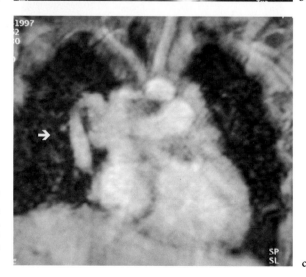

Fig. 5.16a–c. Anomalous right unilateral single pulmonary vein. Axial SE T1-weighted images at two different levels (**a**, **b**) reveal an enlarged and serpiginous right pulmonary vein (*arrows*) draining at the left atrium. **c** Coronal MR GRE 2D demonstrates the huge and tortuous single right pulmonary vein (*arrow*)

the left atrium and a systemic vein. The anomalous vein drains all the pulmonary veins, and MRI shows the pathway of the vein as well as the points where it meets with the systemic vein and the left atrium (Fig. 5.17) (Mata et al. 2000). MRI can demonstrate that there is no gradient between the left atrium and the systemic vein.

5.3.2.4
Congenital Venolobar Syndrome

In congenital venolobar syndrome (CVS), also known as scimitar syndrome, partial anomalous venous return (PAVR) is associated with hypogenetic lung syndrome. This malformation is one of the extremes of the dysmorphic lung continuum. Most patients are asymptomatic. The left–right shunt produced by the anomalous drainage is usually small and has no clinical repercussions, though on rare occasions it can lead to pulmonary hypertension (Haworth et al. 1983). Associated cardiac malformations may cause symptoms in pediatric patients (Canter et al. 1986). CVS occurs almost exclusively in the right hemithorax.

Plain film findings are similar to those of hypogenetic lung. The differential finding is the anomalous vein. The vessel is seen as a widening tubular shadow that extends toward the base of the lung, originating the term scimitar syndrome. The anomalous vein usually drains into the inferior vena cava or the right atrium. The fact there may be more than one vein or that a single vein may be hidden behind the displaced heart, accounts for the fact that the PAVR is not seen on plain film in half of the cases.

CT allows visualization of the anomalous vein and where it drains (Mata et al. 1990; Woodring et al. 1994) (Fig. 5.18), and the absence of inferior pulmonary vein. PAVR is associated with an accessory pulmonary fissure that is visible on CT study (Godwin and Tarver 1986). The anomalous vein can be seen with MRI (Baxter et al. 1990), and in some cases the entire course of the vessel can be followed in a single plane. In our experience, MRI is less useful than CT for this malformation, as it cannot show the bronchial anomaly.

5.3.2.5
Horseshoe Lung

Horseshoe lung is associated with hypogenetic lung syndrome and occurs when a small quantity of right pulmonary tissue arising from the lower lobe crosses

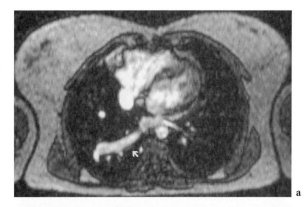

a

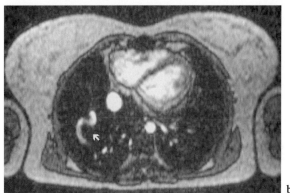

b

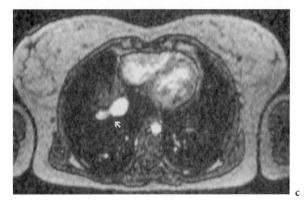

c

Fig. 5.17a–c. Levo-atriocardinal vein in the right lung. Axial MR GRE 2D images at three different levels (**a–c**) show the tortuous vein that goes from the left atrium to the inferior vena cava (*arrows*)

the midline and joins the left lower lung. The right and left lower lobes may fuse, or be separated by a fissure. The isthmus of pulmonary tissue crosses the mediastinum behind the pericardium, in front of the aorta and the esophagus and it is supplied by the right lower lobe vessels and bronchus (Frank et al. 1986; Freedom et al. 1986).

The hest radiograph shows hypogenetic lung syndrome or congenital venolobar syndrome together

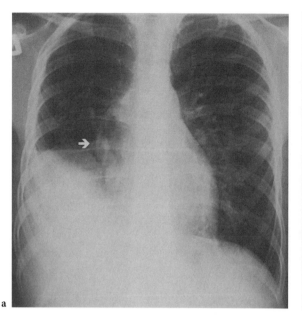

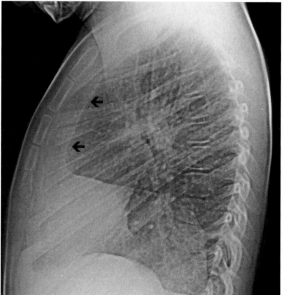

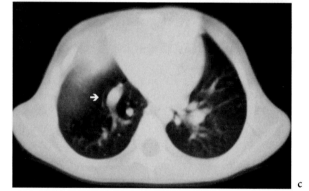

Fig. 5.18a–c. Venolobar syndrome. a Chest plain film shows a tubular image in the right pulmonary base (*arrow*) and an elevation of right diaphragm secondary to diaphragmatic eventration; the right lung is smaller than the left lung. The lateral view (b) shows a retrosternal band (*arrows*). c CT slice reveals the scimitar vein (*arrow*) draining to the inferior vena cava

with an anomalous fissure in the base of the left lung. This finding suggests the correct diagnosis on the PA chest film (FRANK et al. 1986). Sometimes the anomalous fissure can be seen as a thick opacity due to internal fat. CT shows the typical findings of hypogenetic lung, with or without abnormal veins, plus two additional findings: mediastinal discontinuity behind the heart, with the vessels of the right lower lobe crossing the midline and, when present, an anomalous fissure located at the base of the left lung (BEITZKE et al. 1982).

5.3.2.6
Accessory Diaphragm

Accessory diaphragm, also known as diaphragmatic duplication, is a rare congenital anomaly associated with the lobar agenesis–aplasia complex. It does not occur as an isolated malformation. Accessory diaphragm was first described by DRAKE et al. in 1950. These authors postulated that the anomaly is produced in the initial stages of embryonic development when the septum transversum, which gives rise to the diaphragm, is in a very high position. If for some reason the descent of the septum transversum is arrested, part of the primitive lung can be trapped by it. The septum transversum would remain anchored to the posterior wall, creating an additional diaphragmatic leaf.

Accessory diaphragm is a thin fibromuscular membrane fused anteriorly with the diaphragm and coursing posterosuperiorly to join the posterior chest wall. It produces two compartments in the right hemithorax, trapping part of the lung parenchyma (WILLE et al. 1975). The vessels and bronchi that supply the trapped lung pass through a central hole in the accessory diaphragm.

The accessory diaphragm can have two different appearances in the chest radiograph. When the central hiatus is very narrow, the trapped lung is not aerated and appears as a mass. When the trapped lung is aerated, the accessory diaphragm appears in plain film as a thin oblique line in either the posteroanterior or lateral chest view. In some patients a haziness is visible where the duplicated diaphragm joins the normal one.

When the lung is aerated, CT scans show the accessory diaphragm as a fissure-like line with a hole in the center (WOODRING et al. 1994) (Fig. 5.19). Depending upon the size of the central hole, the CT appearance varies. When the hole is large, it may be difficult to identify the accessory diaphragm. When the hole is small, the trapped lung may be opaque or hyperlucent, due to air-trapping. Vessels and bronchi are crowded together when they go through the central hiatus.

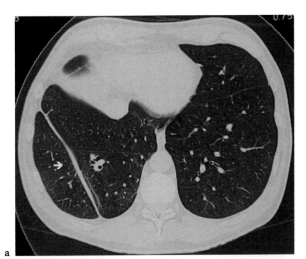

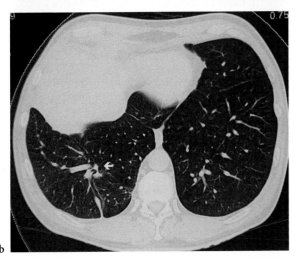

Fig. 5.19a,b. Accessory diaphragm. **a** The accessory diaphragm can be seen by CT as a line, simulating a fissure (*arrow*). **b** The vessels and bronchus are crowded together as they go through the central hole (*arrow*)

References

Ang JGP, Proto A (1984) CT demonstration of congenital pulmonary venolobar syndrome. J Comput Assist Tomogr 8:753–757

Baker EL, Gore RM, Moss AA (1982) Retroperitoneal pulmonary sequestration: computed tomographic findings. Am J Roentgenol 138:956–957

Baker EM (1989) Intrathoracic duplication cysts: a review of 17 patients. J Med Imag 3:127–134

Bankoff MS, Daly BDT; Johnson HA, Carter BL (1985) Bronchogenic cyst causing superior vena cava obstruction: CT appearance. J Comput Assist Tomogr 9:951–952

Baxter R, McFadden PM, Gradman M, Wright A (1990) Scimitar syndrome: cine magnetic resonance imaging demonstration of anomalous pulmonary venous drainage. Ann Thorac Surg 50:121–123

Beitzke VA, Gypser G, Sager WD (1982) Scimitarsyndrom mit Hufeisenlunge. ROFO 136:265–269

Benfield JR, Gots RE, Mills D (1971) Anomalous single left pulmonary vein mimicking a parenchymal nodule. Chest 59:101–102

Boyden EA (1955) Developmental anomalies of the lung. Am J Surg 89:79–89

Braffman B, Keller R, Stein Gendal E, Finkel SI (1988) Subdiaphragmatic bronchogenic cyst with gastric communication. Gastrointest Radiol 13:309–311

Brünner S, Nissen E (1963) Agenesis of the lung. Am Rev Respir Dis 78:103–106

Cachia R, Sobonya RE (1981) Congenital cystic adenomatoid malformation of the lung with bronchial atresia. Hum Pathol 12:947–950

Calenoff L, Friederici HH (1964) Unilateral pulmonary hypoplasia in an adult. Am J Roentgenol 91:265–272

Canter CE, Martin TC, Spray TL, Weldon CS, Strauss AW (1986) Scimitar syndrome in childhood. Am J Cardiol 58:652–654

Ch'in KY, Tang My (1949) Congenital adenomatoid malformation of one lobe of the lung with general anasarca. Arch Pathol 48:221–229

Dische MR, Teixeira ML, Winchester PA, Engle MA (1974) Horseshoe lung associated with a variant of the "scimitar" syndrome. Br Heart J 36:617–620

Drake EH, Portland ME, Lynch JP (1950) Bronchiectasis associated with anomaly of the right pulmonary vein and right diaphragm. J Thorac Surg 19:433

DuMontier C, Graviss ER, Silberstein MJ, McAlister WH (1985) Bronchogenic cysts in children. Clin Radiol 36:431–436

Edwards JE, DuShane JW (1950) Thoracic venous anomalies. Arch Pathol 49:517

Felson B (1979) Mucoid impaction (inspissated secretions) in segmental bronchial obstruction. Radiology 133:9–16

Finck S, Milne ENC (1988) A case report of segmental atresia: Radiologic evaluation including computed tomography and magnetic resonance imaging. J Thorac Imag 3:53–57

Fitch SJ, Tonkin ILD, Tonkin AK (1986) Imaging of foregut duplication cysts. Radiographics 6:189–201

Frank JL, Poole CA, Rosas G (1986) Horseshoe lung: clinical, pathologic, and radiologic features and a new plain film finding. Am J Roentgenol 146:217–226

Frazier AA, Rosado-de-Christenson M, Stocker JT, Templenton PA (1997) Intralobar sequestration: radiologic-pathologic correlation. Radiographics 17:725–745

Freedom RM, Burrows PE, Moes CAF (1986) "Horseshoe" lung: report of five new cases. Am J Roentgenol 146:211–215

Frush DP, Donelly LF (1997) Pulmonary sequestration spectrum: a new spin with helical CT. Am J Roentgenol 169:679–682

Garcia-Peña P, Lucaya J, Hendry GMA et al (1998) Spontaneous involution of pulmonary sequestration in children: a report of two cases and review of the literature. Pediatr Radiol 28:266–270

Gebauer PW, Mason CB (1959) Intralobar pulmonary sequestration associated with anomalous pulmonary vessels: a nonentity. Dis Chest 35:282–287

Godwin JD, Tarver RD (1986) Scimitar syndrome: four new cases examined with CT. Radiology 159:15–20

Griscom NT (1993) Diseases of the trachea, bronchi, and smaller airways. Radiol Clin North Am 31605–615

Hasuo K, Numaguchi Y, Kishikawa T, Ikeda J, Matsuura K (1981) Anomalous unilateral single pulmonary vein mimicking pulmonary varices. Chest 79:602–604

Haworth SG, Sauer U, Bühlmeyer K (1983) Pulmonary hypertension in scimitar syndrome in infancy. Br Heart J 50:182–189

Heitzman ER (1984) The lung: radiologic-pathologic correlations. Mosby, St Louis

Herer B, Jaubert F, Delaisements C, Huchon G, Chretien J (1988) Scimitar sign with normal pulmonary venous drainage and anomalous inferior vena cava. Thorax 43:651–652

Holder PD, Langston C (1986) Intralobar pulmonary sequestration (a nonentity?). Pediatr Pulmonol 2:147–153

Hruban RH, Shumway SJ, Orel SB, Dumler JS, Baker RR, Hutchins M (1989) Congenital pulmonary foregut malformations. Intralobar and extralobar pulmonary sequestration communicating with the foregut. Am J Clin Pathol 91:403–408

Ikezoe J, Murayama S, Godwin JD, Done SL, Verschakelenm JA (1990) Bronchopulmonary sequestration: CT assessment. Radiology 176:375–379

Jederlinic PJ, Sicilian LS, Baigelman W, Gaensler EA (1986) Congenital bronchial atresia. Medicine 65:73–83

Kim WS, Lee KS, Kim IO et al (1997) Congenital cystic adenomatoid malformation of the lung. CT-pathologic correlation. Am J Roentgenol 168:47–53

Kimura A, Makuuchi M, Takayasu K, Sakamoto M, Hiroshashi S (1990) Ciliated hepatic foregut cyst with solid tumor appearance on CT. J Comput Assist Tomogr 14:1016–1018

Kleinman PK (1979) Pleural telangiectasia and absence or a pulmonary artery. Radiology 132:281–284

Knowles S, Thomas RM, Lindenbaum RH, Keeling JW, Winter RM (1988) Pulmonary agenesis as part of the VACTERL sequence. Arch Dis Child 63:723–726

Ko SF, Ng SH, Lee TZ et al (2000) Noninvasive imaging of bronchopulmonary sequestration. Am J Roentgenol 175:1005–1012

Kriss VM, Woodring JH, Cottrill CM (1995) "Meandering" pulmonary veins: report of a case in an asymptomatic 12-year-old girl. J Thorac Imaging 10:142–145

Kwak GL, Stork WI, Greenberg SD (1971) Partial defect of the pericardium associated with a bronchogenic cyst. Radiology 101:287–288

Laurin S, Hägertrand I (1999) Intralobar bronchopulmonary sequestration in the newborn – a congenital malformation. Pediatr Radiol 29:174–178

Lejeune C, Deschildre A, Thumerelle C et al (1999) Pneumothorax revealing cystic adenomatoid malformation of the lung in a 13 year old boy. Arch Pediatr 6:863–866

Lemire P, Trepanier A, Hebert G (1970) Bronchocele and blocked bronchiectasis. Am J Roentgenol 110:687–693

Lyon RD, McAdams HP (1993) Mediastinal bronchogenic cyst demonstration of a fluid-fluid level at MR imaging. Radiology 186:427–428

Lucaya J, García-Conesa JA, Bernadó L (1984) Pulmonary sequestration associated with unilateral pulmonary hypoplasia and massive pleural effusion. Pediatr Radiol 14:228–229

Lucaya J, García-Peña P, Herrera L et al (2000) Expiratory chest CT in children. Am J Roentgenol 174:235–241

Mäkinen EO, Merikanto J, Rikalinen H, Satokari K (1981) Intralobar pulmonary sequestration occurring without alteration of pulmonary parenchyma. Pediatr Radiol 10:237–240

Martin KW, Siegel MJ, Chesna E (1988) Spontaneous resolution of mediastinal cysts. Am J Roentgenol 150:1131–1132

Mata JM, Cáceres J (1996) The dysmorphic lung: imaging findings. Eur Radiol 6:403–414

Mata JM, Cáceres J, Lucaya J, García-Conesa JA (1990) CT of congenital malformations of the lung. Radiographics 10:651–674

Mata JM, Cáceres J, Lucaya X (1991) CT diagnosis of isolated systemic supply to the lung: a congenital broncho-pulmonary vascular malformation. Eur J Radiol 13:138–142

Mata JM, Cáceres J, Castañer E, Gallardo X, Andreu J (2000) The dysmorphic lung: imaging findings. Postgrad Radiol 20:3–15

MacGillivray TE, Harrison MR, Goldstein RB, Adzik SA (1993) Disappearing fetal lung lesions. J Pediatr Surg 28:1321–1325

McAdams HP, Kirejczyk WM, Rosado-de-Christenson ML, Matsumoto S (2000) Bronchogenic cyst: imaging features with clinical and histopathologic correlation. Radiology 217:441–446

Medelli J, Lattaignant JC, Bertoux JP, Goudot B, Remond A (1979) L'atrésie bronchique segmentarie. Poumon 35:53–58

Murphy JJ, Blair GK, Fraser GC et al (1992) Rabdomyosarcoma arising within congenital pulmonary cysts: report of three cases. J Pediatr Surg 27:1364–1367

Naidich DP, Rumancick, Ettenger NA et al (1988) Congenital anomalies of the lung in adults: MR diagnosis. Am J Roentgenol 151:13–19

Nakata H, Egashira K, Warnanake H (1993) MRI of bronchogenic cysts. J Comput Assist Tomogr 17:267–270

Nazarian M, Currarino G, Webb WR, Willis K, Kiphart RJ, Wilson HE (1971) Accessory diaphragm: report of a case with complete physiological evaluation and surgical correction. J Thorac Cardiovasc Surg 61:293

Newman B, Gondor M (1997) MR evaluation of right pulmonary agenesis and vascular airway compression in pediatric patients. Am J Roentgenol 168:55–58

Osborne J, Masel J, McCredie J (1989) A spectrum of skeletal anomalies associated with pulmonary agenesis: possible neural crest injuries. Pediatr Radiol 19:425–432

Partridge JB, Osborne JM, Slaughter RE (1988) Scimitar etcetera: the dysmorphic lung. Clin Radiol 39:11–19

Patcher MR, Lattes R (1963) Mediastinal cysts: a clinicopathologic study of twenty cases. Dis Chest 44:416–422

Pedersen ML, LeQuire MH, Spies JB, Ladd WA (1988) Computed tomography of intralobar bronchopulmonary sequestration supplied from the renal artery. J Comput Assist Tomogr 12:874–875

Pryce DM (1946) Lower accessory pulmonary artery with intralobar sequestration of lung, report of seven cases. J Pathol Bacteriol 58:457–467

Pryce DM, Holmes Sellors T, Blair LG (1947) Intralobar sequestration of lung associated with an abnormal pulmonary artery. Br J Surg 35:18–29

Pugatch RD, Gale ME (1983) Obscure pulmonary masses: bronchial impaction revealed by CT. Am J Roentgenol 141:909–914

Pulpeiro JR, López I, Sotelo T, Ruiz JC, García-Hidalgo E (1987) Congenital cystic adenomatoid malformation of the lung in a young adult. Br J Radiol 60:1128–1130

Reed JC, Sobonya RE (1975) RCP from the AFIP. Radiology 117:315–319

Rees S (1981) Arterial connections of the lung. Clin Radiol 32:1–15

Remy-Jardin M, Remy J, Ribet M, Gosselin B (1989) Bronchial atresia: diagnostic criteria and embryologic considerations. Diagn Interv Radiol 1:45–51

Rogers LE, Osmer JC (1964) Bronchogenic cyst. A review of 46 cases. Am J Roentgenol 91:273–283

Rosado-de-Christenson M, Stocker JT (1991) Adenomatoid malformation. Radiographics 11:865–886

Rosado-de-Christenson M, Frazier AA, Stocker JT, Templenton PA (1993) Extralobar sequestration: radiologic-pathologic correlation. Radiographics 13:425–441

Samuel M, Burge DM (1999) Management of antenatally diagnosed pulmonary sequestrations associated with congenital cystic adenomatoid malformation. Thorax 54:701–706

Savic B, Birtel FJ, Tholen W, Funke HD, Knoche R (1979) Lung sequestration: report of seven cases and review of 540 published cases. Thorax 34:96–101

Senac MO, Wood BP, Isaacs H, Weller M (1991) Pulmonary blastoma: a rare childhood malignancy. Radiology 179:743–746

Stern EJ, Webb WR, Warnock ML et al (2000) Bronchopulmonary sequestration: dynamic, ultrafast, high-resolution CT evidence of air trapping. Am J Roentgenol 74:235–241

Stocker JT, Kagan-Hallet K (1979) Extralobar pulmonary sequestration. Analysis of 15 cases. Am J Clin Pathol 72:917–925

Stocker JT, Madewell JE, Drake RM (1977) Congenital cystic adenomatoid malformation of the lung. Hum Pathol 8:155–171

Ueda K, Gruppo R, Unger F, Martin L, Bove K (1977) Rhabdomyosarcoma of the lung arising in congenital cystic adenomatoid malformation. Cancer 40:383–388

Ward S, Morcos SK (1999) Congenital bronchial atresia. Presentation of three cases and a pictorial review. Clin Radiol 54:144–148

West MS, Donaldson JS, Shkolnik A (1989) Pulmonary sequestration. Diagnosis by ultrasound. J Ultrasound Med 8:125–129

Wille L, Holthusem W, Willich E (1975) Accessory diaphragm: report of 6 cases and a review of the literature. Pediatr Radiol 4:14–20

Winters WD, Effmann EL, Nghiem HV et al (1997) Disappearing fetal lung masses :importance of postnatal imaging studies. Pediatr Radiol 27:535–539

Woodring JH, Howard TA, Kanga JF (1994) Congenital pulmonary venolobar syndrome revisited. Radiographics 14:349

Zumbro GL, Green DC, Brott W, Tresaure RL (1974) Pulmonary sequestration with spontaneous intrapleural hemorrhage. J Thorac Cardiovasc Surg 68:673–674

6 CT of Acute Pulmonary Infection/Trauma

LANE F. DONNELLY

6.1
Introduction

The chest radiograph is the primary initial imaging modality for acute lung disease. When considering means to image acute lung disease, chest radiography, rather than chest computed tomography (CT), comes to mind. Chest radiography is inexpensive, easy to obtain, rapidly processed, low in radiation dose, and available on a ubiquitous basis. However, there are a number of scenarios in which CT is playing an increasing role in evaluating acute lung disease. Because CT of the lung can be performed with tube currents as low as 40 mAs, high quality images can be obtained while minimizing radiation dose. Acute pulmonary processes can be related to infection, trauma, or infarction. Helical CT is playing an increasing role in the evaluation for pulmonary embolism and lung infarction in adults. However, because pulmonary embolism is uncommonly encountered in children and the helical CT techniques differ only slightly from adult protocols, pulmonary infarction will not be discussed. This chapter will review the roles of and findings seen with CT imaging of pulmonary infection and trauma.

LANE F. DONNELLY, M.D.
Department of Radiology, Children's Hospital Medical Center, 3333 Burnet Ave., Cincinnati, OH 45229-3039, USA

6.2
Technical Factors

There are number of technical factors requiring modification when performing CT of the pediatric chest. Considerations include adjustments to adapt to the relatively small size of children, attempts to decrease radiation dose, and the use of intravenous contrast.

In children, in contrast to adults, intravenous contrast is often administered when processes involving the mediastinum are evaluated by CT. In the majority of cases in which the lung is the primary area being evaluated, administration of intravenous contrast is unnecessary. One of the exceptions is evaluation for complications of pneumonia, such as empyema or cavitary necrosis. In these cases, intravenous contrast is an essential part of the CT examination (DONNELLY and KLOSTERMAN 1997b, 1998b).

Concerning minimizing radiation dose from helical CT, the most important parameters are tube current (mA) and pitch. In conventional radiography, the need to tailor tube current (mA) and kVp is visually obvious on the radiograph produced. The penalty for ignoring these details on CT is not apparent on the images produced. This has allowed routine use of unnecessarily high mA settings. In pediatric patients, the mA can be adjusted, or reduced, according the child's size (DONNELLY et al. 2001). It is unacceptable to use mA appropriate for an adult on a child. There have been several investigations that have suggested that mA can be significantly reduced from adult doses within the chest without loss of important diagnostic information (ROBINSON et al. 1986; AMBROSINO et al. 1994; KAMEL et al. 1994; FRUSH and DONNELLY 1998; ROGALLA et al. 1999). With all other technical factors (kVp, time, etc.) held constant, patient radiation dose is directly proportional to tube current (mA). A 50% reduction in mA results in a decrease in radiation dose by 50%. At our institution, we have adjusted CT protocols such that the chosen mA is based on patient weight (Table 6.1) (DONNELLY et al. 2001). This table was created for use on a single slice helical CT scanner (CT/i, General Electric, Milwaukee, WI). The chosen mA is significantly lower than those we have used in the past. By using a tube current of 40 mA in an infant, rather than an mA of 200 (typical mA used in an adult), the radiation dose is reduced by a factor of five.

Table 6.1. Suggested tube current (mA) by weight of pediatric patients undergoing single-detector helical computed tomography

| Weight | | Chest |
lb	kg	mA
10–19	4.5–8.9	40
20–39	9.0–17.9	50
40–59	18.0–26.9	60
60–79	27.0–35.9	70
80–99	36.0–45.0	80
100–150	45.1–69.0	100–120
150+	>70	>140

lb, pounds; *kg*, kilograms.

In addition to mA, the other parameter that can be adjusted to significantly decrease radiation dose in helical scanning is pitch. By doubling the pitch, the radiation dose is reduced by half (VADE et al. 1996; FRUSH and DONNELLY 1998). This is related to the time that the X-ray beam is required to scan the area. If the pitch is increased, the amount of time needed to cover the anatomic area of interest and resultant dose to the patient is decreased. One study showed that by increasing from a pitch of 1:1–1.5:1, the radiation dose is decreased by 33% without loss of diagnostic information (VADE et al. 1996). Our standard pitch for pediatric helical CT is 1.5:1 and we sometimes increase this to 1.7:1 or 2:1 for follow-up examinations or general surveys.

Pediatric helical CT dose can be further reduced by appropriately addressing several additional issues. Firstly, inappropriate referrals for CT can be eliminated. Work ups that can equally be served by an alternative examination with less or no radiation exposure, such as sonography or magnetic resonance imaging (MRI), can be appropriately triaged. Secondly, in most pediatric cases, precontrast images are unnecessary when intravenous contrast material is to be administered. Obtaining both pre- and post-contrast images doubled the radiation dose unnecessarily. If nonenhanced imaging is indicated, every effort should be made to limit the area of non-enhanced scanning.

One CT parameter that has a much less profound effect on dose as compared to mA or pitch is collimation. Small changes in collimation do not largely affect radiation dose (assuming that mA is not increased with smaller collimation to compensate for increased noise). We typically decrease collimation to 5 mm in young children because of their smaller size.

6.3
CT in the Evaluation of Immunocompetent Children with Pneumonia

Respiratory tract infection is the most common cause of illness in children and continues to be a significant cause of morbidity and mortality (CONDON 1991). The roles of imaging in the evaluation of immunocompetent children with community acquired pneumonia are multiple: confirmation or exclusion of pneumonia, characterization and prediction of infectious agents, exclusion of other causes of symptoms, evaluation when there is failure to resolve, and evaluation of related complications (DONNELLY 1999). CT is also used in the follow up for chronic complications of pneumonia, such as bronchiectasis. Radiography of the chest remains the primary imaging modality in the majority of these scenarios and CT plays a secondary role in most of these respects.

Concerning confirmation or exclusion of pneumonia, CT usually plays no role in making the diagnosis of pneumonia and consequently deciding on treatment and patient disposition. This is accomplished with chest radiography (LEVENTHAL 1982; ZUKIN et al. 1986; ALARIO et al. 1987; GROSSMAN and CAPLAN 1988; PETER 1988). Concerning characterization and prediction of infectious agents, the previously described patterns of radiographic and CT findings which suggest a specific infectious agent are rarely of clinical relevance in the previously healthy child who is imaged for suspected pneumonia. The more general issue in the evaluation of the child with suspected pneumonia is whether the infectious agent is likely bacteria or viral. The differentiation between viral and bacterial pneumonia is accomplished through a combination of clinical examination and radiography of the chest (CONTE et al. 1970; OSBORNE 1978; SWISCHUK and HAYDEN 1986; TURNER et al. 1987; BETTENAY et al. 1988; WILDIN et al. 1988; CONDON 1991). CT plays no role.

CT can sometimes play a role in the child who has pneumonia that is recurrent or fails to resolve. Unlike in adults, in whom post obstructive pneumonia secondary to bronchogenic carcinoma is a concern, follow-up radiography to ensure resolution of radiographic findings is not routinely necessary in an otherwise healthy child who has had pneumonia. There is a tendency to obtain follow-up radiographs both too early and too often (HEDLUND et al. 1997). Follow-up radiographs should be reserved for those children who have persistent or recurrent symptoms and those who have an underlying condition such as immunodeficiency. The radiographic findings of pneumonia can persist for 2–4 weeks, even when the patient is clinically recovering appropriately. When follow-up radiographs are indicated, ideally they should not be obtained until at least 2–3 weeks have passed (HEDLUND et al. 1997). Causes of failure of suspected pneumonia to resolve include infected developmental lesions, bronchial obstruction, gastroesophageal reflux and aspiration, and underlying systemic disorders. Developmental lung masses that may become infected and present as recurrent or persistent pneumonia include sequestration, bronchogenic cyst, and cystic adenomatoid malformation. CT may be helpful in confirming and characterizing the presence of these developmental masses. In cases of

sequestration, CT is capable of identifying the characteristic systemic arterial supply (FRUSH and DONNELLY 1997) (Fig. 6.1) and may demonstrate cystic structures in cases of bronchogenic cyst and cystic adenomatoid malformation (Fig. 6.2).

6.3.1
Complications of Pneumonia

The potential uses of CT in the evaluation of complications related to pneumonia can be divided into two clinical scenarios: primary evaluation of parapneumonic effusions and evaluation of the child who has persistent or progressive symptoms despite medical or surgical therapy.

6.3.1.1
Primary Evaluation of Parapneumonic Effusions

Bacterial pneumonia is often complicated by parapneumonic effusions in children. There are multiple

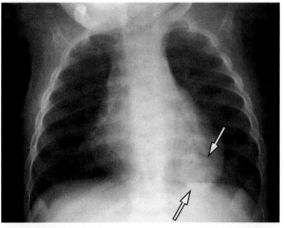

a

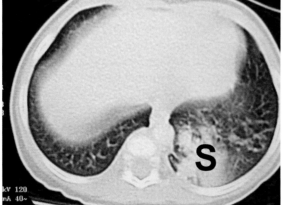

b

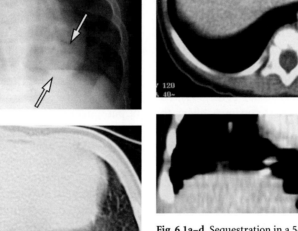

c

d

Fig. 6.1a–d. Sequestration in a 5-month-old girl with persistent left lower lobe opacity on chest radiography. **a** Chest radiograph shows left lower lobe opacity (*arrows*), which was persistent over multiple films. **b** Computed tomography (CT) shown at lung windows shows left lower lobe opacity (*S*). **c** CT shown at mediastinal windows shows anomalous arterial supply as vessel (*arrow*) arising from aorta (*arrowhead*) and coursing towards sequestration (*S*). **d** Reconstructed sagittal oblique CT shows anomalous vessel (*arrow*) arising from descending aorta

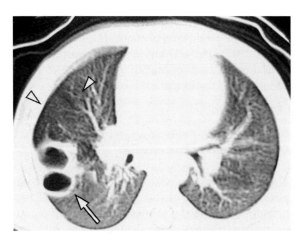

Fig. 6.2. Congenital cystic adenomatoid malformation in an infant. computed tomography (CT) shows air-filled multicystic mass (*arrow*). There is associated abnormal lucent lung (*arrowheads*) adjacent to the cystic mass

therapeutic options available in the management of parapneumonic effusions including antibiotic therapy alone, repeated thoracentesis, chest tube placement, urokinase therapy, and thoracoscopy with surgical debridement (LIGHT 1985; KERN and RODGERS 1993; ROSEN et al. 1993; BOUROS et al. 1994; LIGHT 1995; MOULTON et al. 1995; SILEN and WEBER 1995; STROVROFF et al. 1995; DONNELLY and KLOSTERMAN 1997a). There are great differences of opinion regarding the timing and aggressiveness of the management of parapneumonic effusions. Many investigators advocate antibiotics, drainage tube placement, and thrombolytic therapy (LIGHT 1985; ROSEN et al. 1993; BOUROS et al. 1994; LIGHT 1995; MOULTON et al. 1995; DONNELLY and KLOSTERMAN 1997a). Other investigators advocate early intervention with thoracoscopy and debridement (KERN and RODGERS 1993; SILEN and WEBER 1995; STROVROFF et al. 1995). The indications for imaging these effusions reflect the patterns of management at specific institutions. Traditionally, the aggressiveness of therapy has been based on categorizing parapneumonic effusions as empyema or transudative effusion (LIGHT 1985, 1995; ROSEN et al. 1993; BOUROS et al. 1994; DONNELLY and KLOSTERMAN 1997a). This differentiation has been based on aspiration and analysis of pleural fluid (LIGHT 1985). Traditional wisdom has advocated that parapneumonic effusions that meet the criteria for empyema are unlikely to resolve with antibiotic therapy alone and will often progress to a fibrinopurulent organized stage if left undrained (LIGHT 1985). Multiple attempts have been made to use imaging criteria to differentiate empyema from transudative

effusion, so that every child with a parapneumonic effusion does not have to undergo diagnostic thoracentesis.

CT was previously advocated in the differentiation between empyema and transudative parapneumonic effusion (BABER et al. 1980; STARK et al. 1983; WAITE et al. 1990; MULLER 1993). Initially, the CT findings of empyema were described in the context of differentiating empyema from peripheral pulmonary abscess (BABER et al. 1980; STARK et al. 1983). Later, CT findings of enhancement and thickening of the parietal and visceral pleura, thickening of the extrapleural subcostal tissues, and increased attenuation of the extrapleural subcostal fat (Fig. 6.3) were described as highly accurate in differentiating empyema from transudate (STARK et al. 1983; MULLER 1993) and were advocated as useful in making therapeutic decisions concerning parapneumonic effusions. Enhancement of the parietal pleura was advocated as the most sensitive finding of empyema and thickening of and increase from fat to soft tissue attenuation of the extrapleural space the most specific findings (WAITE et al. 1990; MULLER 1993). However, later studies have shown these findings to be inaccurate in determining which parapneumonic effusions meet the laboratory criteria for empyema in children (DONNELLY and KLOSTERMAN 1997a). No individual CT findings (pleural enhancement, pleural thickening, extrapleural subcostal tissue abnormality, or adjacent chest wall edema) nor a score based on a combination of CT findings accurately separated empyema from effusion (DONNELLY and KLOSTERMAN 1997a). These authors concluded that CT characteristics of parapneumonic effusions do not allow radiologists to accurately predict empyema and that the presence or absence of such CT findings should not influence therapeutic decisions concerning the management of parapneumonic effusions (DONNELLY and KLOSTERMAN 1997a).

A recent study (RAMNATH et al. 1998) advocated the use of sonography to aid in making therapeutic decisions for parapneumonic effusions. In this study, parapneumonic effusions were categorized as low-grade (anechoic fluid without internal heterogeneous echogenic structures) (Fig. 6.4) or high-grade (fibrinopurulent organization demonstrated by the presence of fronds, septations, or loculations). In children whose effusions were high-grade, hospital stays were reduced by nearly 50% when operative intervention was performed (RAMNATH et al. 1998). The length of hospital stay in children with low-grade effusions was not affected by operative intervention (RAM-

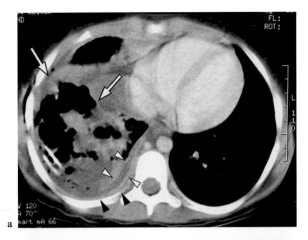

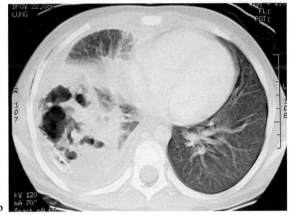

Fig. 6.3a,b. Cavitary necrosis and parapneumonic effusion demonstrating computed tomography (CT) findings classically attributed to empyema in a 7-year-old girl. **a** CT shows enhancement and thickening of the pleura (*white arrowheads*) and thickening and increased attenuation of the extrapleural subcostal space (*black arrowheads*). The extrapleural tissues are those between the ribs and the pleura. CT also shows findings of cavitary necrosis in the right lower lobe (*white arrows*) including decreased enhancement, loss of normal architecture, and multiple air- and fluid-filled cavities without enhancing walls. **b** CT shown at lung windows shows multiple air-filled cavities within the right lower lobe, consistent with cavitary necrosis

NATH et al. 1998). Therefore, sonography may play a more useful role than CT in the early evaluation of parapneumonic effusions.

6.3.1.2
Evaluation of Persistent or Progressive Symptoms

Underlying suppurative complications are often present when children exhibit persistent or progressive symptoms (fever, respiratory distress, sepsis) despite appropriate medical management of pneumonia (DONNELLY and KLOSTERMAN 1997b, 1998b). Potential suppurative complications include parapneumonic effusions, such as empyema, other inadequately drained effusions, or malpositioned chest tubes; parenchymal complications, such as cavitary necrosis or lung abscess; and purulent pericarditis (DONNELLY and KLOSTERMAN 1997b, 1998b; DONNELLY 1999). Although chest radiography is the primary imaging modality to detect such complications, a significant percentage of these complications will not be demonstrated by radiography (DONNELLY and KLOSTERMAN 1997b, 1998b; DONNELLY 1999). In the setting of a child with a non-contributory radiograph who has not responded appropriately to therapy, contrast-enhanced CT has been shown to be useful in detecting clinically significant suppurative complications (DONNELLY and KLOSTERMAN 1998b). In one study of children who were not responding to therapy for pneumonia and had a non-contributory chest radiograph, contrast-enhanced CT revealed the cause of the persistent sepsis in all cases (DONNELLY and KLOSTERMAN 1998b). CT has been shown to be accurate for the identification of lung abscess, the differentiation of lung abscess form empyema, the detection of parapneumonic effusions, the identification of bronchopleural fistulas, and the identification of malpositioned chest tubes or failure of lung re-expansion after chest-tube placement, both of which help to indicate when chest-tube drainage therapy will be unsuccessful (STARK et al. 1983; PUGATCH and SPIRN 1985; HIMELMAN and CALLEN 1986; WAITE et al. 1990; NAIDICH et al. 1991; STERN et al. 1996; DONNELLY and KLOSTERMAN 1997b, 1998b; DONNELLY 1999). CT can help differentiate whether the reason for persistent illness is pleural or related to lung

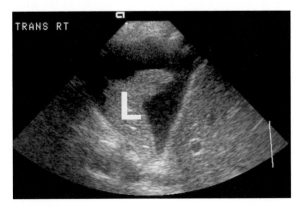

Fig. 6.4. Sonography of low-grade parapneumonic effusion in an infant girl. Longitudinal image shows anechoic effusion without fronds or septa. The right lung (*L*) is collapsed

parenchyma, directing therapy in the appropriate direction (DONNELLY and KLOSTERMAN 1998b).

6.3.1.3
Lung Parenchymal Complications

On contrast-enhanced CT, non-compromised lung parenchyma consolidated with pneumonia typically diffusely enhances (SILEN and WEBER 1995) (Fig. 6.5). This enhancement is not surprising given the degree of inflammation associated with pneumonia. Large areas of decreased or absent enhancement are indicative of underlying parenchymal ischemia or impending infarction (SILEN and WEBER 1995). In one study, the presence of decreased enhancement was associated with a significantly increased rate of admission to the intensive care unit, increased length of hospital stay, and increased incidence of development of cavitary necrosis (SILEN and WEBER 1995). Therefore, the detection of the presence of decreased lung enhancement in this setting yields important prognostic information.

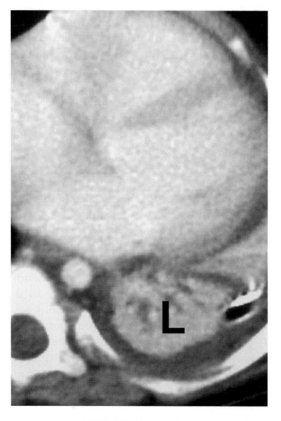

Fig. 6.5. Non-complicated lung parenchyma in a child with left lower lobe pneumonia. Contrast-enhanced computed tomography shows diffuse enhancement of consolidated left lower lobe (*L*)

Historically, there has been some confusion concerning lung enhancement on CT and its relation to pneumonia. Atelectasis demonstrates marked enhancement on contrast-enhanced CT (NAIDICH et al. 1983a,b; LEATHERMAN et al. 1984; KHOURY et al. 1985; DAVIES and TURNER 1990). Initially, it was reported that in adults, when lung was collapsed secondary to an obstructing bronchogenic carcinoma, the degree of enhancement could be used to accurately differentiate enhancing, collapsed lung from non-enhancing neoplasm (NAIDICH et al. 1983a,b). The accuracy of this finding, however, has been debated (LEATHERMAN et al. 1984; KHOURY et al. 1985). Most likely a permutation extending from these publications, a common unsubstantiated radiology teaching has been that opacification secondary to atelectasis enhances and that opacification due to pneumonia does not (DONNELLY and KLOSTERMAN 1997b). However, because uncomplicated pneumonias do enhance, enhancement is not a reliable way to differentiate atelectasis from pneumonia (DONNELLY and KLOSTERMAN 1997b).

Suppurative lung parenchymal complications represent a spectrum of abnormalities and include cavitary necrosis, lung abscess, pneumatocele, bronchopleural fistula, and pulmonary gangrene (DONNELLY and KLOSTERMAN 1997b). The name given to the suppurative process depends on several factors including the severity and distribution of the process, condition of the adjacent lung parenchyma, and temporal relationship with disease resolution (DONNELLY and KLOSTERMAN 1997b).

Cavitary necrosis represents a dominant area of necrosis of a consolidated lobe associated with a variable number of thin-walled cysts (NAIDICH et al. 1991; DONNELLY and KLOSTERMAN 1997b, 1998a). The mechanism of necrosis complicating pneumonia is related to thrombotic occlusion of alveolar capillaries associated with adjacent inflammation, resulting in ischemia and eventually necrosis of the lung parenchyma. Initially on CT, decreased enhancement may be the only finding. The characteristic CT findings of cavitary necrosis include loss of normal lung architecture, decreased parenchymal enhancement, loss of the lung–pleural margin, and multiple thin-walled cavities containing air or fluid and lacking an enhancing border (DONNELLY and KLOSTERMAN 1998a) (Fig. 6.3, 6.6).

Historically, cavitary necrosis has been described as uncommon and usually associated with staphylococcal pneumonias (DANNER et al. 1968; GUTMAN et al. 1973; KNIGHT et al. 1975; O'REILLY et al. 1978;

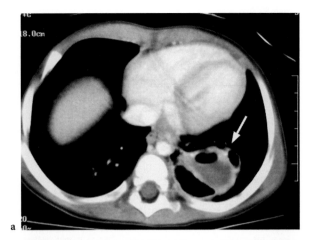

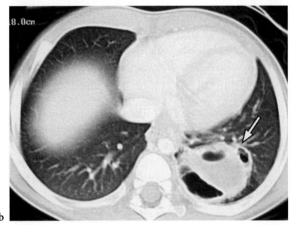

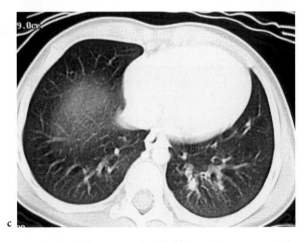

Fig. 6.6a–c. Cavitary necrosis of left lower lobe pneumonia in a 3-year-old girl. **a,b** Computed tomography (CT) shown at mediastinal (**a**) and lung (**b**) windows demonstrates multiple fluid- and air-filled cavities (*arrows*) within the left lower lobe. **c** CT obtained 2 months later after conservative management shows complete resolution of both the lung opacification, as well as of the cavities

YANGCO and DERESINSKI 1980; TORRES et al. 1984; ISAACS 1986; KEREM et al. 1994; DONNELLY and KLOSTERMAN 1998a). However, more recently, cavitary necrosis has become a not uncommon complication of pneumonia and is most commonly encountered in children with *Streptococcus pneumoniae* infection (YANGCO and DERESINSKI 1980; TORRES et al. 1984; ISAACS 1986; DONNELLY and KLOSTERMAN 1998a). Chest radiography is less sensitive than CT in detecting cavitary necrosis (DONNELLY and KLOSTERMAN 1998a). Only 41% of cases of cavitary necrosis identified on CT are seen on chest radiography and of those cases identified on chest radiography, over 90% are visualized later on chest radiography than CT (SILEN and WEBER 1995). When lung first becomes necrotic, the necrotic tissue liquefies and forms fluid-filled cavities (DONNELLY and KLOSTERMAN 1998a). When portions of this necrotic fluid are expectorated via bronchial communications, the cavities may fill with air. Fluid-filled cavities are isodense to adjacent opacified lung on chest radiography. This sequence of progression from fluid-filled to air-filled cavities contributes to the earlier detection and increased sensitivity of CT compared with radiography (DONNELLY and KLOSTERMAN 1998a). Most children with cavitary necrosis are severely ill (DONNELLY and KLOSTERMAN 1997b, 1998a). Such prognostic information helps in patient management decisions concerning intensity of management and, by outlining the patients expected course of illness, decreases unnecessary diagnostic tests and helps in counseling the patient's family. However, unlike in adults in whom the mortality rate of cavitary necrosis is high and early surgical removal of the affected lung has been advocated (DANNER et al. 1968; GUTMAN et al. 1973), the long term outcome of children with cavitary necrosis is favorable with medical management alone (Fig. 6.6) (DONNELLY and KLOSTERMAN 1998a). In children, the presence of cavitary necrosis should not be considered an indication for surgical lung resection unless the patient's condition continues to worsen with medical management. Amazingly, in children with cavitary necrosis, follow-up radiographs obtained at more than 40 days after the acute illness are most often normal, lacking any evidence of chronic scarring, persistent cavity formation, or other sequelae (DONNELLY and KLOSTERMAN 1998a). Therefore, in these patients, resolution should be the expected course and, similar to children with non-complicated pneumonia, long-term follow-up radiographs are not considered routinely necessary (DONNELLY and KLOSTERMAN 1998a).

Lung abscess represents a dominant focus of suppuration surrounded by well-formed fibrous wall (Naidich et al. 1991; Donnelly and Klosterman 1997b). On contrast-enhanced CT, lung abscesses appear as fluid- or air-filled cavities with definable, enhancing walls (Naidich et al. 1991; Donnelly and Klosterman 1997b, 1998b; Donnelly 1999) (Fig. 6.7). Typically there is no evidence of necrosis in the surrounding lung. Pneumatocele is a term given to thin-walled cysts seen at imaging (Fig. 6.8) and may represent a later or less severe stage of resolving or healing necrosis (Donnelly and Klosterman 1997b; Donnelly 1999). On CT, a thin-walled cyst

containing air with or without fluid is identified. The wall does not enhance. The surrounding lung may be opacified but does not demonstrate findings of necrosis. Bronchopleural fistula are identified on CT when a direct communication is visualized between the airspaces of the lung and the pleural space.

6.3.1.4
Pleural Complications

The cause of persistent sepsis in a child being treated for pneumonia may also be related to a pleural complication. This is most often the unrecognized cause of sepsis when previous intervention has been performed to treat a parapneumonic effusion. CT yields helpful information regarding the management of parapneumonic effusions such as depicting a loculated pleural collection not in communication with an indwelling chest tube (Fig. 6.9), poor chest tube placement, or failure of lung re-expansion (Himelman and Callen 1986; Danner et al. 1968; Gutman et al. 1973; Knight et al. 1975; O'Reilly et al. 1978; Baber et al. 1980; Yangco and Deresinski 1980; Naidich et al. 1983a,b; Stark et al. 1983; Leatherman et al. 1984; Torres et al. 1984; Khoury et al. 1985; Pugatch and Spirn 1985; Himelman and Callen 1986; Isaacs 1986; Davies and Turner 1990; Naidich et al. 1991; Muller 1993; Kerem et al. 1994; Stern et al. 1996; Donnelly and Klosterman 1998a; Ramnath et al. 1998). All of these findings suggest a need for a change

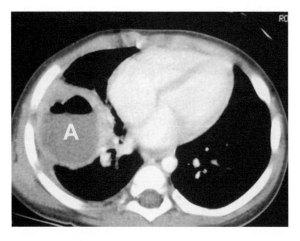

Fig. 6.7. Lung abscess in a 2-year-old child. Computed tomography shows well defined cavity (*A*) containing an air–fluid level. The surrounding lung shows no evidence of necrosis. There is adjacent pleural thickening

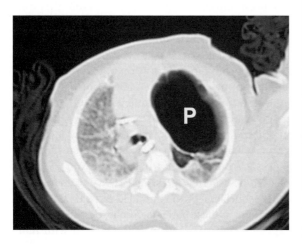

Fig. 6.8. Pneumatocele in an infant. Computed tomography shows a thin-walled cavity (*P*) in the left upper lobe. The adjacent lung is not opacified

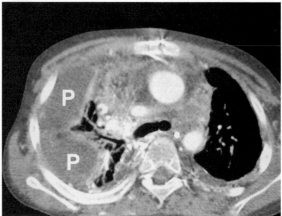

Fig. 6.9. Loculated pleural fluid following chest-tube drainage in a 6-year-old girl. Computed tomography shows bilobed, loculated pleural fluid collection (*P*) in the superior right pleural space. There is a chest tube (not shown) in the more inferior pleura. A second drainage catheter was then placed into the loculated collection under sonographic guidance

in drainage strategy. Drainage catheters may need to be repositioned or replaced with larger bore catheters and thoracoscopic debridement may need to be considered. Finally, on chest radiography, it is often difficult to determine how much of an opacity seen is due to pleural effusion and how much is due to consolidated lung, when both are present. Accurate determination of the amount of pleural fluid provided by CT also affects therapeutic decisions regarding drainage (DONNELLY and KLOSTERMAN 1998b).

6.3.1.5
Purulent Pericarditis

Although rare, purulent pericarditis is fatal if not rapidly diagnosed and treated. Prior to the advent of antibiotics, purulent pericarditis was a common complication of childhood pneumonia and one of the most frequent causes of death (DONNELLY et al. 1999). Although the classic presentation of purulent pericarditis is septicemia and enlarging cardiopericardial silhouette on chest radiograph, cardiac enlargement is often not present in children. In fact, children can progress to cardiac tamponade prior to enlargement of the pericardial silhouette being present on chest radiography (DONNELLY et al. 1999). With the increasing number of antimicrobial resistant bacteria, the incidence of purulent pericarditis may be rising. In one study of children who underwent CT to evaluate for complications of pneumonia, pericardial fluid was present in pericardial effusions in 23% (DONNELLY et al. 1999). Two cases had large effusions and clinically unrecognized cardiac tamponade (DONNELLY et al. 1999). Therefore, it is important to evaluate for pericardial effusion in children being imaged for complications of pneumonia.

6.3.2
Chronic Complications of Pneumonia

There are a number of potential complications from pneumonia that can cause chronic respiratory difficulties. These include parenchymal scarring, fibrothorax, bronchiectasis, and Swyer-James syndrome. Swyer-James syndrome is defined as the presence of a unilateral hyperlucent lung in association with decreased pulmonary vasculature. The lucent lung is typically enlarged and demonstrates air-trapping on fluoroscopy or expiratory CT. It is thought to represent an obliterative bronchiolitis that occurs secondary to viral infection, often with adenovirus.

Bronchiectasis is probably the most common chronic complication of childhood pneumonia. It is defined as dilatation of the bronchi (Fig. 6.10). On high resolution CT, the bronchus is considered dilated if it is larger than the associated companion pulmonary artery. Reversible bronchiectasis can occur during acute pneumonia. Chronic bronchiectasis most commonly occurs secondary to adenovirus or bacterial infection.

6.4
CT in the Evaluation of Immunocompromised Children with Suspected Pneumonia

The number of immunocompromised children continues to increase. Children can be immunocompromised for a variety of reasons including cancer therapy, bone marrow transplantation, solid organ transplantation, primary immunodeficiency, and AIDS. At most tertiary children's medical centers, the

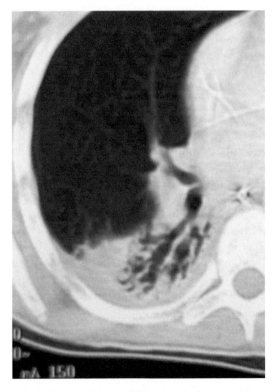

Fig. 6.10. Bronchiectasis following right lower lobe pneumonia in a 14-year-old girl. Computed tomography shows dilatation of the right lower lobe bronchi with chronically opacified adjacent lung

number of CT examinations of the chest performed in immunocompromised children far out number those performed in immunocompetent children. It is also important for those working in imaging departments at community hospitals to have an understanding of those processes as many of these patients receive much of their primary care in their home towns.

Acute pulmonary processes are a common cause of morbidity and mortality in immunocompromised children (Mori et al. 1991; Brown et al. 1994; Winer-Muram et al. 1994; McAdams et al. 1995; Marks et al. 1996; Worthy et al. 1997). Because of the fragile condition of these patients, prompt diagnosis and treatment of pulmonary infections is imperative. When a pulmonary process is suspected on the basis of imaging, invasive diagnostic procedures such as bronchoscopy may be performed or new therapies may be empirically started. In regards to confirmation or exclusion of pneumonia, as in immunocompetent patients, chest radiography is the primary imaging modality. However, because of the poor condition of many of these patients and risk associated with exposure to multiple persons, radiographic evaluation of these patients is often performed with a portable technique. These patients are also often not able to take deep breaths rendering low lung volume radiographic examinations. The negative predictive value of such radiographs is low in comparison to frontal and lateral radiographs obtained at full inspiration. Because of these factors, as well as the greater risk of progressive illness if infection is not promptly diagnosed, CT plays a greater role in the detection and exclusion of pulmonary infection. The detection of pulmonary abnormalities with CT is excellent (Mori et al. 1991). In an immunocompromised child with clinical findings that could be attributed to pneumonia and a non-contributory radiograph, we do not hesitate to perform CT. The amount of disease that is often present on CT but not detected on chest radiograph is continuously surprising. When detected, CT localizes high yield areas for diagnostic procedures such as bronchoscopy or needle aspiration.

In immunocompetent children, the primary characterization of pulmonary infections is determining whether the infectious agent is bacterial or viral. In immunocompromised hosts, the issue is more complex. The array of agents that can cause aggressive infections is great and includes fungal infections such as *Aspergillus* and *Candida*, viral infections such as cytomegalovirus infection, and *Pneumocystis carinii*

(Mori et al. 1991; Brown et al. 1994; Winer-Muram et al. 1994; McAdams et al. 1995; Marks et al. 1996). In addition, there are a variety of non-infectious pulmonary processes that can present with acute or subacute clinical findings mimicking pulmonary infection (Mori et al. 1991). These include alveolar hemorrhage, pulmonary edema, drug reaction, idiopathic pneumonia, lymphoid interstitial pneumonitis, bronchiolitis obliterans, bronchiolitis obliterans with organizing pneumonia, and chronic graft-vs-host disease (Mori et al. 1991; Brown et al. 1994; Winer-Muram et al. 1994; McAdams et al. 1995; Marks et al. 1996).

The CT findings of many of these entities are nonspecific, with overlap of the findings seen between different etiologies. However, the combination of certain CT findings, in conjunction with clinical findings, can be very suggestive of a specific diagnosis. The clinical issue that we most often encounter is whether there are CT findings which suggest the possibility of fungal infection. The hallmark CT finding which is associated with possible fungal infection is the presence of nodules (Mori et al. 1991; McAdams et al. 1995). These nodules are often clustered (Fig. 6.11) and can demonstrate any of the following associated findings: poorly defined margins, cavitation, or a surrounding halo of ground glass opacity (Mori et al. 1991; Brown et al. 1994; Winer-Muram et al. 1994; McAdams et al. 1995; Marks et al. 1996).

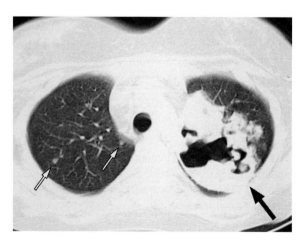

Fig. 6.11. Fungal pneumonia in a 17-year old recipient of both a liver and renal transplant. Computed tomography shows large cavitary mass (*black arrow*) within the left upper lobe. There are poorly defined nodules clustered adjacent to the cavity. In addition, there are several nodules within the right upper lobe (*arrows*)

Pathologically, the central nodular density on CT represents the actual fungal infection and the surrounding halo represents hemorrhagic infarction caused by thrombosis secondary to vascular invasion by the fungus (MORI et al. 1991). These findings are, however, non-specific and can be seen with non-fungal infections such as cytomegalovirus infection (Fig. 6.12) (MORI et al. 1991; BROWN et al. 1994; WINER-MURAM et al. 1994; McADAMS et al. 1995; KANG et al. 1996; MARKS et al. 1996).

6.5
CT in the Evaluation of Pulmonary Trauma

There are a number of causes of lung consolidation in children who have undergone traumatic injury. These include contusion, laceration, aspiration, atelectasis, and pre-existing lung opacification such as from pneumonia (EICHELBERGER et al. 1988; SIVIT et al. 1989a; DONNELLY and KLOSTERMAN 1997c). CT is uncommonly performed for the primary purpose of evaluating for pulmonary trauma. However, the inferior lung is often visualized when CT is performed to evaluate for traumatic injury to the contents of the abdomen and pelvis, and CT of the chest is sometimes performed to evaluate for suspected thoracic aortic injuries. When CT is being performed to evaluate for traumatic injury to either the abdominal contents or mediastinum, it is important to evaluate the lung for lung contusion or other trauma-related lung opacity.

Lung contusion is defined as hemorrhage and edema formation in the alveoli and interstitium secondary to blunt chest trauma, without accompanying parenchymal laceration (WILLIAMS and STEMBRIDGE 1964; KIRSH et al. 1972; SHACKLEFORD 1987; WAGNER et al. 1988; SIVIT et al. 1989a; MANSON et al. 1993; DONNELLY and KLOSTERMAN 1997c). The presence of lung contusion has been reported to be associated with an adverse effect on patient outcome (EICHELBERGER et al. 1988; SIVIT et al. 1989a). In one study, mortality was 1.3% for pediatric trauma victims without lung contusions and 10.8% for those with contusions (SIVIT et al. 1989a). Therefore, accurate identification of lung contusion and differentiation from other causes of lung opacification is helpful when planning management of pediatric trauma patients. Also, the incidence of lower thoracic trauma is not uncommon in battered children (SIVIT et al. 1989b). Accurate identification of lung opacification as contusion when child abuse is suspected may facilitate evidence in criminal proceedings and help in decisions regarding the removal of a child from a high risk environment.

On CT, lung contusions are characteristically non-segmental in distribution, not following segmental or lobar anatomic boundaries (SIVIT et al. 1989a; DONNELLY and KLOSTERMAN 1997c). Contusions are usually located posteriorly (85%), are crescentic (50%) or amorphous (45%) in shape, and are mixed confluent and nodular quality (70%) (DONNELLY and KLOSTERMAN 1997c) (Fig. 6.13). The lung contusions of children may also demonstrate a 1–2 mm region of uniformly non-opacified subpleural lung, separating the area of lung consolidation from the adjacent chest wall (DONNELLY and KLOSTERMAN 1997c) (Fig. 6.13). This finding is referred to as subpleural sparing and is seen with many lung contusions and is not seen with other causes of airspace opacification and is therefore helpful in identifying contusions (McADAMS et al. 1995). The larger the lung contusion, the less likely subpleural sparing is to be present (DONNELLY and KLOSTERMAN 1997c).

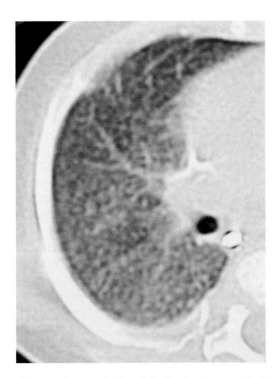

Fig. 6.12. Cytomegalovirus infection in a 3-year-old girl after bone marrow transplant. There are poorly defined nodules (*arrows*) throughout the right lung. The findings are non-specific and similar to those seen with many fungal infections

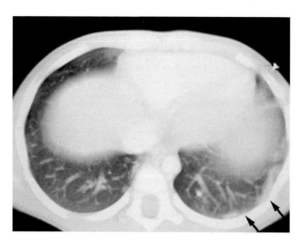

Fig. 6.13. Lung contusion in a 5-year-old boy after a high-speed collision. Computed tomography shows a crescent, peripheral opacity that is predominantly in the posterior left lower lung. The opacity crosses segmental borders and demonstrates subpleural sparing (*arrows*)

The CT appearance of lung contusion in children is related to both the plasticity of the anterior thorax seen in children and the rapid deceleration mechanism encountered in most motor vehicle accidents. In high speed collisions, rib fractures occur much more commonly in adults than in children (WILLIAMS and STEMBRIDGE 1964; KIRSH et al. 1972; EICHELBERGER and RANDOLPH 1981; SHACKLEFORD 1987; WAGNER et al. 1988; SIVIT et al. 1989b; MANSON et al. 1993). The decreased incidence in children is related to increased pliability of the anterior chest wall. This pliability of the anterior chest wall in combination with the contra-coup forces of rapid deceleration injury most likely compresses the relatively fixed posterior lung against the immediately adjacent, less compliant posterior ribs and vertebral column (WILLIAMS and STEMBRIDGE 1964; MANSON et al. 1993). The distribution of the disruptive forces along the least mobile regions of lung explains both the posterior location and crescentic shape of most contusions (DONNELLY and KLOSTERMAN 1997c). The diffuse distribution of force associated with blunt trauma also explains the non-segmental distribution of pulmonary contusions (MANSON et al. 1993).

The exact mechanism explaining the association of subpleural sparing and pulmonary contusion is speculative. Lung contusions are the result of alveolar capillary damage with extravasation of edema and hemorrhage into alveoli and interstitial spaces (WILLIAMS and STEMBRIDGE 1964). Anatomically, terminal arterial branches terminate prior to the subpleu-

ral region of lung. The resultant sparse vascularity of this region may protect the subpleural lung from hemorrhage. Also, when contra-coup forces compress the posterior lung against the chest wall and result in contusion, the subpleural lung may be compressed against the chest wall during the time of injury, "squeezing" the extravasated blood and edema into the more central lung and resulting in a spared zone of aerated subpleural lung (DONNELLY and KLOSTERMAN 1997c). Larger lung contusions are less likely to demonstrate both the characteristic crescentic shape and subpleural sparing than smaller contusions. This may be related to the tendency of larger areas of hemorrhage to extend into the subpleural space and more central lung, related to persistent bleeding after the moment of trauma (DONNELLY and KLOSTERMAN 1997c).

Chest radiography is a relatively insensitive diagnostic test for detecting lung contusions (WAGNER et al. 1988; SIVIT et al. 1989a; MANSON et al. 1993; DONNELLY and KLOSTERMAN 1997c). In one study, 69% of lung contusions were either underestimated (24%) or not identified (45%) by plain radiographs (DONNELLY and KLOSTERMAN 1997c).

Pulmonary laceration differs from contusion in that with laceration there is a frank tear within the lung parenchyma. The characteristic CT finding of pulmonary laceration is the presence of an air- or fluid-filled cavity (TOCINO and MILLER 1987; WAGNER et al. 1988; SIVIT et al. 1989a; MANSON et al. 1993; DONNELLY and KLOSTERMAN 1997c) (Fig. 6.14). The CT findings of atelectasis include triangular shape, segmental distribution, and obvious signs of volume loss (SIVIT et al. 1989a,b).

Traumatic rupture of the bronchi or trachea is rare and has been only sparsely reported in children (MAHBOUBI and O'HARA 1981). The diagnosis is usually questioned in the setting of a pneumothorax that does not resolve with tube placement or an area of persistent collapsed lung (HARVEY-SMITH et al. 1980; MAHBOUBI and O'HARA 1981; WEIR et al. 1988; WAN et al. 1997). The diagnosis is usually confirmed with bronchoscopy or primarily investigated surgically. Because of the low incidence of this traumatic entity and primary evaluation with bronchoscopy, the role of CT is not well defined. CT can demonstrate findings of bronchial rupture. Findings include a discontinuous bronchus in conjunction with pneumothorax or pneumomediastinum (HARVEY-SMITH et al. 1980; WEIR et al. 1988; WAN et al. 1997). Three-dimensional helical CT may be helpful in showing such a discontinuous bronchus.

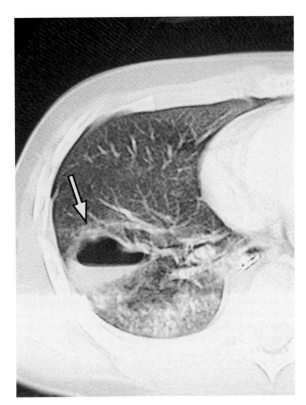

Fig. 6.14. Lung laceration in a 9-year-old boy after a high speed collision in a all terrain vehicle. Computed tomography shows right lower lobe posterior opacity. There is a large cavity (*arrow*) containing an air–fluid level

References

Alario AJ, McCarthy PL, Markowitz R et al (1987) Usefulness of chest radiographs in children with acute lower respiratory tract disease. J Pediatr 111(2):187–193

Ambrosino MM, Genieser NB, Roche KJ et al (1994) Feasibility of high-resolution, low-dose chest CT in evaluating the pediatric chest. Pediatr Radiol 24(1):6–10

Baber CE, Hedlund LW, Oddson TA et al (1980) Differentiating empyemas and peripheral pulmonary abscesses: the value of computed tomography. Radiology 135(3):755–758

Bettenay FA, de Campo JF, McCrossin DB et al (1988) Differentiating bacterial from viral pneumonias in children. Pediatr Radiol 18(6):453–454

Bouros D, Schiza S, Panagou P et al (1994) Role of streptokinase in the treatment of acute loculated parapneumonic pleural effusions and empyema. Thorax 49(9):852–855

Brown MJ, Miller RR, Muller NL et al (1994) Acute lung disease in the immunocompromised host: CT and pathologic examination findings. Radiology 190(1):247–254

Condon VR (1991) Pneumonia in children. J Thorac Imaging 6(3):31–44

Conte P, Heitzman ER, Markarian B et al (1970) Viral pneumonia. Roentgen pathological correlations. Radiology 95(2):267–272

Danner PK, McFarland DR, Felson B et al (1968) Massive pulmonary gangrene. Am J Roentgenol Radium Ther Nucl Med 103(3):548–554

Davies SG, Turner MJ (1990) Enhancement of collapsed lung: a potential pitfall in CT interpretation. Clin Radiol 42(3):192–194

Donnelly LF (1999) Maximizing the usefulness of imaging in children with community-acquired pneumonia. AJR Am J Roentgenol 172(2):505–512

Donnelly LF, Klosterman LA (1997a) CT appearance of parapneumonic effusions in children: findings are not specific for empyema. AJR Am J Roentgenol 169(1):179–182

Donnelly LF, Klosterman LA (1997b) Pneumonia in children: decreased parenchymal contrast enhancement – CT sign of intense illness and impending cavitary necrosis. Radiology 205(3):817–220

Donnelly LF, Klosterman LA (1997c) Subpleural sparing: a CT finding of lung contusion in children. Radiology 204(2):385–387

Donnelly LF, Klosterman LA (1998a) Cavitary necrosis complicating pneumonia in children: sequential findings on chest radiography. AJR Am J Roentgenol 171(1):253–256

Donnelly LF, Klosterman LA (1998b) The yield of CT of children who have complicated pneumonia and non-contributory chest radiography. AJR Am J Roentgenol 170(6):1627–1631

Donnelly LF, Kimball TR, Barr LL et al (1999) Purulent pericarditis presenting as acute abdomen in children: abdominal imaging findings. Clin Radiol 54(10):691–693

Donnelly LF, Emery KH, Brody AS et al (2001) Minimizing radiation dose for pediatric body application of single-detector helical CT: strategies at a large children's hospital. AJR Am J Roentgenol (2001)

Eichelberger MR, Randolph JG (1981) Thoracic trauma in children. Surg Clin North Am 61(5):1181–1197

Eichelberger MR, Mangubat EA, Sacco WJ et al (1988) Outcome analysis of blunt injury in children. J Trauma 28(8):1109–1117

Frush DP, Donnelly LF (1997) Pulmonary sequestration spectrum: a new spin with helical CT. AJR Am J Roentgenol 169(3):679–682

Frush DP, Donnelly LF (1998) State of the art: techical CT: techical considerations and body applications. Radiology 209:37–48

Grossman LK, Caplan SE (1988) Clinical, laboratory, and radiological information in the diagnosis of pneumonia in children. Ann Emerg Med 17(1):43–46

Gutman E, Pongdee O, Park YS et al (1973) Massive pulmonary gangrene. Radiology 107(2):293–294

Harvey-Smith W, Bush W, Northrop C et al (1980) Traumatic bronchial rupture. AJR Am J Roentgenol 134(6):1189–1193

Hedlund GL, Griscom NT, Cleveland RH et al (1997) Respiratory system. In: Kirks DR (ed) Practical pediatric imaging, vol 3. Little, Brown and Company, Bostonpp 619–821

Himelman RB, Callen PW (1986) The prognostic value of loculations in parapneumonic pleural effusions. Chest 90(6):852–856

Isaacs RD (1986) Necrotizing pneumonia in bacteraemic pneumococcal infection. Br J Dis Chest 80(3):295–296

Kamel IR, Hernandez RJ, Martin JE et al (1994) Radiation dose reduction in CT of the pediatric pelvis. Radiology 190(3):683–687

Kang EY, Patz EF, Muller NL et al (1996) Cytomegalovirus pneumonia in transplant patients: CT findings. J Comput Assist Tomogr 20(2):295–299

Kerem E, Bar Ziv Y, Rudenski B et al (1994) Bacteremic necrotizing pneumococcal pneumonia in children. Am J Respir Crit Care Med 149(1):242–244

Kern JA, Rodgers BM (1993) Thoracoscopy in the management of empyema in children. J Pediatr Surg 28(9):1128–1132

Khoury MB, Godwin JD, Halvorsen RA et al (1985) CT of obstructive lobar collapse. Invest Radiol 20(7):708–716

Kirsh MM, Pellegrini RV, Sloan HE et al (1972) Treatment of blunt chest trauma. Surg Annu 4:51–90

Knight L, Fraser RG, Robson HG et al (1975) Massive pulmonary gangrene: a severe complication of Klebsiella pneumonia. Can Med Assoc J 112(2):196–198

Leatherman JW, Iber C, Davies SF et al (1984) Cavitation in bacteremic pneumococcal pneumonia. Causal role of mixed infection with anaerobic bacteria. Am Rev Respir Dis 129(2):317–321

Leventhal JM (1982) Clinical predictors of pneumonia as a guide to ordering chest roentgenograms. Clin Pediatr (Phila) 21(12):730–734

Light RW (1985) Parapneumonic effusions and empyema. Clin Chest Med 6(1):55–62

Light RW (1995) A new classification of parapneumonic effusions and empyema. Chest 108(2):299–301

Mahboubi S, O'Hara AE (1981) Bronchial rupture in children following blunt chest trauma. Report of five cases with emphasis on radiologic findings. Pediatr Radiol 10(3):133–138

Manson D, Babyn PS, Palder S et al (1993) CT of blunt chest trauma in children. Pediatr Radiol 23(1):1–5

Marks MJ, Haney PJ, McDermott MP et al (1996) Thoracic disease in children with AIDS. Radiographics 16(6):1349–1362

McAdams HP, Rosado-de-Christenson ML, Templeton PA et al (1995) Thoracic mycoses from opportunistic fungi: radiologic-pathologic correlation. Radiographics 15(2):271–286

Mori M, Galvin JR, Barloon TJ et al (1991) Fungal pulmonary infections after bone marrow transplantation: evaluation with radiography and CT. Radiology 178(3):721–726

Moulton JS, Benkert RE, Weisiger KH et al (1995) Treatment of complicated pleural fluid collections with image-guided drainage and intracavitary urokinase. Chest 108(5):1252–1259

Muller NL (1993) Imaging of the pleura. Radiology 186(2):297–309

Naidich DP, McCauley DI, Khouri NF et al (1983a) Computed tomography of lobar collapse: 1. Endobronchial obstruction. J Comput Assist Tomogr 7(5):745–757

Naidich DP, McCauley DI, Khouri NF et al (1983b) Computed tomography of lobar collapse: 2. Collapse in the absence of endobronchial obstruction. J Comput Assist Tomogr 7(5):758–767

Naidich DP, Szerhouni EA, Siegelman SS et al (1991) Computed tomography and magnetic resonance of the thorax, 2nd edn. Raven, New York, pp 423–426

O'Reilly GV, Dee PM, Otteni GV et al (1978) Gangrene of the lung: successful medical management of three patients. Radiology 126(3):575–579

Osborne D (1978) Radiologic appearance of viral disease of the lower respiratory tract in infants and children. AJR Am J Roentgenol 130(1):29–33

Peter G (1988) The child with pneumonia: diagnostic and therapeutic considerations. Pediatr Infect Dis J 7(6):453–456

Pugatch RD, Spirn PW (1985) Radiology of the pleura. Clin Chest Med 6(1):17–32

Ramnath RR, Heller RM, Ben-Ami T et al (1998) Implications of early sonographic evaluation of parapneumonic effusions in children with pneumonia. Pediatrics 101(1):68–71

Robinson AE, Hill EP, Harpen MD et al (1986) Radiation dose reduction in pediatric CT. Pediatr Radiol 16(1):53–54

Rogalla P, Stover B, Scheer I et al (1999) Low-dose spiral CT: applicability to paediatric chest imaging. Pediatr Radiol 29(8):565–569

Rosen H, Nadkarni V, Theroux M et al (1993) Intrapleural streptokinase as adjunctive treatment for persistent empyema in pediatric patients. Chest 103(4):1190–1193

Shackleford SR (1987) Blunt chest trauma: the intensivist's perspective. J Intensive Care Med 1:125–136

Silen ML, Weber TR (1995) Thoracoscopic debridement of loculated empyema thoracis in children. Ann Thorac Surg 59(5):1166–1168

Sivit CJ, Taylor GA, Eichelberger MR et al (1989a) Chest injury in children with blunt abdominal trauma: evaluation with CT. Radiology 171(3):815–818

Sivit CJ, Taylor GA, Eichelberger MR et al (1989b) Visceral injury in battered children: a changing perspective. Radiology 173(3):659–661

Stark DD, Federle MP, Goodman PC et al (1983) Differentiating lung abscess and empyema: radiography and computed tomography. AJR Am J Roentgenol 141(1):163–167

Stern EJ, Sun H, Haramati LB et al (1996) Peripheral bronchopleural fistulas: CT imaging features. AJR Am J Roentgenol 167(1):117–120

Strovroff M, Teaque G, Heiss KF et al (1995) Thoracoscopy in the management of pediatric empyema. J Pediatr Surg 30:1211–1215

Swischuk LE, Hayden CK (1986) Viral vs. bacterial pulmonary infections in children (is roentgenographic differentiation possible?). Pediatr Radiol 16(4):278–284

Tocino I, Miller MH (1987) Computed tomography in blunt chest trauma. J Thorac Imaging 2(3):45–59

Torres A, Gn Agusti A, Rodriguez-Roisin R et al (1984) Cavitation in bacteremic pneumococcal pneumonia. Am Rev Respir Dis 130(3):533–534

Turner RB, Lande AE, Chase P et al (1987) Pneumonia in pediatric outpatients: cause and clinical manifestations. J Pediatr 111(2):194–200

Vade A, Demos TC, Olson MC et al (1996) Evaluation of image quality using 1 : 1 pitch and 1.5 : 1 pitch helical CT in children: a comparative study. Pediatr Radiol 26(12):891–893

Wagner RB, Crawford WO, Schimpf PP et al (1988) Classification of parenchymal injuries of the lung. Radiology 167(1):77–82

Waite RJ, Carbonneau RJ, Balikian JP et al (1990) Parietal pleural changes in empyema: appearances at CT. Radiology 175(1):145–150

Wan YL, Tsai KT, Yeow KM et al (1997) CT findings of bronchial transection. Am J Emerg Med 15(2):176–177

Weir IH, Muller NL, Connell DG et al (1988) CT diagnosis of bronchial rupture. J Comput Assist Tomogr 12(6):1035–1036

Wildin SR, Chonmaitree T, Swischuk LE et al (1988) Roentgenographic features of common pediatric viral respiratory tract infections. Am J Dis Child 142(1):43–46

Williams JR, Stembridge VA (1964) Pulmonary contusion secondary to nonpenetrating chest trauma. AJR Am J Roentgenol 91:284–290

Winer-Muram HT, Rubin SA, Fletcher BD et al (1994) Childhood leukemia: diagnostic accuracy of bedside chest radiography for severe pulmonary complications. Radiology 193(1):127–133

Worthy SA, Flint JD, Muller NL et al (1997) Pulmonary complications after bone marrow transplantation: high-resolution CT and pathologic findings. Radiographics 17(6):1359–1371

Yangco BG, Deresinski SC (1980) Necrotizing or cavitating pneumonia due to Streptococcus Pneumoniae: report of four cases and review of the literature. Medicine (Baltimore) 59(6):449–457

Zukin DD, Hoffman JR, Cleveland RH et al (1986) Correlation of pulmonary signs and symptoms with chest radiographs in the pediatric age group. Ann Emerg Med 15(7):792–796

7 Pediatric Tuberculosis

Pedro Daltro and Eloá Nunez-Santos

CONTENTS

7.1
Introduction and Historical Aspects

Tuberculosis (TB) is a transmittable chronic bacterial disease caused by infection with the *Mycobacterium tuberculosis* complex. Pathologically it is characterized by the formation of granulomas. Clinical signs and symptoms depend upon the location of the lesions. TB can affect every organ in the body, but pulmonary infection is by far the most common.

Tuberculosis has been known to affect man as far back as historical data can record. Skeletal remains of prehistoric humans dating back to 8000 BC and Egyptian mummies dating from between 2500 and 1000 BC have revealed clear evidence of the disease in the spine (CREMIN and JAMIESON 1995). The best-documented confirmation of TB infection has come from DNA studies of an 8-year-old male Inca mummy who lived in around 700 AD. Radiographic study of his lumbar spine showed evidence of Pott's disease and smears of the lesion revealed acid-fast bacilli, most likely *Mycobacterium bovis* (DUTT and STEAD 1999).

Jean Antoine Villemin (1827–1892) was the first to prove the infectious nature of tuberculosis by passing it from humans to cattle, and from cattle to rabbits. The actual agent of TB, the tubercle bacillus, was identified by Robert Koch, in Germany, in 1882. The vaccination against tuberculosis [(bacille Calmette-Guérin (BCG)] was developed in the early part of the 20th century by the French researchers Calmette and Guérin. Effective therapy against tuberculosis became available in 1943 with Waksman's discovery of streptomycin, the first antituberculosis drug.

7.2
Epidemiology

Mycobacterium tuberculosis is the most devastating bacterial pathogen of all time. Approximately one-third of the world's population is infected with this bacteria and therefore at risk of developing the disease (CREMIN and JAMIESON 1995). In 1993, more than a century after the TB causal agent discovery, followed by decades of research on and implementation of appropriate chemical therapy, the World Health Organization (WHO) declared tuberculosis a global emergency. This was the first time in the history of the organization that such a document was issued. According to WHO records, 3.3 million cases of tuberculosis were reported during the year of 1995 alone. Without treatment, tuberculosis is often fatal. It is estimated that 50%–60% of the untreated patients

PEDRO DALTRO, MD
Instituto Fernandes Figueira-Fiocruz and Clinica de Diagnóstico por Imagem – Barrashopping – Av. Ataulfo de Paiva 226/301, Leblon, Rio de Janeiro, Rj-Brasil-22440-030, Brazil
ELOÁ NUNEZ-SANTOS, MD
Instituto Fernandes Figueira-Fiocruz, Av. Ataulfo de Paiva, 226/301, Leblon, Rio de Janeiro, Rj-Brasil-22440-030, Brazil

are likely to die within 5 years after diagnosis (MAHER and RAVIGLIONE 1999).

Tuberculosis has always been a public health problem in developing countries, especially among young people. In total, 95% of the estimated tuberculosis cases and 98% of estimated tuberculosis deaths occur in developing countries (RAVIGLIONE et al. 1995). There are neither age nor gender safeguards against tuberculosis and children also pay a heavy tribute to the disease: an estimation of 100 000 child deaths per year was acknowledged by the WHO in 1998.

The alarming worldwide resurgence of tuberculosis is due to many reasons. Poverty and poor living conditions (resulting in malnutrition and crowding), associated with lack of appropriate anti-tuberculosis drugs and sometimes governmental lack of interest in the control of tuberculosis are the most important causes in many developing countries.

In developed countries, tuberculosis has also proven burdensome. The disease has been mainly reported in HIV-positive patients, intravenous drug users, groups of people living in enclosed, crowded settings (prisons, shelters and nursing homes) and, last but not least, in outer unsanitary city areas, as well as among immigrants or refugees from countries where tuberculosis is endemic (CREMIN and JAMIESON 1995).

The worldwide distribution of registered tuberculosis cases mapped by WHO (from the 1997 Global Tuberculosis Programme: Global Tuberculosis Control) is as follows: 42% in the South-East Asian region, 24% in the Western Pacific Region, 14% in the African Region, 9% in the European Region, 4% in the Eastern Mediterranean Region and 7% in the American Region.

The most recent factor allowing for the increase of tuberculosis is the HIV pandemic, affecting both developed and developing countries. In African countries and South-East Asia, the association between tuberculosis and HIV has progressively increased.

Multidrug-resistant tuberculosis is a new face of the disease. Drug resistance results from inappropriate drug treatment or patient non-adherence to treatment and has a potentially dramatic impact on the epidemiology and control of tuberculosis worldwide (WHO/IUATLD Global Project on Anti-Tuberculosis Drug Resistance Surveillance 1997–2000). In the USA, about 13% of the cases are resistant to at least one antituberculosis drug, and 3.2% are resistant to both isoniazid and rifampicin (COSTELLO and ROOK 1995).

In 1997, in response to the growing concern about global tuberculosis control, the WHO adopted a new strategy, DOTS (Directly Observed Treatment Short Course), based on five pillars:

- Governmental political support
- Microscopic detection of the cases by sputum-smear examination
- Short and supervised therapy
- Regular supply of antituberculosis drugs
- A standardized recording and reporting system for program supervision and evaluation.

The aims of this program are to prevent the emergence of resistant strains of *M. tuberculosis* and to detain their spread.

Since tuberculosis is a global emergency, the disease will be only defeated by a global alliance, bringing together public health agencies, the pharmaceutical industry and the academia. Effective control programs must foster private–public partnership in order to succeed.

7.3
Pathogenesis

7.3.1
Infection

Humans are the only species in which *M. tuberculosis* is a self-perpetuating pathogen. The only epidemiologically important mode of transmission is air borne with infection occurring through inhalation of viable bacilli in an enclosed space. Pediatric tuberculosis infection almost invariably occurs by contact with an adult or adolescent with cavitary pulmonary tuberculosis, most often at home, but also at school or in the day care center. In outside air the bacilli are rapidly killed by ultraviolet light and viable bacilli are so widely dispersed that inhalation of even a single bacillus is extremely improbable.

Tuberculosis spreads more easily among family members or among people who share the same facilities. However, contact alone is not bound to develop the disease. Immunologic and genetic factors affect the child's response to the initial infection (STARKE 1999). Children under 5 years of age, and especially those under two, are less resistant to the organism and, therefore, disseminated forms of the disease are more common in this age group. There is less risk of progressive primary disease in later childhood, between 6 and 12 years of age.

Child-to-child transmission is virtually unknown, mainly because children do not show the tussive force of an adult and have only sparse secretions. However, they play a peculiar role in the transmission of tuberculosis because they may harbor a partially healed infection that lies dormant, only to be reactivated as infectious pulmonary TB many years later (STARKE 1999). Thus, children constitute a long-lasting reservoir of tuberculosis in the population from which future generations will be infected (CREMIN and JAMIESON 1995).

In more than 95% of cases, the entrance door of tuberculous infection is the lung, by inhalation of bacilli. Infection through the oro-pharynx, throat, eye or skin rarely occurs. The exposed child inhales aerosolized particles containing 1–3 bacilli. These bacillary particles can be moved up the bronchial tree by cilia and might eventually be swallowed, causing no infection. They can also reach the alveoli, where they will be ingested by the alveolar macrophages. The bacilli can be killed or inhibited by these cells. If the bacilli are quite virulent, they grow and multiply inside the alveolar macrophage until it bursts, releasing a greater number of pathogens. These bacilli will be then ingested by other alveolar and blood macrophages (i.e. monocytes), forming the *tubercle*, which consists of an aggregation of macrophages, epithelioid cells and lymphocytes. Central necrosis inside the tubercle is formed by destruction of macrophages. This immune response is mainly tissue-damaging delayed-type hypersensitivity, and at this time, usually 3–8 weeks after infection, the tuberculin skin test will usually be positive. Eventually, sclerosis and calcification of the lesion may develop (DANNENBERG 1999).

In the next stage, cell-mediated immunity is very important. If only poor cell-mediated immunity develops, bacilli escape from the edge of the caseous necrosis, multiply again and spread from the tubercle to nearby mediastinal lymph nodes. These three items together – the alveolar site of infection, the infected lymph nodes and associated lymphangitis – form the "primary (Ranke's) complex".

7.3.2
Disease

From the infected lymph nodes, bacilli can travel via the lymphatics or bloodstream to many parts of the body, such as the liver, spleen, kidneys, bone metaphysis, brain and other organs, or return to the lungs causing secondary lung lesions. Infants and young children have poor cell-mediated immunity. So, when infected, they show a higher incidence of

tuberculosis than adults or older children. Lesions in the lymph nodes and extrapulmonary sites are common. Sometimes a pulmonary lesion spreads locally causing pneumonitis and pleural disease. Occasionally the caseous center of the granuloma progresses to liquefaction and is expelled through a bronchus, leaving a cavity and leading to bronchogenic spread, following the pattern of adult pulmonary tuberculosis (Fig. 7.1).

In children, the disease usually develops soon after the primary infection (primary tuberculosis) but the bacilli can also lie dormant in tissue macrophages for many years, only to develop the disease some decades later (secondary tuberculosis). Complete eradication of the bacillus by the immune system never occurs, and it is still very difficult even with the use of effective antituberculosis therapy (EHLERS 1999). Calcified lesions are sterile in 85% and fibrotic lesions in 86%. In contrast, solid caseous lesions are sterile in only 50% (MOULDING 1999).

It is important to always bear in mind that tuberculosis-infected children, left untreated, will house the bacilli for longer periods of time than adults and can become a source of tuberculosis in future years (INSELMAN 1996).

7.4
Clinical Aspects

Most cases of infection with *M. Tuberculosis* do not result in disease, but the risk of developing disease is higher for children than for adults. Children under 6 years of age have the highest case rates and the most serious disease (COSTELLO and ROOK 1995).

The risk of a child acquiring tuberculous infection is environmental, depending on whether the child has had contact with an adult or adolescent with pulmonary TB. Not all infected children have the same risk of developing the disease; the patient's immunocompetence, age, and certain genetic factors all play a part. The virulence of the bacillus is also important (STARKE 1999).

The high-risk categories for exposed children to develop tuberculous disease are infants and children under 4 years of age who have had close contact with a person with smear-positive TB, children with HIV disease or some other immunodeficiency, and those receiving high-dose corticosteroids.

Most infants and children who become infected with *M. tuberculosis* are completely asymptomatic

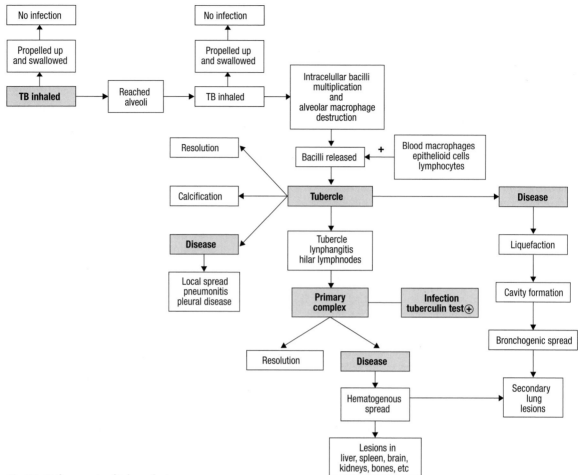

Fig. 7.1. Pathogenesis of tuberculosis

and will never develop disease. Those who do, demonstrate few symptoms or signs of pulmonary disease at the outset. Fewer than half develop non-specific symptoms such as fever, anorexia and weight loss. Most develop cough and many wheeze. If untreated, symptoms and signs of pulmonary bronchopneumonia and extrapulmonary disease may become apparent. Tuberculous infection is defined by a reactive tuberculin skin test. During the period of infection (3–8 weeks), usually the child has no symptoms and the chest radiograph is normal.

For the absolute diagnosis of TB the demonstration on culture of *M. tuberculosis* in secretions or tissue of the patient is required. A positive tuberculin skin test demonstrates that the individual has been infected with *M. tuberculosis* but it cannot tell whether the bacilli are living in a quiescent latent state or actively replicating and causing disease. When the pathology is virtually confined to the lungs, as is usu-

ally the case in adults with pulmonary TB, it is relatively easy to confirm the diagnosis by sputum culture. When the principle focus of infection is the intrathoracic lymph nodes, as often is the situation in infants and young children, the organisms are inaccessible and it becomes difficult to prove that the patient has TB. Furthermore, children produce little sputum, which, in addition, contains few microorganisms, and they generally swallow it. Because of these factors and the difficulties associated with obtaining adequate samples of swallowed sputum from the stomach, the diagnosis of TB is confirmed bacteriologically in considerably less than half (range 10%–75%) of infants and young children who are treated for TB (KLEIN and ISEMAN 1999). Thus, the triad of a positive tuberculin skin test, abnormal chest radiographs and a history of exposure to an adult with TB remains the most effective method for diagnosing TB in children.

Primary TB has been used to describe pediatric pulmonary disease that arises as a complication of the tuberculous infection. In children, disease frequently complicates the initial infection immediately, making the distinction between the two stages impossible. Miliary and meningeal TB can develop any time, but they are more likely to occur during the initial 3 months following the primary infection. Endobronchial TB can also develop at this time. Tuberculosis of the pleura and peritoneum characteristically occurs 3–7 months after demonstration of a positive skin test (INSELMAN 1996) (Table 7.1).

Table 7.1. Clinical types of pulmonary tuberculosis in children (adapted from INSELMAN 1996)

Infection
Positive tuberculin skin test reaction without clinical, radiographic or laboratory evidence of disease

Pulmonary disease
Primary pulmonary tuberculosis (hilar adenopathy with or without primary parenchymal disease)   Progressive pulmonary tuberculosis (pneumonia, endobronchial disease)   Chronic pulmonary tuberculosis (cavitary, fibrosis, tuberculoma)   Acute disseminated disease   Tuberculous pleural and pericardial effusion   Unusual presentations

Imaging methods such as chest X-ray, chest US and chest CT are extremely important tools for the diagnosis of pediatric pulmonary TB. In some instances, particularly in difficult cases, they offer the only way to reach a correct diagnosis and a thorough evaluation of the extent of the disease.

7.5
Imaging: Technique and Features

7.5.1
Chest X-Ray

Chest radiography (AP-PA and lateral X-rays) remains the first and most widely used imaging technique for the evaluation of pulmonary TB in children. It is usually very effective for detecting parenchymal lesions and lymphadenopathy in most of the cases.

7.5.2
Computed Tomography (CT)

CT is the examination of choice in unusual, complicated or disseminated presentations of the disease. It is also helpful for the evaluation of infants with positive skin test and normal chest X-rays, and for older children with either a history of recent exposure to TB or a positive skin test and inconclusive chest X-ray findings. In small children with miliary TB, head CT should always be performed as well. Recognition of brain lesions, which commonly occur in these patients, can influence therapy.

The advantages of CT over conventional radiographs in defining the extent of the disease and its possible complications (bronchial, pleural, pericardiac and chest wall involvement) have been well documented in the literature (W. S. KIM et al. 1997).

When evaluating TB by CT we prefer to use the helical technique without contrast followed by contrast-enhanced scans, using 5–10 mm slice collimation. Multiplanar and 3D reconstructions are helpful in some cases, particularly in the evaluation of tracheobronchial disease. High Resolution CT (HRCT) using limited thin slices (1–1.5 mm) and edge-enhancing reconstruction algorithms are useful when assessing parenchymal lesions, such as bronchogenic and miliary nodules, and bronchiectasis.

7.5.3
Magnetic Resonance Imaging (MRI)

MRI is an excellent method for detecting mediastinal lymph node involvement and has the advantage of multiplanar imaging capacity. However, high cost, need for sedation in most cases and poor visualization of the lung parenchyma limits its use.

7.5.4
Ultrasound (US)

US is an easy-to-use, inexpensive, non-aggressive technique that is useful for identifying mediastinal lymph nodes and differentiating them from a large normal thymus in patients who present mediastinal widening. It is also helpful for detecting pleural and pericardial effusion (see Chap. 1).

7.5.5
Infection – The Primary Complex

The primary (Ranke's) complex consists of the primary parenchymal lesion, draining lymphatic vessels and regional lymph nodes. It can develop in any part of the lung, although the middle lobe has a lower frequency of occurrence (INSELMAN 1996). At the onset of hypersensitivity to tuberculin, most often 4–8 weeks after mycobacterial inoculation, the primary complex may become visible on the chest X-ray or CT. (Fig. 7.2).

Of infected children, 95% will not develop disease. In these cases the primary complex becomes fibrotic, calcifies or resolves completely and the chest radiograph appears normal or demonstrates calcifications (Fig. 7.3). Viable mycobacteria can persist for decades even within calcified lesions.

7.5.6
Primary Pulmonary Tuberculosis

The hallmark and most constant feature of pulmonary TB in infancy and childhood is mediastinal and/or hilar lymphadenopathy, and most radiologists would be reluctant to consider the diagnosis of TB in its absence. Whenever this feature is observed in the chest radiograph, particularly in infants, tuberculin skin testing should be considered The right side is more commonly affected than the left because of the usual pattern of lymphatic circulation within the lungs. A left-sided parenchymal focus often leads to bilateral hilar adenopathy, whereas a right-sided focus is usually associated only with right-sided lymphadenitis (STARKE 1999).

Lymphadenopathy is not always easy to detect on conventional radiographs. Computed tomography has a higher sensitivity. On chest plain films lymphadenopathy usually presents as asymmetrically distributed paratracheal, hilar and/or sub-carinal lobulated nodes with sharp or ill-defined borders The enlarged lymph nodes can compress and stretch the bronchi (Fig. 7.4), or compress and displace the trachea. Sub- carinal lymph node involvement can cause splaying of the mainstem bronchi. Shift of the mediastinum may not occur because of the fixed nature of these lymph nodes (INSELMAN 1996).

On CT, the enlarged nodes can be partially or completely calcified or appear as soft tissue density masses. In our experience heavily calcified nodes indicate long-standing infection. Following contrast

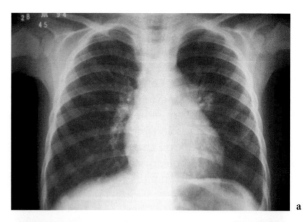

a

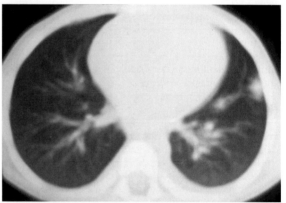

b

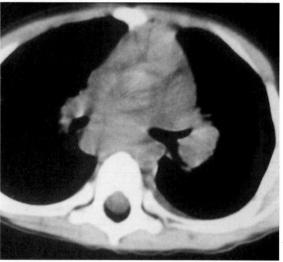

c

Fig. 7.2. a Chest X-ray of an 8-year-old boy shows slight enlargement of the left hilum. **b** Unenhanced CT of the same patient demonstrates peripheral pulmonary focus in the left lower lobe and lymphangitis. **c** Mediastinal window shows left hilar adenopathy

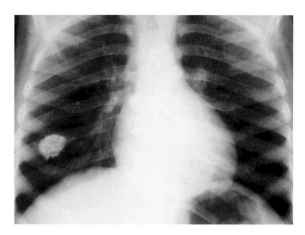

Fig. 7.3. Primary complex with calcified pulmonary focus in a 6-year-old child

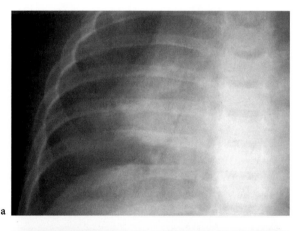

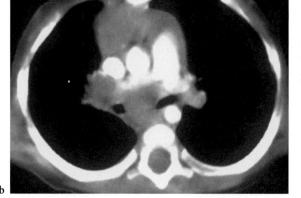

Fig. 7.4. a An 11-month-old boy. Chest X-ray shows a "stretched bronchus" sign. **b** CT demonstrates that it corresponds to the intermediate bronchus encased by two large lymph nodes

administration, nodes that are not completely calcified will enhance homogeneously or present ring-like enhancement with low-attenuation centers due to internal caseous material (Figs. 7.5 and 7.10c). Delayed images can be extremely helpful for differentiating paratracheal lymph nodes from normal retrocaval thymus.

Enlarged and edematous hilar, paratracheal and sub-carinal lymph nodes may encroach upon the regional bronchus. This compression can cause bronchial stenosis and lead to hyperinflation in the distal lung secondary to air-trapping, (Fig. 7.6) or completely occlude an airway and produce lung collapse.

7.5.7
Progressive Primary Pulmonary Tuberculosis

Inflamed nodes sometimes erode a bronchial wall and discharge caseous material into the bronchus (Fig. 7.7), leading to bronchogenic spread. On HRCT this will manifest as poorly defined nodules or rosettes of nodules, 2–10 mm in diameter that can be identified as centrilobular or branching centrilobular opacities mimicking the "tree in bud" image. Coalescence of the centrilobular opacities results in focal areas of bronchopneumonia (WEBB et al. 1996). Extensive bronchogenic spread can cause other patterns, such as pulmonary consolidation, or multiple nodules throughout the lungs (Fig. 7.8). Occasionally, the primary parenchymal lesion continues to enlarge, resulting in focal pneumonitis or lobar pneumonia with thickening of the overlying pleura without distinct hilar lymphadenopathy (Fig. 7.9).

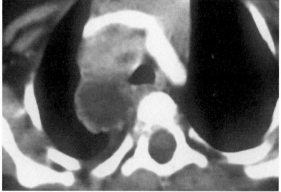

Fig. 7.5. A 12-month-old boy with TB. Contrast enhanced CT shows enhancement of the anterior node while the posterior remains centrally hypodense

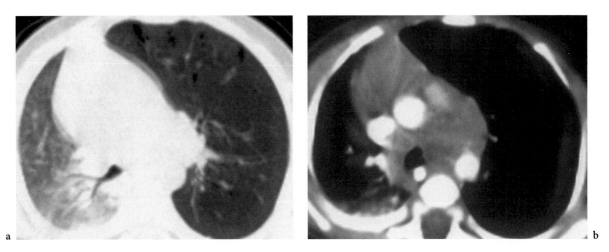

Fig. 7.6a,b. CT of a 4-month-old boy with obstructive emphysema of the left lung caused by hilar adenopathy

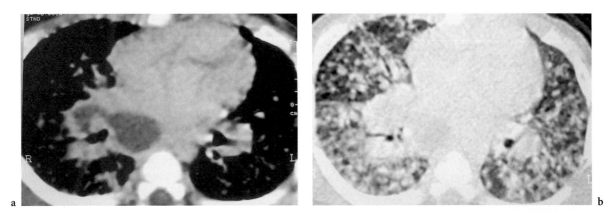

Fig. 7.7a,b. Unenhanced CT (mediastinal window) in a 6-month-old boy shows right hilar lymph node with hypodense center (caseum) with fistulous tract to the right main bronchus, causing bronchogenic spread with multiple pulmonary nodules of different sizes

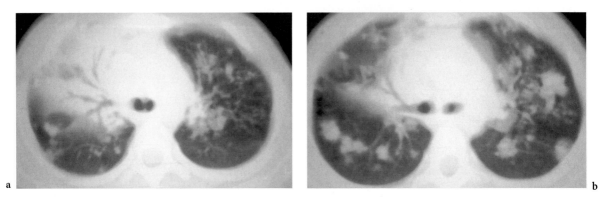

Fig. 7.8a, b. CT of a 10-year-old girl shows alveolar consolidation of the right upper lobe and bilateral confluent, nodular opacities

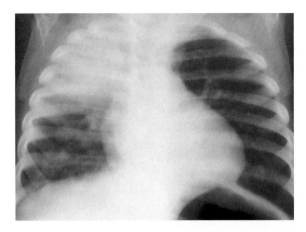

Fig. 7.9. Chest X-ray of a 3-year-old boy shows extensive consolidation of the right upper lobe, without evident lymphadenopathy

When tuberculosis is progressively destructive, liquefaction of lung parenchyma leads to formation of a primary tuberculous cavity (Fig. 7.10). Hematogenous spread can also develop, though it is less frequent (INSELMAN 1996).

Another rare complication is the appearance of bullous or cystic lesions in the lung. These have been reported to occur during treatment (MATSANIOTIS et al. 1967), but we have observed them before therapy was initiated (Fig. 7.11). Occasionally peripheral bullous lesions will lead to pneumothorax.

7.5.8
Chronic and Postprimary Pulmonary Tuberculosis

It is very common for tuberculous lymph nodes to affect the adjacent airways by compression from without or by infiltration of the wall and eventual erosion

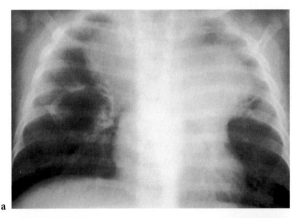

a

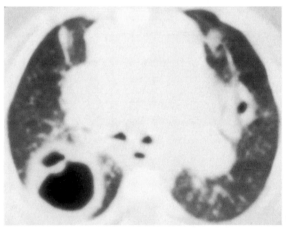

b

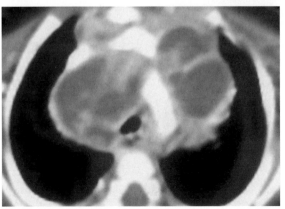

c

Fig. 7.10. a Chest X-ray in a 2-month-old boy with a huge mediastinal and hilar lymphadenopathy with a cavitary lesion in the right lung. **b** HRCT better demonstrates the cavity in the right lung. **c** Enhanced CT shows widened superior mediastinum due to large, rim-enhancing TB lymph nodes

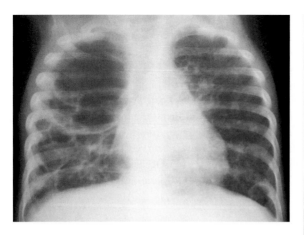

Fig. 7.11. Chest X-ray in a 6-year-old boy with multiple bullous tuberculous lesions in both lungs that appeared prior to receiving antituberculosis therapy

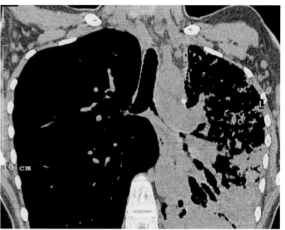

a

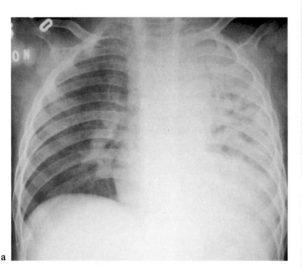

a

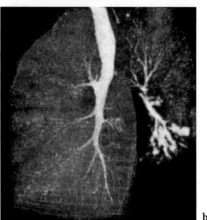

b

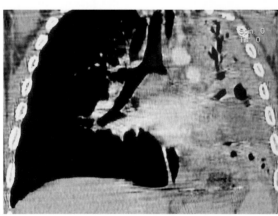

b

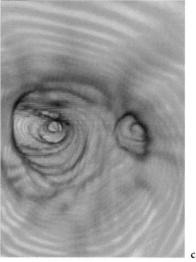

c

Fig. 7.12. a Chest X-ray of a 1-year-old boy with consolidation and loss of volume of the left lung. **b** CT coronal reconstruction shows obstruction of the left main bronchus causing the lung opacity. Moderate bronchial dilatation can also be observed

Fig. 7.13. a, b Coronal reconstruction and volume rendered image from multidetector-row CT in a 16-year-old girl shows complete opacification of the left lung caused by total occlusion of the left main bronchus. Bronchiectasis can be observed in the left lung. **c** Virtual bronchoscopy in the carinal view well demonstrates the complete obstruction of the left main bronchus

into the lumen. Epituberculosis is one of the terms applied to the radiographic consequences of this event. Airway involvement can cause bronchial stenosis, bronchiectasis or collapse, which may be segmental, lobar or involve the entire lung. Helical CT with multiplanar and 3D reconstructions are particularly helpful for examining the airways (Figs. 7.12 and 7.13).

Tuberculosis disease that occurs more than 1 year after the primary infection is thought to be secondary to endogenous regrowth of persistent bacilli from the primary infection and subclinical dissemination. Exogenous reinfection is very rare.

Postprimary tuberculosis occurs in patients previously sensitized to *Mycobacterium tuberculosis*. Reactivation of dormant bacilli occurs during periods of immunosuppression, malnutrition and debilitation. Postprimary tuberculosis in the pediatric age group mainly occurs in adolescents and most commonly involves the apical and posterior segments of the upper lung lobes, and the superior segments of the lower lobes. The lesions are often smaller in adolescents than adults and lordotic views or even CT may be necessary to demonstrate small lesions (STARKE 1999). The CT findings of active post-primary tuberculosis include centrilobular nodules, tree-in-bud, lobular consolidation, cavitation and bronchial wall thickening (Fig. 7.14).

Dissemination during postprimary tuberculosis is rare among immunocompetent adolescents, but is very common in HIV-infected or immunocompromised adolescents.

7.5.9
Acute Disseminated Disease

Miliary spread complicating the primary infection occurs most often in infants and small children, usually no later than 3–6 months after the infection. The organs most commonly seeded are the lungs, liver, spleen, meninges, peritoneum, lymph nodes, pleura and bones. Pulmonary dissemination leads to the formation of pulmonary nodular interstitial granulo-

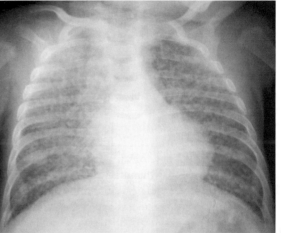

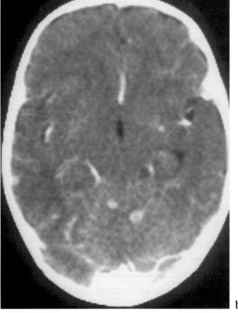

Fig. 7.15. a Chest X-ray in a 3-month-old boy shows a typical bilateral miliary pattern, with widespread tiny nodules in both lungs. **b** In the same patient, enhanced head CT shows a small brain granuloma

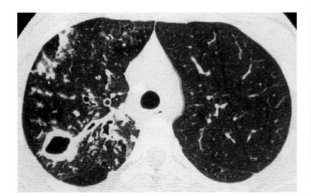

Fig. 7.14. A 10-year-old girl with secondary apical tuberculosis. CT demonstrates nodules (some with a hazy halo), ground-glass opacities and a cavity

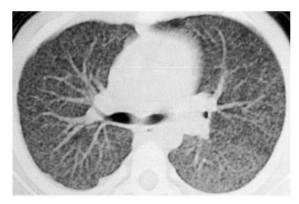

Fig. 7.16. HRCT of an 8-year-old boy shows a typical miliary pattern with tiny, widespread, randomly distributed nodules in both lungs

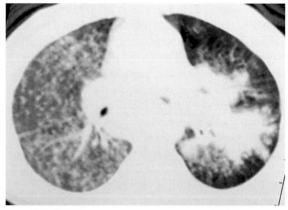

a

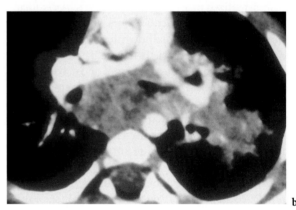

b

Fig. 7.17a,b. Chest CT of a 1-year-old boy with miliary spread mostly in the right lung. This asymmetrical involvement was due to obstructive emphysema with decreased perfusion of the left lung secondary to marked compression of the left bronchus by huge subcarinal and left hilar lymph nodes

mas, usually 1–2 mm in size, widely disseminated throughout the lungs.

On chest radiographs, the lungs usually show a miliary pattern. Brain involvement is common in miliary TB (SCHUIT 1979). Therefore, head CT should be performed in all children with miliary tuberculosis even if they do not show neurological symptoms (Fig. 7.15).

On CT, miliary tuberculosis appears as numerous small, well-defined nodules of up to several millimeters in diameter uniformly distributed through the lungs. A random distribution of nodules with respect to the lobule is observed (WEBB et al. 1996) (Fig. 7.16). In addition, CT can reveal hilar or mediastinal lymph nodes (Fig. 7.17) and occasionally small pleural effusions (OH et al. 1994). Exceptionally, pulmonary involvement by the miliary nodules will be asymmetrical (Fig. 7.17).

7.5.10
Pleural and Pericardial Effusions

Tuberculous pleural effusion results from rupture of a subpleural lesion into the pleural space, spread from caseous lymph nodes or an adjacent spinal lesion (HULNICK et al. 1983). Tuberculous pleural effusion is infrequent in children under 6 years of age and rare in those under 2. The fluid is usually unilateral to the primary parenchymal lesion, but may occur in both pleural spaces with bilateral primary complexes and with miliary dissemination (Fig. 7.18) (INSELMAN 1996). However, in our experience pleural effusion is exceedingly rare in miliary tuberculosis. Even without treatment, the fluid usually resorbs without sequelae, but empyema can ensue.

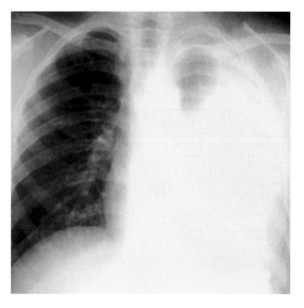

Fig. 7.18. A 14-year-old girl. Chest X-ray depicts unilateral pleural effusion. Pleural fluid culture yielded *M. tuberculosis*

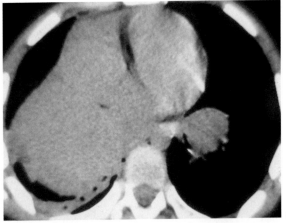

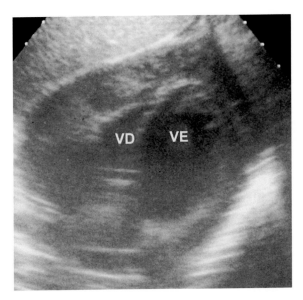

Fig. 7.19. Ultrasound of an 8-year-old boy shows pericardial effusion. *VD*, right ventricle; *VE*, left ventricle

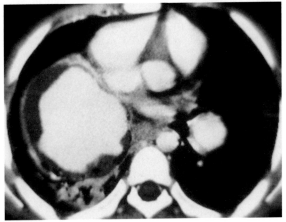

Fig. 7.20a. a Unenhanced CT performed in an 11-year-old girl demonstrates extensive opacity in the right hemithorax and a small nodular lesion on the left. b Following contrast enhancement, opacification of a huge right pulmonary artery with parietal thrombosis can be seen. There is a smaller aneurysmal dilatation of the left pulmonary artery. The patient died 15 days later due to severe hemoptysis (Courtesy of Dr. Alexandre Kalil; Hospital São Rafael, Salvador, Brazil)

Pericarditis and pericardial effusion are complications resulting from secondary extension of infected peribronchial nodes to the pericardium. Ultrasound and CT are very useful in the diagnosis of pericardial tuberculous lesions (Fig. 7.19).

7.5.11
Unusual Presentations and Complications

Pneumothorax, hemothorax, and bronchopleural or bronchoesophageal fistulas are unusual complications of pulmonary tuberculosis. Aortic rupture, which can result from spread of lymph nodes into the vessel, is even rarer (INSELMAN 1996).

Rasmussen aneurysm is an exceedingly unusual complication of tuberculosis in children. It corresponds to a pseudoaneurysm caused by erosion of a peripheral pulmonary artery branch by an adjacent tuberculous cavity lesion. It is almost exclusively seen in advanced pulmonary cavitary forms of tuberculosis in adults and can occur despite adequate treatment. The typical Rasmussen aneurysm is a peripheral, solitary lesion in the upper lobes, but uncommon presentations can also be seen (Fig. 7.20).

7.6
Conclusions

Diagnosis of pulmonary tuberculosis presents a continuing challenge to pediatricians and radiologists. Careful clinical history, tuberculin skin testing, and chest radiography remain the basic elements for establishing diagnosis. Chest US, MRI and particularly chest CT can provide information not available with conventional imaging, and thereby clarify diagnosis and influence therapy.

Acknowledgements. The authors thank Dr. Laurinda Higa for her contribution to the clinical aspects of TB.

References

Costello AM, Rook G (1995) Tuberculosis in children. Curr Opin Pediatr 7:6–12

Cremin BJ, Jamieson DH (1995) Imaging of pulmonary tuberculosis. In: Cremin BJ, Jamieson DH (eds) Childhood tuberculosis: modern imaging and clinical concepts. Springer, Berlin Heidelberg New York, pp 19–50

Dannenberg AM Jr (1999) Pathophysiology: basis aspects. In: Schlossberg D (ed) Tuberculosis and nontuberculous mycobacterial infections, 4th edn. Saunders, Philadelphia, pp 17–47

Dutt AK, Stead WW (1999) Epidemiology and host factors. In: Schlossberg D (ed) Tuberculosis and nontuberculous mycobacterial infections, 4th edn. Saunders, Philadelphia, pp 3–16

Ehlers S (1999) Immunity to tuberculosis: a delicate balance between protection and pathology. FEMS Immun Med Microbiol 23:149–158

Hulnick DH, Naidich DP, McCauley DI (1983) Pleural tuberculosis evaluated by computed tomography. Radiology 149:759–765

Inselman LS (1996) Tuberculosis in children: an update. Pediatr Pulmonol 21:101–120

Kim WS, Moon WK, Kim IO et al (1997) Pulmonary tuberculosis in children: evaluation with CT. AJR 168:1005–1009

Kim Y, Lee K, Yoon J et al (1997) Tuberculosis of the trachea and main bronchi: CT findings in 17 patients. AJR:168:1051–1056

Klein M, Iseman MD (1999) Mycobacterial infections. In: Taussig LM, Landau LI (eds) Pediatric respiratory medicine. Mosby, St Louis, pp 702–732

Maher D, Raviglione MC (1999) The global epidemic of tuberculosis: a World Health Organization Perspective. In: Schlossberg D (ed) Tuberculosis and nontuberculous mycobacterial infections, 4th edn. Saunders, Philadelphia, pp 104–115

Matsaniotis N, Kattamis C, Economou-Mavrou C et al (1967) Bullous emphysema in childhood tuberculosis. J Pediatr 71:703–707

Moulding T (1999) Pathogenesis, pathophysiology, and immunology: Clinical orientations. In: Schlossberg D (ed) Tuberculosis and nontuberculous mycobacterial infections, 4th edn. Saunders, Philadelphia, pp 48–56

Oh YW, Kim YH, Lee NJ et al (1994) High-resolution CT appearance of miliary tuberculosis. J Comput Assist Tomogr 18:862–866

Raviglione MC, Snider DE, Kochi A (1995) Global epidemiology of tuberculosis: morbidity and mortality of a worldwide epidemic. JAMA 273:220–226

Schuit KE (1979) Miliary tuberculosis in children. Clinical and laboratory manifestations in 19 patients. Am J Dis Child 133:583–585

Starke JR (1999) Tuberculosis in infants and children. In: Schlossberg D (ed) Tuberculosis and nontuberculous mycobacterial infections, 4th edn. Saunders, Philadelphia, pp 303–324

Webb R, Muller N, Naidich D (1996) High resolution CT of the lung, 2nd edn. Lippincott-Raven, Philadelphia

World Health Organization, Global Tuberculosis Programme (1997) Global tuberculosis control. WHO, Geneva, WHO/TB/97.225

8 Pulmonary Manifestations of AIDS

Leena Grover and Jack O. Haller

CONTENTS

8.1 Introduction

Since the advent of the AIDS epidemic in 1981, multiple opportunistic infections, lymphoproliferative disorders, and lung neoplasms are noted in AIDS patients. Pulmonary manifestations are a significant source of morbidity and mortality in HIV-infected patients in whom the lungs remain the chief target organ (HALLER 1993). AIDS is the sixth leading cause of death in children aged 1–4 years and seventh leading cause of death in children aged 5–14 years (MILLER 1997).

Chest infection is the presenting symptom in more than 50% of children with AIDS and is the cause of death in the majority of these patients (HALLER et al. 1997). It is also noted to be one of the most frequent disease pro-

cesses encountered throughout the course of the child's illness. Infections commonly seen in children with the HIV virus are *Pneumocystis carinii pneumonia* (PCP), lymphocytic interstitial pneumonitis (LIP) and bacterial pneumonias. The most frequent bacterial organisms seen are *Streptococcus pneumoniae* and *Hemophilus influenzae*. Additional opportunistic organisms including *Mycobacterium tuberculosis, Mycobacterium avium-intracellulare*, cytomegalovirus, toxoplasmosis, cryptococcus, and fungal infections such as aspergillus are identified. Malignancies involving the thorax are less commonly noted in the pediatric AIDS population. However, a greater variety of neoplasms have recently been observed in these patients, the most common type being B cell lymphoma. A recent emergence of smooth muscle tumors has also been documented. Kaposi's sarcoma is seen in less than 5% of pediatric cases, which is in contrast to its occurrence in adults.

In recent years, there has been a decrease in the incidence of PCP, which is attributed to prophylaxis in these patients. An increased frequency of mycobacterial tuberculosis has been identified in HIV-infected adults, but to a lesser extent in the pediatric age group. There is also a slight increase in the occurrence of malignancies in the AIDS patient; however, these are unusual in affected children. In order of frequency, the most common AIDS defining illnesses involving the lungs in a child are PCP, LIP, and recurrent bacterial pneumonias. The latter two illnesses are not considered index diseases in adults. High-grade lymphoma also classifies as an AIDS defining illness.

8.2 Infections

8.2.1 *Pneumocystis carinii* Pneumonia

Pneumocystis carinii pneumonia (PCP) (Fig. 8.1a–c) is the most common and serious opportunistic infec-

Leena Grover, MD, Jack O. Haller, MD
Department of Radiology, Long Island College Hospital, 339 Hicks Street, Brooklyn, NY 11201, USA

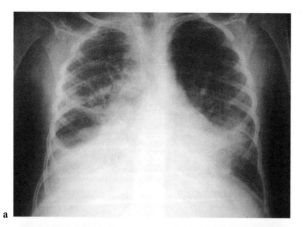

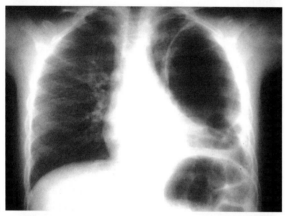

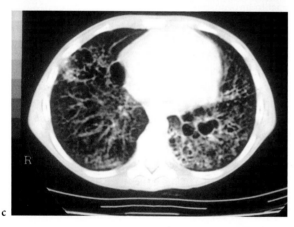

Fig. 8.1a–c. *Pneumocystis carinii* pneumonia (PCP). **a** An anteroposterior chest film reveals bilateral diffuse fine reticulonodular densities, which are characteristic of PCP. A thin walled cystic cavity is noted at the right base. **b** A large pneumatocele occupying almost two thirds of the left hemithorax is visualized on a radiograph of another patient. **c** Computed tomography demonstrates multiple bilateral thin wall cysts with some ground glass attenuation

tion seen in the HIV population. It occurs in approximately 50% of children with AIDS; however, there has been a decline in this infection due to widespread routine prophylaxis (MILLER 1997). This disease is often lethal when occurring in infants aged 3–6 months. Classically the patient presents with a tetrad of tachypnea, dyspnea, cough, and fever.

The majority of patients have an abnormal chest film; up to 10% may have a normal radiograph. Usual roentgenographic findings include fine reticular or reticulonodular infiltrate involving the perihilar region in a bilaterally symmetrical manner (ZIMMERMAN et al. 1987). This progresses from a heterogeneous to a diffuse homogeneous pattern involving the alveoli. Occasionally, lobar consolidation or a nodular pattern may be seen. These findings are very similar to those seen in adults and those we have been familiar with in the past with other immunodeficiency states (WOOD 1992; SUSTER et al. 1986).

Atypical presentations on chest radiographs include focal parenchymal lesions or cavitary nodules, which are often bilateral but in an asymmetric or unilateral pattern. Lymphadenopathy and pleural fluid are so rare with this disease that if noted it should virtually exclude PCP. However, studies have shown that patients on aerosolized pentamidine prophylaxis often demonstrate lymphadenopathy. There is also a predominance of PCP pneumonia in the upper lobes of these patients. Occasionally, patients with a negative chest radiograph will show abnormal uptake on a gallium scan in 85%–100% of cases of PCP; however, this is nonspecific as it can invariably be positive in patients with LIP. Chest radiographs and clinical findings help to distinguish between these two disease entities (AMBROSINO et al. 1992).

Computed tomographic (CT) scans of the chest in patients with PCP demonstrate a ground glass pattern which is secondary to the accumulation of fluid, organisms, fibrin, and debris within the alveolar spaces (MCGUINNESS 1997). The most common CT appearance of PCP is a patchwork or mosaic pattern, characterized by bilateral, asymmetric, and patchy involvement. There maybe segmental or subsegmental sparing. This appearance is most characteristic of PCP (KUHLMAN et al. 1990). Another pattern identified is interstitial involvement, which could be asymmetric or symmetric, with thickening of the secondary lobular septa. Atypical CT features noted are the presence of nodules or cavities; however, when such findings are noted, a mixed infection or secondary disease process should be considered (WOLLSCHLANGER et al. 1984).

A complication exclusively noted with PCP are pneumatoceles which can rupture and lead to spontaneous pneumothorax (BELMAN et al. 1988; BERDON et al. 1993). Two mechanisms are suggested for this process: (1) The macrophages produce elastase, which weakens the alveolar wall, and (2) a check valve process by intraalveolar PCP (HALLER et al. 1997; EFFEREN and HENDLER 1991).

Patients who are treated show partial clearance of infection within 3–4 days and complete resolution within 2 weeks. Since there is a delay between clinical improvement and roentgenographic clearance, blood gases are more accurate in confirming early response to treatment (WOOD 1992).

Nowadays, as a result of prophylaxis, PCP is not seen as frequently as before. When it is diagnosed, it is usually in an unidentified HIV-positive child or a breakthrough of prophylaxis.

8.2.2
Lymphocytic Interstitial Pneumonitis or Pulmonary Lymphoid Hyperplasia

Lymphocytic interstitial pneumonitis (LIP) or pulmonary lymphoid hyperplasia (PLH) (Fig. 8.2a–c) is part of a generalized diffuse interstitial lymphocytosis syndrome (DILS). DILS causes a stimulation of CD8 T cells resulting in the clustering of lymphocytes, which infiltrate the alveolar and interlobular septa and lead to usual interstitial pneumonitis and, finally, chronic interstitial pneumonitis of AIDS. Lymphocytosis also invades the hilar and paratracheal lymph nodes, which are an important feature of this disorder in HIV-infected children.

LIP is seen in 40% of children with perinatally acquired HIV infection and in only 12% of those having received contaminated blood products. The exact etiology of this disease process is unclear, however it may represent an increased response to bacterial antigens or primary pulmonary infection with Epstein-Barr virus (EBV) or HIV itself (JOSHI 1991).

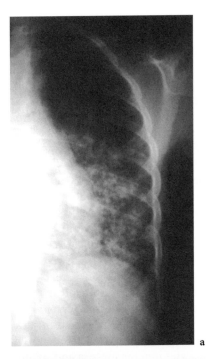

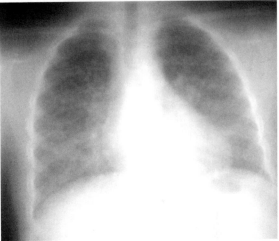

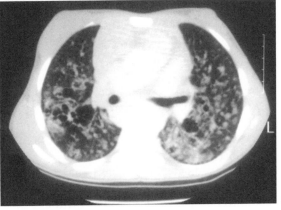

Fig. 8.2a–c. Lymphocytic interstitial pneumonitis (LIP). **a** Cone-down view of left lung shows multiple small coarse nodular opacities. **b** An anteroposterior chest radiograph reveals fine reticulonodular opacities bilaterally. **c** Computed tomography of another patient shows ill-defined nodules, some of which are in peribronchiovascular distribution. Bronchiectasis is seen predominantly in the right upper lobe; this occurs with increased frequency in LIP

In many cases, LIP/PLH may be the first presentation of HIV infection. If this is histologically proven in a child less than 13 years old, then it is considered diagnostic for AIDS. Usually, these patients present with cough and mild hypoxia and, unlike PCP, these children commonly display clubbing of the fingers. The presence of DILS is a good prognostic indicator, as the AIDS related complications are delayed in these children (WINCHESTER 1992; ITESCU et al. 1989; LEONIDAS et al. 1996).

The typical chest film demonstrates bilateral reticular or reticulonodular opacities predominantly at the bases or the periphery. This imaging characteristic is similar to miliary tuberculosis. Another pattern observed is homogeneous densities, which may be secondary to atelectasis or the filling of alveoli with lymphocytes or plasma cells. Besides parenchymal changes, hilar and mediastinal adenopathy is noted. In addition, bronchiectasis and air filled cysts, which may progress to pneumothorax, are noted in these patients. AMOROSA et al. (1990) postulated that infiltration of lymphocytes into the mucosa and submucosa of the respiratory bronchi causes parenchymal destruction, fibrosis, atelectasis, and bronchial dilatation. CT better demonstrates these findings of bronchiectasis than chest radiography. A definitive diagnosis can be obtained by lung biopsy.

8.2.3
Mycobacterial Infections

The incidence of mycobacterial infection in the pediatric AIDS patient has increased in the past decade. This occurs in approximately 10% of the HIV-infected population. These children with dysfunctional macrophages and CD4 cells are at increased risk of this infection (MEDILENSKY et al. 1989; SHAFER et al. 1991).

8.2.3.1
Mycobacterium tuberculosis

In the pediatric AIDS population, tuberculosis (Fig. 8.3a–c) is probably due to active primary disease, in contrast to adults where it is thought to be secondary to the reactivation of latent infection (BARNES et al. 1991; KEIPER et al. 1995).

Specific radiographic findings in HIV-positive patients are the same as those in children without HIV infection (HALLER et al. 1997; KHOURI et al. 1992; DALEY et al. 1992). These include ill-defined

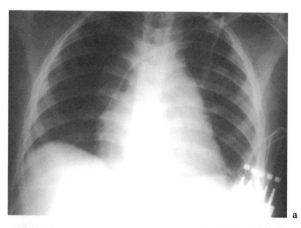

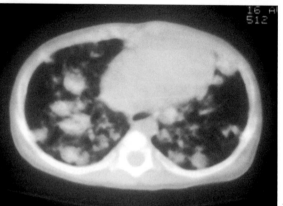

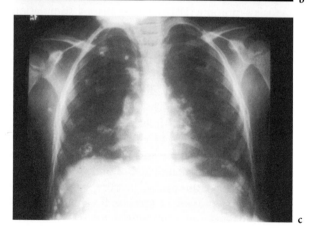

Fig. 8.3a–c. *Mycobacterium tuberculosis* (MTB). **a** Bilateral hilar and right paratracheal adenopathy is identified on this chest radiograph. **b** Computed tomography reveals bilateral extensive coarse nodular infiltrates. **c** Frontal view of the left chest in another patient shows multiple calcified densities in the left paratracheal, hilar region, left lung base and overlying

densities involving upper and lower lobes, lobar collapse, pleural effusion, and extensive adenopathy. The
thoracic imaging appearance of tuberculosis depends
on the stage of HIV infection (BAKSHI et al. 1993).
Early in the course of the disease, these findings
reveal coarse linear and nodular opacities with and
without cavitations in the apical and posterior segments of the upper lobes and superior segments of
the lower lobes. In late stages, the roentgenographic
findings demonstrate diffuse symmetric, bilateral,
coarse reticulonodular opacities. This pattern is difficult to distinguish from fungal infections (MURRAY
and MILLS 1990; GUTMAN et al. 1994).

Contrast CT examination of tuberculous lymph
nodes reveals low-density masses with peripheral
rim enhancement (NAIDICH et al. 1991). This may be
seen in fungal infections; however, it is distinct from
adenopathy of lymphoma or Kaposi's sarcoma. CT
appearance of parenchymal disease is non-specific
but may be valuable in revealing cavitary lesions
(GOODMAN 1990).

Children infected with HIV may present with atypical findings for tuberculosis such as diffuse infiltrates on chest film; these may also be seen in PCP or
LIP (HALLER et al. 1997).

The incidence of disseminated disease and extrapulmonary manifestations of tuberculosis is higher in
AIDS patients than in non-HIV-infected hosts (BRAUN
et al. 1993; CHAN et al. 1996). Disseminated infection
is noted frequently in pediatric populations, compared
with adult hosts (NOEL 1991; SMALL et al. 1991).

8.2.3.2
Mycobacterium avium-intracellulare Complex

In HIV disease, *Mycobacterium avium-intracellulare*
causes multisystem disease and is usually disseminated at the time of diagnosis. The major risk factor
for this infection in the AIDS population is immune
dysfunction with a CD4 count of less than 60/mm³.

Radiologic imaging in pediatric AIDS patients
with *Mycobacterium avium-intracellulare* complex
(MAC) (Fig. 8.4a–c) infection demonstrates massive
adenopathy (PURSNER et al. 2000). This not only
includes the retroperitoneal and mesenteric lymph
nodes, as seen in adults, but hilar and posterior mediastinal nodes are also involved in more than one
third of the patients. There may be central necrosis of
these nodes; however, this is less commonly seen than
with *Mycobacterium tuberculosis*. Rarely these lymph
nodes may break down and lead to an esophagobron-
chial fistula.

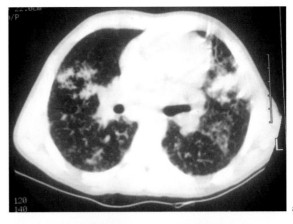

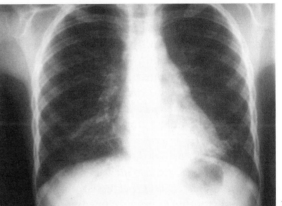

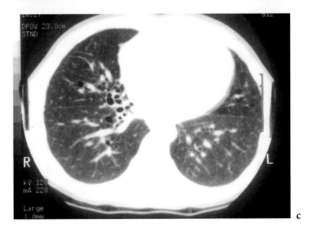

Fig. 8.4a–c. *Mycobacterium avium-intracellulare complex*
(MAC). **a** This child with MAC shows diffuse coarse nodular
densities bilaterally. Mediastinal adenopathy is also noted. **b**
Chest film in another patient shows dilation of the bronchi at
the bases, with "tram track" appearance of bronchiectasis. **c**
Computed tomography in the same patient demonstrates the
"signet ring" sign; the bronchi have a larger diameter than the
accompanying pulmonary arteries

CT appearances of MAC reveal cavitations, bronchiectasis, and diffuse reticulonodular densities which are non-specific. These manifestations are also seen with LIP, as well as with *Mycobacterium tuberculosis*, and therefore do not exclude the diagnosis of *Mycobacterium avium-intracellulare* (HARTMAN et al. 1993).

8.2.4
Other Infections

8.2.4.1
Bacterial Infection

Besides PCP and LIP, bacterial pneumonias are also one of the most common AIDS defining illnesses encountered in children. Pyogenic pneumonia occurs more commonly in the pediatric AIDS population than in their adult counterpart (GOODMAN 1993). The organisms commonly involved secondary to B cell defects are *Streptococcus pneumoniae*, and *Hemophilus influenzae*. With the progression of immune deficiency, *Staphylococcus aureus*, as well as gram-negative organisms such as *Escherichia coli, Klebsiella*, and *Pseudomonas*, are also identified. Rarely, *Salmonella, Nocardia, Listeria,* pertussis, *and Legionella* have been reported to produce pneumonia.

Chest film imaging reveals homogeneous segmental or lobar consolidation, nodules, or infiltrates with or without pleural effusion, similar to that seen in the general population. Radiologically, these focal lung opacities are typical findings of pyogenic pulmonary infection and unusual in patients with PCP. CT can further help in the evaluation of cavitation or necrosis in these patients. Treatment with the appropriate antibiotics results in rapid radiographic and clinical improvement.

8.2.4.2
Fungal Infection

Fungal pneumonias are unusual, occurring in 5% of adult AIDS patients and with less frequency in HIV-infected children, probably due to their lack of exposure to these organisms. The most common opportunistic fungi noted in the AIDS population include *Candida* species, *Cryptococcus neoformans* and *Aspergillus* (Fig. 8.5a,b). Other fungi include histoplasmosis and coccidioidomycosis. *Candida* rarely causes pneumonia in the absence of disseminated disease. Mucosal candidiasis is the most common fungal infection in the pediatric AIDS population.

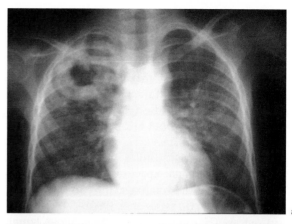

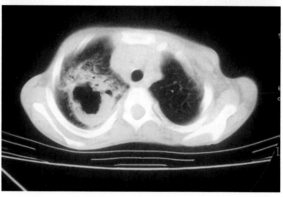

Fig. 8.5a,b. *Aspergillus.* **a** Chest radiograph demonstrates a large, irregularly thick-walled cavity in the right upper lobe. Multiple small nodules are seen in both lung fields. **b** Axial computed tomography in the same patient, with known tuberculosis, shows aspergilloma in the central cavity

Pulmonary candidiasis is uncommon and usually results from either aspiration of fungi from upper airways or hematogenous spread from the gastrointestinal tract or infected central venous catheters. Chest film shows scattered air space disease in the lower lobes. Less commonly, diffuse reticular or reticulonodular opacities and/or pleural effusions are reported.

C. neoformans is the most important fungal infection and is the AIDS defining illness in 40%–45% of affected children. This more commonly involves the brain and meninges than the lungs, even though the lung is the portal of entry for these organisms. Radiographically, they manifest with mediastinal/hilar adenopathy and/or diffuse nodular interstitial infiltrates. Isolated pleural effusion has been reported. Other findings associated with pulmonary cryptococcosis in immunocompetent hosts and immunocompromised patients without AIDS, are nodules, with or without cavitations and alveolar infiltrates that are rarely encountered in HIV-infected children. Cryptococcal pneumonia in AIDS patients often represents disseminated cryptococcosis and, therefore, should prompt a search for clinically silent cryptococcal meningitis.

Invasive pulmonary aspergillosis occurs at the end stage of AIDS (HERBERT and BAYER 1981; POTENTE 1989). Its appearance on chest radiographs ranges from multiple ill-defined peripheral nodules of varying sizes to larger masses or areas of consolidation. On CT, a rim of ground glass opacity surrounding the nodule (CT halo sign) is an early finding, though non-specific (CONNOLLY et al. 1999; KUHLMAN et al. 1985). A total of 40% of the affected patients demonstrate cavitations within the nodules, which is radiographically characteristic of an "air crescent sign". This is due to sloughed lung tissue surrounded by a rim of air within the cavitary mass (STAPLES et al. 1995; CURTIS et al. 1979; LIBSHITZ and PAGANI 1981). Other findings on CT include non-cavitary nodules, consolidation, and pleural effusions. Adenopathy is rare. Aspergillosis is seen in preexisting cavities and cysts in HIV-positive children with prior PCP or TB infection. Many of these cavities have a thick wall and a preference for the upper lobes (SHAH and SALAZAR 1998; KLEIN and GAMSU 1980; KUHLMAN et al. 1987).

In endemic areas, an increased incidence of pneumonia secondary to *Histoplasma capsulatum* and *Coccidioides immitis* is noted in AIDS patients. Disseminated histoplasmosis is commonly the initial AIDS defining illness, particularly in infants younger than 1 year old. The most frequent chest radiographic findings seen are diffuse nodular opacities, nodules measuring 3 mm or less. Linear and irregular opacities may be another roentgenographic presentation. Other findings such as focal air space opacities, pleural effusions and adenopathy, which are commonly identified in acute pulmonary histoplasmosis, are infrequent in patients with disseminated disease.

Similar to histoplasmosis, patients with HIV infection are prone to develop disseminated coccidioidomycosis. This may represent progressive primary infection or reactivation of dormant infection. Diffuse reticulonodular or nodular infiltrates are the most frequent radiographic pattern. These may be associated with thin walled cavities. Less commonly, focal alveolar opacities, a solitary nodule, pleural effusions, and hilar adenopathy are encountered on chest films. As with other fungal infections, definitive diagnosis is made by culture or tissue biopsy.

8.2.4.3
Viral Infections

Several viruses, including the HIV (human immunodeficiency virus) itself, CMV (cytomegalovirus), varicella, and HSV (herpes simplex virus) are implicated in the AIDS population.

CMV is an uncommon cause of pneumonia, even though this virus was detected in 80% of AIDS patients on autopsy. CMV pneumonia is rare in the pediatric AIDS population. This disease entity should be considered after PCP and TB are excluded. A variety of pulmonary findings are seen, none are pathognomonic. Bilateral alveolar infiltrates are commonly noted both on chest X-ray and CT and are indistinguishable from PCP. Less frequently, dense consolidation, nodules, or masses may be present. CT findings similar to small vessel airway disease including bronchiectasis, bronchial wall thickening, and bronchial impaction ("tree in bud" appearance) were diagnosed in about 30% of HIV-positive patients with CMV pneumonia, which, in some cases, manifested as the primary presentation of this disease.

Varicella may occasionally cause respiratory involvement in the pediatric AIDS population, but the course of the infection is not as severe as seen with other immunocompromised illness such as leukemia. Radiographic features encountered with varicella pneumonia are not the usual miliary pattern but nodular masses (MILLER 1997).

There is rare involvement of the lungs by the HSV in HIV-infected patients. It occurs only in advanced stages of AIDS. Focal disease is described as necrotizing tracheobronchitis, which is the most common presentation. When diffuse, it presents as disseminated interstitial pneumonitis with diffuse or patchy consolidation. Imaging findings cannot establish a diagnosis of this unusual pneumonia; positive culture and tissue confirmation is needed.

8.2.5
Rare Infections

Toxoplasma gondii mainly causes opportunistic infections in the central nervous system of HIV-positive patients. This parasite is now implicated as a cause of pneumonia in a few AIDS cases. Thoracic imaging reveals a diffuse bilateral, symmetric, predominantly coarse nodular pattern, which is indistinguishable from tuberculosis, histoplasmosis, and coccidioidomycosis. In most cases, it has been noted that neurologic symptoms may not precede pulmonary abnormalities even when the organism has multiplied in the brain and spread to the lungs (GOODMAN and SCHNAPP 1992). *T. gondii* infections manifest lymph node enlargement in other hosts; however, in AIDS patients, no definite hilar or mediastinal adenopathy is identified (THEOLOGIDES and KENNEDY 1966). Pleural fluid has occasionally been noted on chest radiograph.

8.3
Neoplasms

It is well established that immunodeficiency increases the risk of malignancy (GROOPMAN and BRODER 1989). With the advent of AIDS, there is a high incidence of cancer such as aggressive B cell lymphoma and Kaposi's sarcoma; however, these are unusual in children. The most common thoracic neoplasm in these children is non-Hodgkin's lymphoma. This presents as either a systemic disease or primary central nervous system tumor (ARICO et al. 1991; DICARLO et al. 1990; DOUECK et al. 1991). Smooth muscle tumors (including leiomyoma and leiomyosarcoma) of the airways are reported with great frequency. Diminished immune surveillance and proliferation of viruses associated with neoplasia predispose patients to malignancy (ROBINSON 1993).

8.3.1
Lymphoma

B cell lymphoma is the most common chest malignancy seen in the pediatric AIDS population. This should be suspected in patients with sudden increase in adenopathy or a mediastinal mass (KAPLAN 1994).

There are multiple hypotheses for the mechanism by which HIV-1 infection affects the B cell. The first of these is that the outcome of chromosome translocation is oncogene activation, and ultimately results in uncontrolled growth of B cells and their transformation. The second is that HIV-1 induced immunosuppression causes the emergence of EBV-infected immortalized B cells. Lastly, chronic antigenic or mitogenic stimulation results in B cell activation and hence increases their own numbers and that of the circulating immunoglobulins. Impairment of T cell suppressor function due to HIV infection is also associated with this process (MCGRATH 1994; PRITZKER et al. 1970).

Although B cell malignancies are commonly seen in the central nervous system, they occur throughout the body. Non-Hodgkin's lymphoma (Fig. 8.6a,b), as well as Burkitt's lymphoma, have also been described in the HIV-infected pediatric population (KAMANIAN et al. 1988). In contrast to immunocompetent patients, AIDS patients have high-grade lymphoma, which are usually B cell type, whereas those occurring in the normal population could be either B or T cell type (NOEL 1991; HASKAL et al. 1990). The known imaging features of thoracic lymphoma include pleural effusion, a reticulonodular interstitial pattern, or alveolar consolidation; hilar or mediastinal adenopathy; and parenchymal nodules which may cavitate. Many of the patients present with a mediastinal mass (GRATTAN-SMITH et al. 1992). Extranodal disease in children is noted frequently involving the gastrointestinal tract, central nervous system, bone marrow,

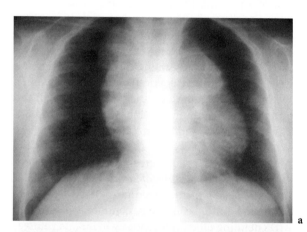

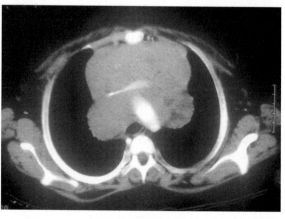

Fig. 8.6a,b. Non-Hodgkin's lymphoma. **a** Frontal projection of chest X-ray shows marked adenopathy involving paratracheal, anteroposterior window and hilar nodes bilaterally. **b** Contrast-enhanced computed tomography in the same patient demonstrates multiple nodular densities adjoining the pulmonary vessels and aorta

and liver. On CT, these lesions appear well circumscribed and low in attenuation. Differential diagnoses in children include mycobacterial infection and, rarely, Kaposi's sarcoma. Approximately 25% of pediatric patients with lymphoma have secondary bone involvement (SISKIN et al. 1995).

8.3.2
Smooth Muscle Tumors

These rare tumors include leiomyoma, leiomyosarcoma, and rhabdomyosarcoma, which are increasingly being reported in children with AIDS. It is postulated that these tumors may be due to EBV infection of the smooth muscle cells (McCLAIN et al. 1995). Another school of thought proposes that immunocompromised patients, such as transplant patients, have altered immune mechanisms, which allows the tumor to develop unchecked.

Leiomyosarcoma comprise less than 2% of all childhood soft tissue sarcomas. These are also noted in non-HIV immunocompromised children such as post-transplant patients or in acute lymphocytic leukemia (ALL) remission (CHADWICK et al. 1990; SHEN and YUNIS 1976; WALKER et al. 1991).

These myogenic tumors usually involve the viscera; however, other commonly affected sites are the tracheobronchial tree, pulmonary and hepatobiliary system, gastrointestinal tract, and bone (McLOUGHLIN et al. 1991).

In the published reports, there is no relationship between the mode of transmission and the development of these malignancies (HA et al. 1993). It is noted that girls are affected more frequently than boys (SCULLY et al. 1986).

On CT, these smooth muscle tumors are usually well circumscribed and easily visualized. They appear as low-attenuation lesions with slight enhancement, occasionally with some central necrosis (BALSAM and SEGAL 1992). Sonographic examination of leiomyomas and leiomyosarcomas demonstrates solid masses with low-level echoes within.

Leiomyosarcomas metastasize early and diffusely, commonly involving the lymph nodes. Sometimes, cannon ball type metastases are identified in the lungs.

8.3.3
Kaposi's Sarcoma

Kaposi's sarcoma (KS) (Fig. 8.7a,b) is the most common malignancy in adults, rarely seen in chil-

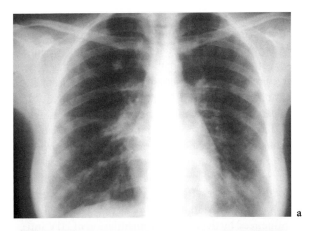
a

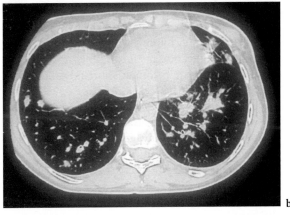
b

Fig. 8.7a,b. Kaposi's sarcoma. **a** Posteroanterior chest view demonstrates ill-defined nodular opacities with central or basilar predominance. **b** Computed tomography shows scattered, ill-defined nodules along the bronchovascular distribution. (Courtesy of Michele Spina, MD, Istituto Nazionale Tumori Centroeuropeo, Italy)

dren. There is a risk of AIDS associated KS in homosexuals and bisexuals; however, exact etiology in children is unclear (DE JARLAIS et al. 1984). Needle infection has contributed to the largest number of HIV-infected children with KS. Others acquired it as a vertical transmission in the perinatal period or, rarely, via blood transfusion (SAFAII et al. 1985). Studies have shown that KS is an AIDS defining illness in 0.5% of children in the United States (HALLER 1997; SERRANO and FRANCESCHI 1996).

KS is noted to appear three times more often in black than white children. It has no predilection for either sex in the pediatric age group, in contrast to adults where there is a higher incidence noted in males.

HIV associated KS has been described in several clinical forms (NORTHFELT 1994; SCHWARTZ 1996); firstly, a nodular form of disease represented by cutaneous nodular lesions of variable sizes. In children it is predominantly visualized in the mucous membranes and draining lymph nodes in the head and neck or inguinal and genital regions. A second form of KS is the lymphadenopathic type, which causes massive enlargement of the lymph nodes with associated lymphedema. There is associated involvement of the spleen, liver, lungs, and gastrointestinal tract. These findings are non-specific and diagnosis can be confirmed by fine needle aspiration cytology. A third type of oral HIV associated KS lesions are seen as large hemorrhagic patches or nodules. These predominantly involve the gastrointestinal and pulmonary systems.

It is suggested that the clinical appearance of KS is influenced by the mode of transmission of HIV infection. The lymphadenopathic, cutaneous, and mucosal forms are frequently seen in vertically transmitted HIV cases. In children with blood transfusion acquired HIV infection, cutaneous or lymphocutaneous disease is more common (MALEKZADEH et al. 1987; RIDOLFO et al. 1996).

With thoracic imaging, ill-defined nodular densities are noted along the central bronchovascular interstitium. As the disease advances, there is evidence of peripheral nodularity, pleural effusion, Kerley B lines, and lymphadenopathy (KHALIL et al. 1995). CT evaluations of these patients reveal endobronchial lesions, multinodular densities, and tumoral masses. Occasionally, in a few cases, ground glass opacities may be seen.

8.3.4
Hodgkin's Disease

It is unclear at this time whether Hodgkin's disease (Fig. 8.8a,b) in an AIDS patient is secondary to HIV, or a coincidental occurrence of this disease. When occurring in an HIV-infected patient, it presents at an advanced stage, with unfavorable histologic tumor types, frequent bone marrow involvement at presentation, and a poor therapeutic outcome. There is not enough data available for a detailed discussion of this disease entity in children; however, it is felt that when a child under 9 years of age is diagnosed with Hodgkin's disease, HIV should be suspected (SCHEIB and SIEGEL 1987).

8.3.5
Other Malignancies

A variety of other malignancies are noted in HIV-infected patients; these, however, are documented in

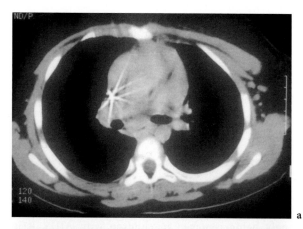
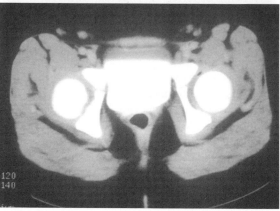

Fig. 8.8a,b. Hodgkin's disease. **a** Computed tomography (CT) of the chest shows multiple nodular densities in both hilar, subcarinal, and left axillary regions in this HIV-positive patient with Hodgkin's disease. **b** CT of the pelvis reveals bilateral inguinal adenopathy

small series or case reports. Many feel these may represent normal incidence of neoplasms seen in the general population, occurring incidentally in AIDS patient. In adults, these include lung cancer, papilloma virus induced neoplasia. and anogenital cancers.

An association between HIV infection and cervical disease in women with a more rapid course and metastatic spread is seen. Human papilloma virus is one of the most frequent organisms affecting the pediatric AIDS population. It manifests as condyloma acuminatum, non-venereal warts, and, rarely, respiratory papillomatosis, which is acquired perinatally. Widespread cutaneous flat warts or severe perineal condylomata are encountered in HIV-positive children. Sexually active teenagers are particularly susceptible to human papilloma virus (MUELLER et al. 1994).

Given the advances in treatment with antiretroviral therapy, there will be an overall increase in life expectancy, as well as in the number of new infections; this, in turn, will increase the incidence of secondary malignancies in the pediatric HIV population (REYNOLDS et al. 1993).

References

Ambrosino MM, Genieser NB, Krasinski K et al (1992) Opportunistic infections and tumors in immunocompromised children. Radiol Clin North Am 30:639–659

Amorosa JK, Nahass RG, Nosher JL, Gocke DJ (1990) Radiologic distinction of pyogenic pulmonary infection from PCP in AIDS patients. Radiology 175:721–724

Arico M, Caselli D, D'Argenio P et al (1991) Malignancies in children with human immunodeficiency virus type I infections. Cancer 68:2473–2477

Bakshi SS, Alvarez D, Hilfer CL et al (1993) Tuberculosis in human immunodeficiency virus infected children, a family infection. Am J Dis Child 147:320–324

Balsam D, Segal S (1992) Two smooth muscle tumors in the airway of an HIV-infected child. Pediatr Radiol 22:522–553

Barnes P, Blotch AB, Davison PT, Snider DE (1991) Tuberculosis in patients with human immunodeficiency virus infection. N Engl J Med 324:1644–1650

Belman AL, Diamond G, Dickson D et al (1988) Pediatric acquired immunodeficiency syndrome: neurologic syndromes. Am J Dis Child 142:29–357

Berdon WE, Mellins R, Abramson SJ et al (1993) Pediatric HIV infection in the second decade: the changing pattern of lung involvement (clinical and plain film and CT findings). Radiol Clin North Am 31:453–463

Braun MM, Cote TR, Raskin CS (1993) Trends in death with tuberculosis during the AIDS era. JAMA 269:2865–2868

Chadwick EG, Connor EJ, Hanson CG et al (1990) Tumors of smooth-muscle origin. JAMA 263:3182–3184

Chan SP, Birnbaum J, Rao M, Steiner P (1996) Clinical manifestation and outcome of tuberculosis in children with acquired immunodeficiency syndrome. Pediatr Infect Dis J 15:443–447

Connolly JE, McAdams HP, Erasmus JJ et al (1999) Opportunistic fungal infections. J Thor Imag 14:51–62

Curtis AM, Smith GJW, Ravin CE (1979) Air crescent sign of invasive aspergillosis. Radiology 133:17–21

Daley CL, Small P, Schecter GF et al (1992) An outbreak of tuberculosis with accelerated progression among persons with the human immunodeficiency virus. N Engl J Med 326:231–235

De Jarlais D, Marmor M, Thomas P et al (1984) Kaposi's sarcoma among four different AIDS risk groups. N Engl J Med 310:1119

Dicarlo FJ, Joshi W, Oleske JM, Connor EM (1990) Neoplastic disease in children with acquired immunodeficiency syndrome cases. Prog AIDS Pathol 2:163–185

Doueck P, Bertrand Y, Tran-Minh VA et al (1991) Primary lymphoma of the CNS in an infant with AIDS: imaging findings. AJR Am J Roentgenol 156:1037–1038

Efferen LS, Hendler JM (1991) Pneumatoceles. NY State J of Med 91:311–314

Goodman PC (1990) Pulmonary tuberculosis in patients with acquired immunodeficiency syndrome. J Thorac Imaging 5:38-I5

Goodman PC (1993) The chest radiograph in AIDS: infections and neoplasms. In: Thrall JH (ed) Current practice of radiology. Mosby-Year Book, St Louis, pp 1–8

Goodman PC, Schnapp LM (1992) Pulmonary toxoplasmosis in AIDS. Radiology 184:791–793

Grattan-Smith D, Harrison LF, Singleton EB (1992) Radiology of AIDS in the pediatric patient. Curr Prob Diagn Radiol 21:79–109

Groopman JE, Broder S (1989) Cancer in AIDS and other immunodeficiency states. In: Devita VT Jr, Hellman S, Rosenberg SA (eds) Cancer: principles and practice of oncology. Lippincott, Philadelphia, pp 1953–1970

Gutman LT, Moye J, Zimmer B, Tian C (1994) Tuberculosis in human immunodeficiency virus exposed or infected United States children. Pediatr Infect Dis J 13:963–968

Ha C, Haller JO, Rollins NK (1993) Smooth muscle tumor in immunocompromised (HIV negative) children. Pediatr Radiol 23:413–414

Haller JO (1993) Radiologic manifestations of AIDS in children. In Thrall JH (ed) Current practice of radiology. Mosby-Year Book, St Louis, pp 687–693

Haller JO (1997) AIDS related malignancies in pediatrics. Radiol Clin North Am 35:1517–1527

Haller JO, Ginsberg KJ (1997) Tuberculosis in children with acquired immunodeficiency syndrome. Pediatr Radiol 27:186–188

Haller JO, Vu VN, Cohen HL et al (1997) Diagnostic imaging in pediatric AIDS. Pediatr Clin North Am 44:721–729

Hartman TE, Swensen SJ, Williams DE (1993) Mycobacterium avium-intracellulare complex: evaluation with CT. Radiology 187:23–26

Haskal ZJ, Lindan CE, Goodman PC (1990) Lymphoma in the immunocompromised patient. Radiol Clin North Am 28:885–899

Herbert PA, Bayer AS (1981) Fungal pneumonia: invasive pulmonary aspergillosis. Chest 80:220–5

Itescu S, Brancato LJ, Wincester R (1989) A sicca syndrome in HIV infection: association with HLA-DR5 and CD4 lymphocytosis. Lancet ii:466–468

Joshi W (1991) Pathology of childhood AIDS. Pediatr Clin North Am 38:97–120

Kamanian N, Kennedy J, Brandsma J (1988) Burkitt lymphoma in a child with human immunodeficiency virus infection. J Pediatr 112:241–244

Kaplan LD (1994) Lymphoma: clinical characteristics and diagnosis. In: Cohen PT, Sande MA, Volberding PA (eds) The AIDS knowledge base, 2nd edn. Little Brown, Boston, pp 7.5-1–7.5-5

Keiper MD, Beaumont M, Elshami A, Langlotz CP, Miller WT (1995) CD4 lymphocyte counts and the radiographic presentation of pulmonary tuberculosis. A study of the relationship between these factors in patients with human immunodeficiency virus infection. Chest 107:74–80

Khalil AM, Carette MF, Cadranel JL et al (1995) Intrathoracic Kaposi's sarcoma: CT findings. Chest 108:1622–1626

Khouri YF, Mastrucci MT, Hutto C, Mitchell C, Scott G (1992) Mycobacterium tuberculosis in children with human immunodeficiency virus type 1 infection. Pediatr Infect Dis J 11:950–955

Klein DL, Gamsu G (1980) Thoracic manifestations of aspergillosis. AJR Am J Roentgenol 134:543–552

Kuhlman JE, Fishman EK, Siegelman SS (1985) Invasive pulmonary aspergillosis and acute leukemia: characteristic findings on CT, the CT halo sign, and the role of CT in early diagnosis. Radiology 157:611

Kuhlman JE, Fishman EK, Burch PA, Karp JE, Zerbouni EA, Siegelman SS (1987) Invasive pulmonary aspergillosis in acute leukemia: the contribution of CT to early diagnosis and aggressive management. Chest 92:95–99

Kuhlman JE, Kavuru M, Fishman EK, Siegelman SS (1990) Pneumocystis carinii pneumonia: spectrum of parenchymal CT findings. Radiology 175:711–714

Leonidas JC, Berdon WE, Valderrama E et al (1996) Human immunodeficiency virus infection and multilocular thymic cysts. Radiology 198:377–379

Libshitz HI, Pagani JJ (1981) Aspergillosis and mucormycosis: two types of opportunistic fungal pneumonia. Radiology 140:301–306

Malekzadeh MH, Church JA, Mitchell WG et al (1987) Human immunodeficiency virus associated Kaposi's sarcoma in a pediatric renal transplant recipient. Nephron 42:62–65

McClain KL, Leach CL, Jenson HB et al (1995) Association of Epstein-Barr virus with leiomyosarcomas in young people with AIDS. N Engl J Med 332:12–18

McGrath MS (1994) Pathogenesis of HIV associated lymphoma. In: Cohen PT, Sande MA, Volberding PA (eds) AIDS knowledge base, 2nd edn. Little Brown, Boston, pp 7.4-1–7.4-9

McGuinness G (1997) Changing trends in pulmonary manifestations of AIDS. In: Goodman PC (ed) The radiologic clinics of North America, vol 35, no 5. Saunders, Philadelphia, pp 1044–1049

McLoughlin LC, Nord KS, Joshi VV et al (1991) Disseminated leiomyosarcoma in a child with acquired immune deficiency syndrome. Cancer 67:2618–2621

Medilensky T, Sattler FR, Barnes PF (1989) Mycobacterial disease in patients with immunodeficiency virus infection. Arch Intern Med 6:633–634

Miller CR (1997) Pediatric aspects of AIDS. In: Goodman PC (ed) The radiologic clinics of North America, vol 35, no 5. Saunders, Philadelphia, pp 1191–2000

Mueller BV, Shad AT, Magrath IT, Horowitz ME (1994) Malignancies in children with HIV infection. In: Pizzo PA, Wilfert CM (eds) Pediatric AIDS, 2nd edn. Williams and Wilkins, Baltimore, pp 603–622

Murray JF, Mills J (1990) Pulmonary infectious complications of human immunodeficiency virus infection, part I. Am Rev Respir Dis 141:1356–1372

Naidich DP, McGuinness G (1991) Pulmonary manifestations of AIDS. Radiol Clin North Am 29:999–1017

Noel GJ (1991) Host defense abnormalities associated with HIV infection. Radiol Clin North Am 38:37–42

Northfelt DW (1994) Other neoplasms. In: Cohen PT, Sande MA, Volberding PA (eds) AIDS knowledge base. Little Brown, Boston, pp 7.10-1–7.10-4

Pritzker KPH, Huang SN, Marshall KG (1970) Malignant tumors following immunosuppressive therapy. Can Med Assoc J 103:1362–1365

Potente G (1989) Computed tomography in invasive pulmonary aspergillosis. Acta Radiol 30:587–90

Pursner M, Haller JO, Berdon WE (2000) Imaging features of MAC in children with AIDS. Pediatr Radiol 30:426–429

Reynolds P, Saunders LD, Layefsky ME et al (1993) The spectrum of acquired immunodeficiency (AIDS): associated malignancies in San Francisco, 1980–1987. Am J Epidemiol 137:19–30

Ridolfo AL, Santambrogio S, Mainini F et al (1996) High frequency of non-Hodgkin's lymphoma in patients with HIV-associated Kaposi's sarcoma. AIDS 10:181–185

Robinson LL (1993) General principles of the epidemiology or childhood cancer. In: Pizzo PA, Poplack DG (eds) Principle and practice of pediatric oncology, 2nd edn. Lippincott, Philadelphia, pp 3–10

Safaii B, Johnson KG, Myskowski PL et al (1985) The natural history of Kaposi's sarcoma in the acquired immunodeficiency syndrome. Am Intern Med 103:744–750

Scheib RG, Siegel RS (1987) Atypical Hodgkin's disease and the acquired immunodeficiency syndrome (letter). Ann Intern Med 107:112

Schwartz RA (1996) Kaposi's sarcoma: advances and prospective. J Am Acad Dermatol 34:804–814

Scully RE, Mark EJ, McNeely Bu (1986) Case records of the Massachusetts General Hospital: case 9–1986. N Engl J Med 314:629–640

Serrano D, Franceschi S (1996) Kaposi's sarcoma and non-Hodgkin's lymphomas in children and adolescents with AIDS. AIDS 10:643–647

Shafer RW, Chirgwin KD, Glatt AE et al (1991) HIV prevalence, immunosuppression and drug resistance in patients with tuberculosis in an area endemic for AIDS. AIDS 5:399–405

Shah RM, Salazar AM (1998) CT manifestations of HIV related pulmonary infections. Semin US CT MRI 19:167–174

Shen CS, Yunis EJ (1976) Leiomyosarcoma developing in a child during remission of leukemia. J Pediatr 89:780–782

Siskin GP, Haller JO, Miller J, Sundaram MD (1995) AIDS related lymphoma: radiologic features in pediatric patients. Radiology 196:63–63

Small PM, Schecter GF, Goodman PC, Sande MA, Chaisson RE, Hopewell PC (1991) Treatment of tuberculosis in patients with advanced human immunodeficiency virus infection. N Engl J Med 324:289–294

Staples CA, Kang EY, Wright JL et al (1995) Invasive pulmonary aspergillosis in AIDS: radiographic, CT and pathologic findings. Radiology 196:409–414

Suster B, Akerman M, Orenstein M et al (1986) Pulmonary manifestations of AIDS: review of 106 episodes. Radiology 161:87–93

Theologides A, Kennedy BJ (1966) Clinical manifestations of toxoplasmosis in the adult. Arch Intern Med 117:536–540

Walker D, Gill TJ, Corson JM (1991) Leiomyosarcoma in renal allograft recipient treated with immunosuppressive drugs. JAMA 215:2084–2086

Winchester R (1992) Invited commentary. Pediatr Radiol 22:606–607

Wollschlanger CM, Kahn FA, Chitkara RK et al (1984) Pulmonary manifestations of acquired immunodeficiency syndrome (AIDS). Chest 85:197–202

Wood BP (1992) Children with acquired immunodeficiency syndrome: radiographic features. Prog Clin Radiol 27:964–970

Zimmerman BL, Haller JO, Price AP et al (1987) Children with AIDS – is pathologic diagnosis possible based on chest radiographs? Pediatr Radiol 17:303–307

9 Advanced Techniques for Imaging the Pediatric Airway

Lane F. Donnelly and Janet L. Strife

CONTENTS

9.1 Introduction

Imaging of diseases affecting the central airways has been one of the unique areas in pediatric radiology. There have been marked advances in this field from the description of the findings of vascular rings on radiographs and fluoroscopic barium studies beginning in the 1950s to the development of advanced imaging studies such as magnetic resonance (MR) and computed tomography (CT) arteriography (BERDON and BAKER 1972; BERDON 2000; NEUHAUSER 1945).

The various advanced imaging techniques that can be used to image the airway are highly useful for different clinical scenarios. A simple categorization of airway pathology that frequently leads to imaging in children includes acute upper airway compromise,

chronic upper airway compromise, and chronic lower airway compromise. Acute upper airway compromise in children can be secondary to inflammatory conditions including croup, epiglottitis, and exudative tracheitis, or secondary to foreign body aspiration. With the exception of using CT to evaluate for retropharyngeal abscess, imaging in children with acute upper airway compromise is limited to radiography. Advanced imaging techniques play little or no role in the evaluation of children with acute upper airway compromise. The group of children with chronic upper airway compromise includes those with obstructive sleep apnea. In selective patients with obstructive sleep apnea, imaging with dynamic sleep fluoroscopy, and more recently with MR imaging (MRI) cine sleep studies, has been shown to influence management in over 50% of cases (GIBSON et al. 1996). Finally, children who present with symptoms of lower airway obstruction and are suspected of having extrinsic airway compression are often imaged with MRI or CT. This chapter will evaluate the following advanced imaging techniques: dynamic sleep fluoroscopy, MRI cine sleep studies, MRI (including MR arteriography), and helical CT (including CT arteriography).

9.2 Dynamic Sleep Fluoroscopy in Children with Obstructive Sleep Apnea

The first advanced imaging technique to be discussed is dynamic sleep fluoroscopy. It is estimated that up to 3% of all children, approximately 2 million in the US alone, are affected by obstructive sleep apnea syndrome (BROUILLETTE et al. 1982; OWENS et al. 1998). The most common cause of obstructive sleep apnea is enlarged adenoid and palatine tonsils in otherwise healthy children. In such children, the information most required can be obtained from the patient's history, a physical examination, and a lateral radiograph

LANE F. DONNELLY, MD, JANET L. STRIFE, MD
Department of Radiology, Children's Hospital Medical Center, 3333 Burnet Ave., Cincinnati, OH 45229-3039, USA

of the airway to evaluate the size of the adenoids and tonsils. Advanced imaging is typically not required in these patients. However, other causes of obstructive sleep apnea include craniofacial anomalies, congenital syndromes (particularly Down syndrome and achondroplasia), mucopolysaccharidosis, as well as prior surgery on the airway (GIBSON et al. 1996), and many of these patients are predisposed to airway obstruction at multiple sites (GIBSON et al. 1996). Polysomnography is helpful in differentiating between central versus obstructive causes of sleep apnea (ROSEN 1999; COLEMAN 1999). However, it provides no accurate information concerning the anatomic level of obstruction in children with obstructive sleep apnea. In cases of obstructive sleep apnea in which there is a complicated medical history or persistent sleep apnea following a surgical procedure performed to treat sleep apnea, dynamic sleep fluoroscopy has been shown to be a useful adjunct to endoscopic evaluation, affecting management decisions in over 50% of cases (GIBSON et al. 1996; DONNELLY et al. 2001a). It is particularly helpful in identifying dynamic abnormalities of the airway, such as functional collapse, as compared to static, fixed obstructions. Despite this, dynamic sleep fluoroscopy in children has received little attention in the imaging literature. In 1979, FELMAN et al. described their cinefluoroscopic technique in nine children using sleep deprivation. We have performed over 100 dynamic sleep fluoroscopy procedures in children utilizing sedation. The following describes the indications and technique for dynamic sleep fluoroscopy and the anatomic sites and common causes of airway obstruction.

9.3
Indications

When children present with symptoms of obstructive sleep apnea, any imaging evaluation typically includes frontal and lateral radiographs of the airway and chest, as well as flexible fiberoptic laryngoscopy. If extrinsic tracheal compression is suspected, cross sectional imaging with CT or MRI is usually performed. If an intrinsic or dynamic problem of the trachea is suspected, direct laryngoscopy and bronchoscopy under general anesthesia is usually performed.

One of the advantages of dynamic sleep fluoroscopy over flexible fiberoptic laryngoscopy is the ability to evaluate the entire airway simultaneously when the child is sleeping. We use sleep fluoroscopy to evaluate those children with complex medical histories who are at increased risk of multi-level airway obstruction. There are multiple disease processes that are associated with an increased risk of multi-level airway obstruction. In Down syndrome, airway obstruction can occur secondary to macroglossia, lymphoid hyperplasia, congenitally narrow nasopharynx, laryngomalacia, congenital subglottic stenosis, tracheobroncomalacia, or tracheal stenosis (JACOBS et al. 1996). Clinical evidence of airway obstruction may be secondary to any, or all, of these potential sites. Children with neuromuscular disorders are also at risk for airway collapse at multiple levels secondary to muscular hypotonia (ARNOLD and ALLPHIN 1993). Other children at risk for multilevel airway obstruction include those with congenital craniofacial anomalies, such as Pierre Robin syndrome, or metabolic disorders, such as the mucopolysaccharidoses (GIBSON et al. 1996). In children who have had previous surgery and have persistent sleep apnea, the problem may be related to residual obstruction secondary to the original cause or secondary to sequelae of the surgical manipulation of the airway (TOM et al. 1993). In some patients who have had tracheotomies, there may be difficulty with decannulation. These children may have episodes of apnea or respiratory distress during sleep secondary to development of granulation tissue or localized tracheomalacia at the surgical site or recurrence of the primary problem.

At our institution, indications for evaluation with dynamic sleep fluoroscopy include: (1) persistent symptoms of sleep apnea despite normal findings on flexible fiberoptic laryngoscopy, (2) persistent symptoms of sleep apnea after a single site of obstruction has been identified and appropriately treated, (3) potential for obstruction at more than one site within the upper airway because of either previous surgery or an underlying abnormality, and (4) difficulty decannulating a patient following tracheotomy (DONNELLY et al. 2001a).

9.3.1
Technique

The study is performed and monitored by a pediatric radiologist. Patients are prepared for the procedure according to our departmental sedation program guidelines (EGELHOFF et al. 1997). Although airway compromise is a relative contraindication to conscious sedation, we have not had a complication related to sedation in over 100 studies that we have performed. During the procedure, a radiologist, radiology technologist, and radiology nurse are present. Food and drink are withheld for 4–8 h prior to the examination to decrease the risk of aspiration. Patients are sedated with either oral chloral hydrate (70–100 mg/kg) or intravenous pentobarbital (3 mg/kg, with repeat dosing up to a total of 7 mg/kg) depending upon patient age. During the entire procedure and sedation recovery, respiratory rate, heart rate and rhythm, and blood oxygen saturation are monitored using transcutaneous pulse oximetry. The child's parents are allowed and encouraged to attend the procedure both to reduce the child's anxiety and to verify if the sleep patterns observed are typical of those which occur at home.

The studies are performed with lateral fluoroscopy. The children are imaged in supine position with lateral fluoroscopy. The fluoroscopic portions of the examinations are videotaped with simultaneous audiotaping so that fluoroscopic findings can be correlated with episodes of oxygen desaturation or noisy breathing. Physical observations, which are noted and correlated with fluoroscopic findings, include respiratory effort, thoracic wall motions, and episodes of apnea. Fluoroscopic evaluation is performed for approximately 10–20 s at areas of anatomic interest when signs of airway occlusion occur. The fluoroscopic evaluation of a child with sleep apnea should be performed at three specific sites: the level of the base of the tongue (oropharynx), the hypopharynx, and the intrathoracic trachea. Rarely, these three areas may be seen simultaneously. In larger children, the intrathoracic trachea may need to be evaluated separately from the hypopharynx. Evaluation of the oropharynx and hypopharynx are performed with the arms positioned at the child's sides. Downward pulling on the arms improves visualization of the neck. Evaluation of the intrathoracic trachea is best performed with the arms extended above the child's head.

Certain maneuvers may be performed during sleep fluoroscopy to further evaluate the obstruction. When present, tracheotomy tubes may be capped in order to see if the patient develops sleep apnea when the artificial airway is bypassed. The tracheotomy tube may also be removed to evaluate for underlying tracheomalacia, which can be masked when the tracheotomy tube is present and physically prevents the trachea from collapsing. In cases in which a child has a tracheotomy tube, which is to be intentionally removed or occluded during the study, an otolar-

yngologist is present to perform these maneuvers. When an area of airway obstruction is encountered, the effect of treatments, such as positive pressure breathing, on decreasing or eliminating the obstruction can be evaluated fluoroscopically.

9.3.2
Commonly Encountered Abnormalities

One of the advantages of sleep fluoroscopy is the evaluation of dynamic motion abnormalities in addition to static fixed causes of obstruction. In the normal sleeping child, there is little or no motion of the pharynx and trachea. Any significant dynamic motion of these structures encountered during sleep should be considered abnormal. Commonly encountered dynamic abnormalities include glossoptosis, pharyngeal collapse, laryngomalacia, and tracheomalacia. It must be stressed that such dynamic abnormalities can occur at multiple sites or in conjunction with fixed causes of airway obstruction.

The first line of treatment for many of these dynamic causes of obstructive sleep apnea is the use of positive pressure airway devices during sleep (Bower and Gungor 2000). Some of these types of obstructive sleep apnea will decrease with increasing age. Therefore, if positive pressure ventilation can relieve the symptoms, it may be the only necessary therapy until the child outgrows the condition. Knowledge of the specific abnormality is important as the odds of positive pressure therapy being helpful and the odds of the child outgrowing the condition are different for each specific entity. Therefore, the length of trial for conservative therapy may be influenced. In addition, when conservative management fails, there are specific types of surgery that can be performed which differ for each of the types of airway obstruction.

9.3.2.1
Adenoid Size

Enlargement of the adenoid tonsils is one of the more common components of obstructive sleep apnea in children (Fig. 9.1). However, determining what size constitutes an abnormally enlarged adenoid has been a subject of debate. Several studies have addressed the range of normal sizes of the adenoid tissues during childhood (Jaw et al. 1999; Vogler et al. 2000). The expected size of the adenoid tonsils changes with age. In newborns, no adenoid tissue may be appreci-

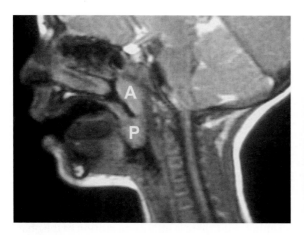

Fig. 9.1. Enlarged adenoid and palatine tonsils in a 2-year-old boy. Midline, sagittal fast gradient echo image shows the adenoid tissues (*A*) to be enlarged and almost obstructing the nasopharynx. The palatine tonsils (*P*) are also enlarged and seen abutting each other on this midline image

ated at imaging (JAW et al. 1999). There is a rapid proliferation of the adenoid tissues during infancy with a plateau in size varying from two to 14 years of age (JAW et al. 1999). The most typical age of maximal size is 7–10 years at which time the adenoid tissues may range from 10–15 mm in diameter on a lateral (or sagittal) image (VOGLER et al. 2000). Beginning in the second decade, the adenoids begin to decrease in size and continue to do so throughout adulthood (VOGLER et al. 2000).

9.3.2.2
Glossoptosis

Glossoptosis is defined as abnormal posterior motion of the tongue during sleep. It is seen most commonly in children with neuromuscular abnormalities, because of an abnormal decrease in muscular tone (DONNELLY et al. 2000a). It can also be associated with macroglossia such as in patients with Down syndrome (JACOBS et al. 1996; DONNELLY et al. 2000b; MARCUS et al. 1991) and micrognathia (such as occurs in patients with Pierre Robin syndrome; RODIGUEZ and DOGLIOTTI 1998; COZZI and PIERNO 1985) . On fluoroscopy, the tongue "falls" posteriorly during sleep, abutting the velum (soft palate) and posterior wall of the pharynx, obstructing the airway (DONNELLY et al. 2000a; Fig. 9.2). The posterior pharyngeal wall remains in a stationary position. Glossoptosis can be difficult to detect with endoscopic evaluation. Surgical interventions to either reduce the volume of the tongue or reposition the mandible have

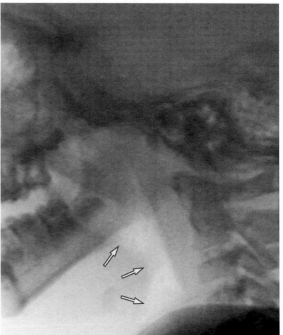

a

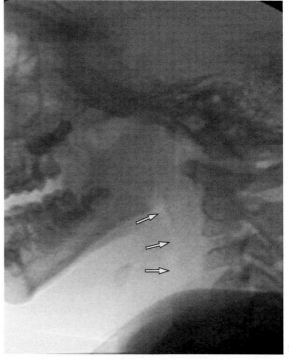

b

Fig. 9.2a,b. Glossoptosis in a 1-year-old boy with cerebral palsy. **a** Video-captured fluoroscopic image shows air within posterior pharynx between base of tongue (*arrows*) and posterior wall of pharynx. **b** Video-captured fluoroscopic image during an episode of oxygenation desaturation shows tongue to have moved posteriorly, such that posterior base of tongue (*arrows*) abuts posterior wall of pharynx obstructing airway. (Used with permission from DONNELLY et al. 2000a)

been described for those cases refractory to medical management (RODIGUEZ and DOGLIOTTI 1998; CHABOLLE et al. 1999).

9.3.2.3
Pharyngeal Collapse

Pharyngeal collapse is another commonly encountered cause of obstruction in this population and, like glossoptosis, can be difficult to detect endoscopically. On fluoroscopy, the anterior wall of the pharynx moves posteriorly and the posterior wall moves anteriorly (DONNELLY et al. 2001a; Fig. 9.3). This differs from glossoptosis in which only the tongue moves posteriorly. With pharyngeal collapse, the posterior pharyngeal wall, velum, and tongue oppose each other causing naso- and oropharyngeal obstruction. Pharyngeal collapse can be a primary abnormality related to decreased structural integrity of the supportive muscular and connective tissue elements of the pharynx, or may be a secondary phenomena related to increased negative pressure generated secondary to an additional site of airway obstruction. For example, a patient with airway obstruction secondary to enlarged palatine tonsils may demonstrate pharyngeal collapse secondary to the negative pressure created relative to the tonsilar obstruction.

9.3.2.4
Laryngomalacia and Tracheomalacia

Laryngomalacia and tracheomalacia are defined by abnormal collapse of the larynx or trachea during breathing secondary to a lack of normal structural integrity of the underlying cartilage. With both, the collapse typically occurs during inspiration. Both the larynx and trachea should be relatively still during sleep and any motion should be considered abnormal (DONNELLY et al. 2001a). With laryngomalacia, there is inferior indrawing of the pharynx and the epiglottis buckles and infolds over the tracheal inlet (Fig. 9.4), secondary to a lack of adequate cartilaginous support (DONNELLY et al. 2001a). Tracheomalacia can be focal or diffuse. With tracheomalacia, the trachea cyclically decreases in caliber (DONNELLY et al. 2001a; Fig. 9.5). Typically, the anterior wall of the trachea bows and collapses posteriorly more prominently than the posterior wall moves anteriorly. Tracheomalacia can occur as a primary weakness of the tracheal cartilage or secondary to extrinsic compression, such as by anomalous vascular structures or masses.

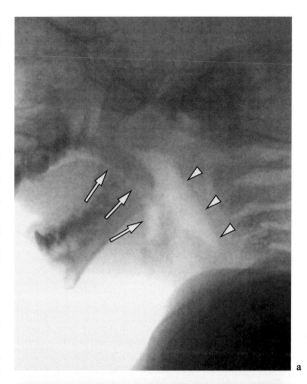

a

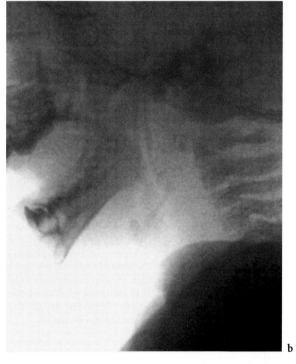

b

Fig. 9.3a,b. Pharyngeal collapse in a 1-year-old boy. **a** Video-captured fluoroscopic image shows normal air-filled space in posterior pharynx between posterior tongue (*arrows*) and posterior wall of pharynx (*arrowheads*). **b** Video-captured fluoroscopic image during an episode of oxygenation desaturation shows posterior motion of base of tongue and anterior motion of posterior wall of pharynx such that the hypopharynx is non-aerated

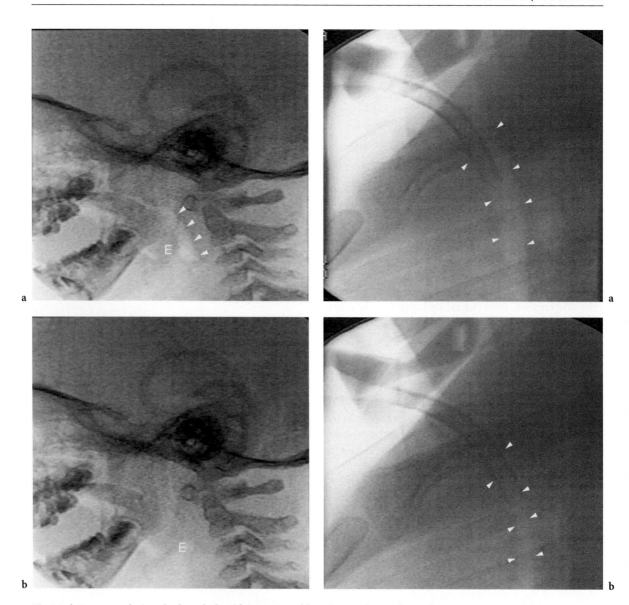

Fig. 9.4a,b. Laryngomalacia and enlarged adenoids in a 7-year-old girl with Down syndrome. **a** Video-captured fluoroscopic images obtained during sleep shows epiglottis (*E*) to be normally positioned with air-filled pharynx between epiglottis and posterior pharyngeal wall (*arrowheads*). The adenoid tonsils are enlarged. **b** Video-captured fluoroscopic image obtained during same respiratory cycle shows epiglottis (*E*) to have buckled, infolded over tracheal inlet, and moved posteriorly obliterating the air-filled pharynx and resulting in intermittent airway obstruction

Fig. 9.5a,b. Tracheomalacia in an 8-year-old boy with persistent sleep apnea despite tracheotomy placement. **a** Video-captured fluoroscopic images with tracheotomy tube in place shows normal caliber tracheal lumen between anterior (*arrows*) and posterior (*arrowheads*) walls of trachea. **b** Video-captured fluoroscopic image with tracheotomy tube in place during same respiratory cycle shows decreased caliber tracheal lumen between anterior (*arrows*) and posterior (*arrowheads*) walls of trachea

9.4
Dynamic Sleep MR Fluoroscopy in Children with Obstructive Sleep Apnea

In adults, there have been several publications suggesting that cine images created from fast gradient MR sequences can be utilized to dynamically evalu-ate the airway during sleep (SUTO et al. 1993, 1996; SHELOCK et al. 1992; JAGER et al. 1992). Little has been published in children. The advantages of using an MRI cine technique over conventional fluoroscopy include no radiation exposure, improved visualization, and evaluation of the airway dimensions in multiple plains. Disadvantages include cost and decreased access to a sedated child with a compromised airway.

One of the difficulties that we have when performing dynamic fluoroscopic sleep studies is that normal variations in motion of the upper airway during sleep have never been well defined. Very little has ever been published on the subject. At times, it is difficult to determine whether mild motion of the airway is pathologic or within the range of normal motion. It is unlikely that an X-ray fluoroscopy study of normal sleeping children would ever be performed because of the associated radiation dose. At the Children's Hospital Medical Center, we began using MR cine to evaluate physiologic motion of the normal airway in asymptomatic children during sleep (Fig. 9.6). To

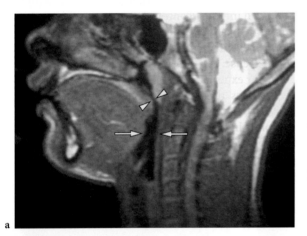

a

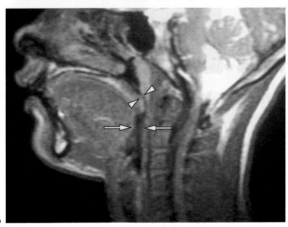

b

Fig. 9.6a,b. Variations in respiratory motion in an asymptomatic 5-year-old boy. **a,b** Sagittal midline fast gradient images (cine) show changes in the caliber of the hypopharynx (*arrows*) and posterior nasopharynx (*arrowheads*), between the soft palate and adenoid tonsils, at different points during the respiratory cycle. Such variations in caliber of the airway are not uncommonly encountered

perform MR cine studies, a single midline, sagittal fast gradient echo image was obtained in those children who were referred for MRI of the brain and required sedation for the examination. The airway images were obtained after the brain imaging was complete and additional sedation was not administered. We found that dynamic motion is commonly encountered in the nasopharynx (36%) and hypopharynx (49%) (Fig. 9.6). However, in no asymptomatic patients was intermittent, complete collapse of the hypopharynx present, as would be seen in symptomatic patients with hypopharyngeal collapse or glossoptosis.

Because of the superior quality of the images that we were obtaining in the studies using MR cine in the asymptomatic patients, our sleep apnea specialists began to request dynamic sleep MR fluoroscopy studies on patient's with obstructive sleep apnea. We our now performing these studies often in place of standard dynamic sleep fluoroscopy. When performing these studies, the child is placed in the head, neck, or torso array coil, depending on the size of the patient. Sedation is implemented in conjunction with our departmental guidelines. We obtain MR cine images in the sagittal midline plain as well as in the axial plain at the level of the hypopharynx and at the level of any abnormalities seen on the sagittal images. T1-weighted images are also obtained in the sagittal and axial plains. The cine images utilize a fast gradient echo sequence (flip angle 80, TR 8.2, TE 3.6, slice thickness 8 mm, 128 consecutive images obtained). The series takes approximately 2 min to obtain. The images are then loaded and displayed as a movie in cine format. Dynamic motion and changes in airway caliber can be evaluated in the sagittal and axial plains. Changes in airway cross-sectional area are calculated.

The clinical indications that we use for sleep MR cine studies are similar to those for dynamic sleep fluoroscopic studies: (1) persistent symptoms of sleep apnea despite normal findings on flexible fiberoptic laryngoscopy, (2) persistent symptoms of sleep apnea after a single site of obstruction has been identified and appropriately treated, and (3) potential for obstruction at more than one site within the upper airway because of either previous surgery or an underlying abnormality. The most commonly encountered entities are glossoptosis, pharyngeal collapse, and tracheomalacia. Criteria for these diagnoses are similar to those seen on dynamic fluoroscopic studies.

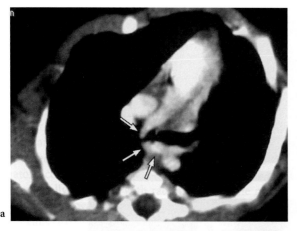

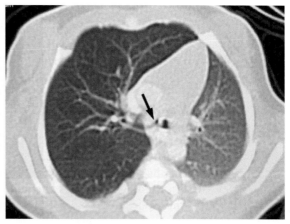

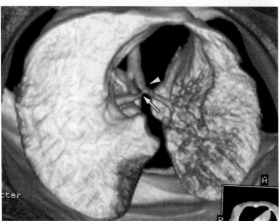

Fig. 9.8a–c. Anomalous origin of the pulmonary artery in a 2-week-old infant girl. The patient weighed 4 kg. For IV contrast injection, 8 cc of contrast were administered via a power injector at a rate of 3 cc/s. **a** Oblique axial computed tomography (CT) image shows an anomalous left pulmonary artery (*arrows*) passing from right to left posterior to the airway. **b** CT image shown at the lung windows demonstrates compression of the right main bronchus (*arrow*) just inferior to the level of the carina. There is asymmetric volume and density with the right lung larger than the left. **c** Surface rendered three-dimensional image shows compression of the right main bronchus (*arrow*) and narrowing of the distal trachea (*arrowhead*). Note asymmetrically larger right lung

tion, even in neonates. One of the most crucial parts of obtaining an optimally enhanced CT arteriogram is the timing of the onset of scanning in relationship to the administration of the contrast bolus. We initiate scanning approximately 10–15 s after administration of the contrast bolus is complete. We have found this timing to be conducive to obtaining images during the arterial rather than venous phase of imaging (FRUSH et al. 1998, 1999).

After images are obtained, they are evaluated in axial format as well as transferred to a work station. On the workstation, coronal and sagittal reformations and 3-D images are created tailored to the imaging findings seen on the axial images (Fig. 9.8). We find the 3-D and reformatted images are very helpful in communicating the imaging findings to the referring clinicians.

9.5.2
MRI for the Evaluation of Children with Suspected Airway Compression

For MRI evaluation of suspected airway compromise, the majority of our patients are evaluated under conscious sedation performed in compliance with our defined sedation program. However, the issue of conscious sedation in a child with a potentially compromised airway is always a consideration. In patients in whom we are not comfortable sedating ourselves, other options include performing the examination under general anesthesia or switching the examination to be performed with helical CT rather than with MRI. We have successfully performed a large number of MRI for airway evaluation under conscious sedation without adverse events.

Either the head coil or torso array coil is used according to patient size. We obtain T1-weighted images in the axial, coronal, sagittal, and sagittal oblique (in the plain of the aortic arch) plains. Most of these images are obtained with 3-mm slice thickness and 1-mm gap. In

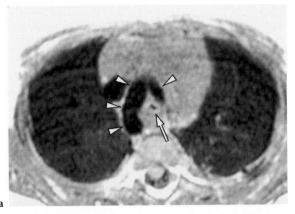

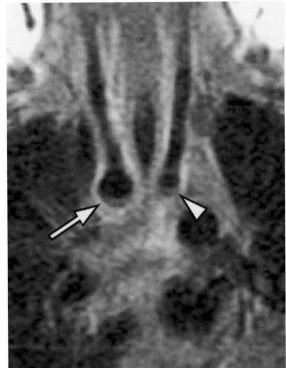

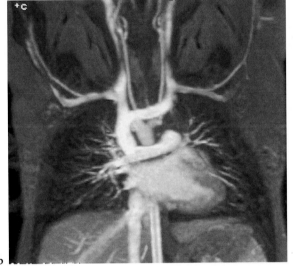

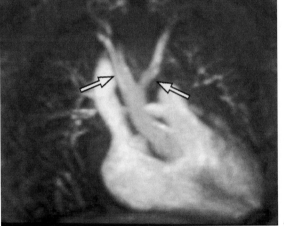

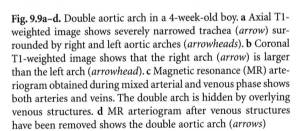

Fig. 9.9a–d. Double aortic arch in a 4-week-old boy. **a** Axial T1-weighted image shows severely narrowed trachea (*arrow*) surrounded by right and left aortic arches (*arrowheads*). **b** Coronal T1-weighted image shows that the right arch (*arrow*) is larger than the left arch (*arrowhead*). **c** Magnetic resonance (MR) arteriogram obtained during mixed arterial and venous phase shows both arteries and veins. The double arch is hidden by overlying venous structures. **d** MR arteriogram after venous structures have been removed shows the double aortic arch (*arrows*)

addition to the T1-weighted images, we obtain a double dose gadolinium enhanced MR arteriogram (Fig. 9.9). A 3-D spoiled gradient-recalled echo (SPGR) imaging sequence is utilized. The amount of gadolinium utilized is 4 ml/kg up to a total volume of 20 ml. We administer our gadolinium with hand injection. Imaging parameters for the 3-D SPGR sequence include: TR 500, TE full, bandwidth 31, field of view 36 cm, slice thickness 2.4 mm, number of locations 28, matrix 256×160, number of excitations 1, frequency superior to inferior, and true coronal plane. It takes 33 s to

obtain this sequence. We perform a test run prior to the administration to ensure that our anatomic locations are correct. We then obtain this sequence repeated with three phases (total of 139 s) with the initiation of imaging starting at the onset of contrast administration. Repeating the series three times ensures that we will obtain at least one series during the arterial phase of enhancement and one series during the mixed arterial and venous phases. Obtained images are evaluated as well as processed with a computer work station to create 3-D and reconstructed images.

9.5.3
Encountered Abnormalities in Children with Extrinsic Airway Obstruction

There are a number of well described vascular rings that can cause extrinsic airway compression in children. In addition, however, there are a large number of other causes of extrinsic compression that can also occur. Almost any structure in the superior mediastinum that is malpositioned or enlarged can cause compression of the central airways.

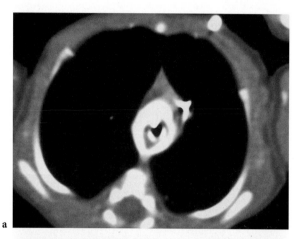

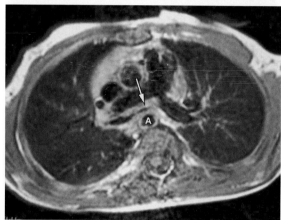

Fig. 9.10a,b. Double aortic arch in a 1-month-old boy. The patient then presented with recurrent symptoms at 17 months of age related to airway compression from midline descending aorta. **a** Computed tomography at 1 month of age demonstrates a double aortic arch. The child had an endotracheal tube in place. **b** Magnetic resonance imaging (axial, T1-weighted image) at 17 months of age shows the descending aorta (*A*) to be anterior to the vertebral bodies, rather than in the normal paraspinal area. The malpositioned descending aorta results in compression of the left main bronchus (*arrow*) between the aorta itself and the pulmonary artery

9.5.3.1
Well Described Vascular Cause of Airway Compression

The most commonly encountered vascular causes of tracheal compression include double aortic arch, other aortic arch anomalies, anomalous origin of the left pulmonary artery, and innominate artery compression syndrome.

Double aortic arch occurs secondary to persistence of both the right and left fourth aortic arches (BERDON and BAKER 1972; BERDON 2000; NEUHAUSER 1945) . The ring caused by the two arches causes compression, typically severe, of the trachea and sometimes esophagus (BERDON and BAKER 1972; BERDON 2000; NEUHAUSER 1945). Because of the severe nature of the tracheal compression, patients typically present with this condition early in life. Double aortic arch is typically an isolated lesion without other associated anomalies. On cross-sectional imaging, the right and left aortic arches are readily apparent as is the severe narrowing of the trachea just above the carina (Figs. 9.9, 9.10). Important presurgical information includes the relative sizes of the two aortic arches. The thoracotomy and surgical ligation will be performed on the side of the smaller aortic arch. Typically, the right arch is the larger and more superior located than the left arch (BERDON and BAKER 1972; BERDON 2000; NEUHAUSER 1945).

With anomalous origin of the left pulmonary artery (pulmonary sling), the left pulmonary artery arises from the right pulmonary artery rather than the typical origin off the main pulmonary artery (BERDON and BAKER 1972; BERDON et al. 1984). The abnormal origin leads to the left pulmonary artery passing between the trachea and esophagus as it courses leftward, rather the normal position anterior to the trachea (BERDON and BAKER 1972; BERDON et al. 1984). The left pulmonary artery results in compression of the posterior aspect of the distal trachea and anterior compression of the esophagus. It is the only vascular anomaly to compress the trachea posteriorly. Patients typically present prior to 6 months of age and there are often associated cardiac anomalies (BERDON et al. 1984). It is the only vascular ring that is associated with asymmetric aeration of the lungs seen on chest radiography or CT. On cross-sectional imaging, the anomalous course of the pulmonary artery and resultant tracheal compression are identified (see Fig.9. 8). Pulmonary sling can also be associated with complete tracheal rings (BERDON et al. 1984). On cross-sectional imaging, in areas of complete tracheal rings, the trachea appear small in caliber and round, as compared to the normal oval configuration.

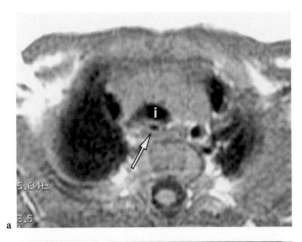

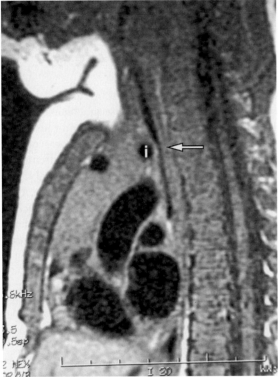

Fig. 9.11a,b. Innominate artery compression syndrome in a 4-month-old girl. **a,b** Axial (**a**) and sagittal (**b**) T1-weighted images show compression of the trachea (*arrow*) at the level of the innominate artery (*arrowhead*). *i*, Innominate artery

Innominate artery compression syndrome is a controversial diagnosis that is related to narrowing of the trachea at the level of the artery (BERDON et al. 1969). The finding represents a spectrum from normal asymptomatic children with slight compression of the trachea at this level to those infants who are severely symptomatic. The airway compromise related to this disorder tends to decrease with time,

as the infant grows. Because of this, surgical therapy is reserved for only the most severe cases. On cross-section imaging, narrowing of the trachea from its anterior aspect is identified at the level of the innominate artery (Fig. 9.11).

9.5.3.2
Other Causes of Airway Compression

As stated above, there are a number of other causes of airway compression that do not occur uncommonly in children. Because of the confined space of the superior mediastinum, almost any abnormally enlarged structure, malpositioned structure, or mediastinal mass has the potential to cause airway obstruction (DONNELLY et al. 1997). In many tertiary centers, where children with multiple medical problems are commonly referred, these other causes of airway compression may be encountered at rates similar to the classic vascular rings. The more commonly encountered other causes of airway compression include: enlarged ascending aorta, malpositioned descending aorta, enlarged pulmonary arteries, enlarged left atrium, nonvascular mediastinal masses, and abnormalities of chest wall configuration (DONNELLY et al. 1997; DONNELLY and BISSET 1998; DONNELLY and FRUSH 1999).

Enlargement of the ascending aorta can cause anterior compression of the distal airway (CAPITANIO et al. 1983). Causes include aneurysms, such as in Marfan's syndrome or cystic medial necrosis, post-stenotic aortic dilatation, and disorders which increase cardiac stroke volume such as tetralogy of Fallot (CAPITANIO et al. 1983).

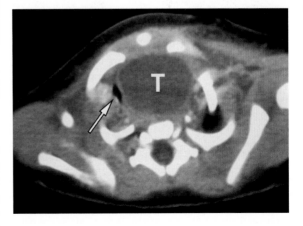

Fig. 9.12. Thymic cyst presenting as airway compression in a 5-day-old male infant. Computed tomography shows a cystic mass (*T*) displacing and compressing the trachea (*arrow*)

When the descending aorta is abnormally located immediately anterior to the spine instead of the normal left intraspinal location, there is abnormal stacking of mediastinal structures in the confined space between the anterior chest wall and spine. This leads to compression of the distal airway between the pulmonary artery and the malpositioned descending aorta (DONNELLY et al. 1995; see Fig. 9.10). Causes include midline descending aorta–carina compression syndrome (DONNELLY et al. 1995), right aortic arch with left descending aorta (ERGIN et al. 1981), left aortic arch with right descending aorta, and unilateral hypoplastic right lung (DOHLEMANN et al. 1991).

Enlarged pulmonary arteries can compress the airway against the descending aorta/spine (DITCH-FIELD and CULHAM 1995). Causes include left-to-right shunts, pulmonary arterial hypertension, and congenital absence of the pulmonic valve (DITCHFIELD and CULHAM 1995). Left atrial enlargement can compress the left main bronchus. Causes of left atrial enlargement in children include cardiomyopathy, myocarditis, large left-to-right shunts, and mitral insufficiency.

In children, diagnostic considerations include chronic esophageal foreign bodies, enteric duplication cysts, or other middle mediastinal masses (Fig. 9.12) such as bronchogenic cysts or lymphadenopathy. Anterior or posterior mediastinal masses can also compress the middle mediastinum and airway, if they are large enough (AURINGER et al. 1991; DONNELLY et al. 1997).

Abnormal thoracic configuration can be associated with a narrow anterior–posterior chest diameter that can directly compress the trachea between the manubrium and spine. Also, abnormal thoracic configuration can lead to alteration in the anatomic relationship between the airway and adjacent structures resulting in abnormal anterior to posterior "stacking" of mediastinal structures and resultant tracheal compression (Fig. 9.13). The most common locations of airway obstruction related to abnormal thoracic configuration includes the trachea at the thoracic inlet and the proximal left main bronchus (DONNELLY et al. 1997; DONNELLY and BISSET 1998; DONNELLY and FRUSH 1999).

9.6 Summary

There a number of clinical scenarios in children with central airway compromise in which advanced imaging techniques currently can play a role. These include the use of dynamic sleep fluoroscopy or dynamic MR sleep fluoroscopy in children with obstructive sleep apnea and the use of helical CT or MRI in children with lower airway compromise. All of the techniques require intensive physician participation in relation to the technical parameters of the studies as well issues related to the use of sedation in children with airway compromise.

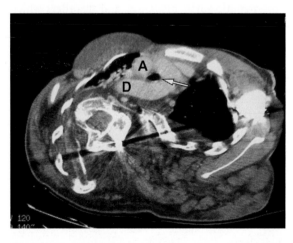

Fig. 9.13. Thoracic deformity leading to airway compression in a 19-year-old with severe scoliosis. Computed tomography shows severe deformity of the thorax with small right hemithorax and vertebral bodies oriented to the right. This resulted in the descending aorta (*D*) being positioned extremely rightward. As a result, the ascending aorta (*A*) and aortic arch form a sling around the trachea (*arrow*) leading to its compression

References

Arnold JE, Allphin AL (1993) Sleep apnea in the neurologically-impaired child. Ear Nose Throat J 72:80–81

Auringer ST, Bisset GS III, Myer CM III (1991) Magnetic resonance imaging of the pediatric airway. Pediatr Radiol 21:329–332

Berdon WE (2000) Rings, slings, and other things: vascular compression of the infant trachea updated from midcentury to the millennium – the legacy of Robert E. Gross, MD and Edward B. D. Neuhauser, MD. Radiology 216:624–632

Berdon WE, Baker DH (1972) Vascular anomalies and the infant lung: rings, slings, and other things. Semin Roentgenol 7:39–63

Berdon WE, Baker DH, Bordiuk J, Mellins R (1969) Innominate artery compression of the trachea in infants with stridor and apnea. Radiology 92:272–278

Berdon WE, Baker DH, Wung JT et al (1984) Complete cartilage ring tracheal stenosis associated with anomalous left pulmonary artery: "the ring sling complex". Radiology 15:57–64

Bower CM, Gungor A (2000) Pediatric obstructive sleep apnea syndrome. Otolaryngol Clin North Am 33:49–75

Brouillette RT, Fernbach SK, Hunt CE (1982) Obstructive sleep apnea in infants and children. J Pediatr 100:31–40

Capitanio MA, Wolfson BJ, Faerber EN, Williams JL, Balsara RK (1983) Obstruction of the airway by the aorta: an observation in infants with congenital heart disease. AJR 140:675–679

Chabolle F, Wagner I, Blumen MB, Sequert C, Fleury B, De Dieuleveult T (1999) Tongue base reduction with hyo-epiglottoplasty: a treatment for severe obstructive sleep apnea. Laryngoscope 109:1273–1280

Coleman J (1999) Disordered breathing during sleep in newborns, infants, and children. Symptoms, diagnosis, treatment. Otolaryngol Clin North Am 32:211–222

Cozzi F, Pierno A (1985) Glossoptosis–apnea syndrome in infancy. Pediatrics 75:836–843

Ditchfield MR, Culham JAG (1995) Assessment of airway compression by MR imaging in children with aneurysmal pulmonary arteries. Pediatr Radiol 25:190–191

Dohlemann C, Mantel K, Schneider K et al (1991) Deviated trachea in hypoplasia and aplasia of the right lung: airway obstruction and its release by aortopexy. J Pediatr Surg 25:290–293

Donnelly LF, Bisset GS III (1998) Airway compression in children with abnormal thoracic configuration. Radiology 206:323–326

Donnelly LF, Frush DP (1999) Abnormalities of the chest wall in pediatric patients. AJR 173:1595–1601

Donnelly LF, Bisset GS III, McDermott B (1995) Anomalous midline location of the descending aorta: a cause of compression of the carina and left mainstem bronchus in infants. AJR 165:705–707

Donnelly LF, Strife JL, Bisset GS III (1997) The spectrum of extrinsic lower airway compression in children: MR imaging. AJR 168:59–62

Donnelly LF, Strife JL, Myer CM (2000a) Glossoptosis (posterior displacement of the tongue) during sleep: a frequent cause of sleep apnea in pediatric patients referred for dynamic sleep fluoroscopy. AJR 175:1557–1559

Donnelly LF, Jones BV, Strife JL (2000b) Imaging of pediatric tongue abnormalities. AJR 175:489–493

Donnelly LF, Strife JL, Myer CM (2001a) Dynamic sleep fluoroscopy in children with obstructive sleep apnea. Appl Radiol (in press)

Donnelly LF, Emery KH, Brody AS, Laor T, Gylys-Morin VM, Anton CG, Thomas SR, Frush DP (2001b) Minimizing radiation dose for pediatric body application of single-detector helical CT: strategies at a large children's hospital. AJR 176:303–306

Egelhoff HC, Ball WS, Koch BL, Parks TD (1997) Safety and efficacy of sedation in children using a structured sedation program. AJR 168:1259–1262

Ergin MA, Jayaram N, LaCorte M (1981) Left aortic arch and right descending aorta: diagnostic and therapeutic implications of a rare type of vascular ring. Ann Thorac Surg 31:82–85

Felman AH, Louhlin GM, Leftridge CA, Cassisi NJ (1979) Upper airway obstruction during sleep in children. AJR 133:213–316

Frush DP, Donnelly LF (1998) State of the art. Spiral CT: technical consideration and applications in children. Radiology 209:37–48

Frush DP, Spencer EB, Donnelly LF, Zheng JY, Delong DM, Bisset GB III (1999) Optimizing contrast-enhanced abdominal CT in infants and children using bolus tracking. AJR 172:1007–1013

Gibson SE, Myer CM III, Strife JL, O'Connor DM (1996) Sleep fluoroscopy for localization of upper airway obstruction in children. Ann Otol Rhinol Laryngol 105:678–683

Jacobs IN, Gray RF, Todd NW (1996) Upper airway obstruction in children with Down's syndrome. Arch Otolaryngol Head Neck Surg 9:945–950

Jaffe R (1990) MRI of vascular rings. Semin Ultrasound CT MRI 11:206–220

Jager L, Gunther E, Gauger J, Reiser M (1998) Fluoroscopic MR of the pharynx in patients with obstructive sleep apnea. Am J Neuroradiol 19:1205–1214

Jaw TS, Sheu RS, Lie GC, Lin WC (1999) Development of adenoids: a study by measurement with MR images. Kao Hsiung I Hsueh Ko Hsueh Tsa Chih 15:8–12

Katz M, Konen E, Rozenman J, Szeinberg A, Itzchak Y (1995) Spiral CT and 3D image reconstruction of vascular rings and associated tracheobronchial anomalies. J Comput Assist Tomogr 19:564–568

Marcus CL, Keens TG, Bautista DB, von Pechmann WS, Ward SL (1991) Obstructive sleep apnea in children with Down syndrome. Pediatrics 88:132–139

Neuhauser EBD (1945) The roentgen diagnosis of double aortic archa nd other anomalies. AJR 56:1–12

Owens J, Opipari L, Nobile C, Spirito A (1998) Sleep and daytime behavior in children with obstructive sleep apnea and behavioral sleep disorders. Pediatrics 102:1178–1184

Pappas JN, Donnelly LF, Frush DP (2000) Reduced frequency of sedation of young children with multisection helical CT. Radiology 215:897–899

Rodriguez JC, Dogliotti P (1998) Mandibular distraction in glossoptosis-micrognathic association: preliminary report. J Craniofac Surg 9:127–129

Rosen CL (1999) Clinical features of obstructive sleep apnea hypoventilation syndrome in otherwise healthy children. Pediatr Pulmonol 27:403–409

Shelock FG, Schatz CJ, Julien P, Steinberg F, Foo TKF, Hopp MK, Westbrook PR (1992) Occlusion and narrowing of the pharyngeal airway in obstructive sleep apnea: evaluation by ultrafast spoiled GRASS MR imaging. AJR 158:1019–1024

Suto Y, Matsuo T, Kato T et al (1993) Evaluation of the pharyngeal airway in patients with sleep apnea: value of ultrafast MR imaging. AJR 160:311–314

Suto Y, Masuda E, Inoue Y, Suzuki T, Ohta Y (1996) Sleep apnea syndrome: comparison of MR imaging of the oropharynx with physiologic indexes. Radiology 201:393–398

Tom LW, Miller L, Wetmore RF, Handler SD, Potsic WP (1993) Endoscopic assessment in children with tracheotomies. Arch Otolaryngo Head Neck Surg 119:321–324

Vogler RC, Ii FJ, Pilgram TK (2000) Age specific size of the normal adenoid pad on magnetic resonance imaging. Clin Otolaryngol 25:392–395

10 Imaging of Foreign Body Aspiration in the Respiratory Tract

Jacob Bar-Ziv, Benjamin Ze'ev Koplewitz, Ronit Agid

CONTENTS

10.1
Introduction

Aspiration of foreign bodies into the respiratory tract can occur at any age, but is most common in young children and in the elderly population. Foreign body aspiration is the most frequent pediatric domestic accident, and has serious and sometimes fatal sequelae (BLACK et al. 1994; FITZPATRICK and GUARISCO 1998). Most cases occur under the age of 4 years (MANTEL and BUTENANDT 1986; ESCLAMADO and RICHARDSON 1987; PIEPSZ 1988; OGUZ et al. 2000). When the history of a foreign body aspiration is definite, bronchoscopy is the modality of choice for both diagnosis and management. Until recently, rigid or flexible bronchoscopy was used for diagnosis, while removal of foreign bodies was carried out by rigid bronchoscopy only (FRIEDMAN 2000). With

JACOB BAR-ZIV, MD
Professor and Chairman, Department of Radiology, Hadassah Medical Organization, Faculty of Medicine, The Hebrew University, Jerusalem, P.O.Box 12000, Jerusalem 91120, Israel
BENJAMIN ZE'EV KOPLEWITZ, MD, BSc
Department of Radiology, Hadassah Medical Organization, Clinical Instructor, Faculty of Medicine, The Hebrew University, P.O. Box 12000, Jerusalem 91120, Israel
RONIT AGID, MD
Department of Radiology, Hadassah Medical Organization, Clinical Instructor, Faculty of Medicine, The Hebrew University, P.O. Box 12000, Jerusalem 91120, Israel

the advance of technology, removal of foreign bodies can now be done by flexible bronchoscopy, which is a shorter and safer procedure. The complication rate of bronchoscopy varies between 1%–8 % (BLACK et al. 1984; STEEN and ZIMMERMANN 1990; ZERELLA et al. 1998), and the mortality rate is as low as 0.25%–1% (MU et al. 1990; STEEN and ZIMMERMANN 1990; HOEVE and ROMBOUT 1992).

In many cases, however, the aspiration event is not witnessed, and the classical triad of choking, cough and wheeze is missing. Diagnosis is then delayed or overlooked, and many children present with unresolved pneumonia, atelectasis or other complications. The role of the radiologist in cases of foreign body aspiration is not only to confirm a clinically suspected diagnosis, but also to suggest the diagnosis in patients with non-specific clinical symptoms and radiologic features that could be related to long-standing foreign bodies. Often the radiologist is the first to raise the possibility of foreign body aspiration.

This chapter discusses imaging techniques and findings related to the various types and mechanisms of obstruction and to the complications of foreign body aspiration.

10.2
Etiology/Types of Foreign Bodies

Most cases of foreign body aspiration occur between the age of 6 months and 3 years, with the highest incidence during the second year of life (MANTEL and BUTENANDT 1986; PIEPSZ 1988; FITZPATRICK and GUARISCO 1998). Infants and toddlers in this age group are already ambulatory and can therefore "disappear" from parent or guardian supervision for varying periods of time. They tend to act as "vacuum cleaners", and examine new objects of any size or shape by inserting them into their mouth. The combination of natural curiosity, lack of posterior dentition, inadequate control of deglutition and a startle response facilitates entry of solids into the larynx (WITT 1985; BYARD 1994). The size and variety of objects that can pass through the vocal cords are quite astonishing (Fig. 10.1).

Food particles and organic materials constitute the vast majority of aspirated objects (BLAZER et al. 1980; KEITH et al. 1980; TEIXIDOR DE OTTO et al. 1980; SVENSSON 1985; MANTEL and BUTENANDT 1986; PIEPSZ 1988; MU et al. 1990; LINEGAR et al. 1992; BLACK et al. 1994; BAHARLOO et al. 1999; METRANGELO et al. 1999). The nature of the aspirated material varies according to geographic and sociologic circumstances. Peanuts are the most common aspirated particles in North America, Europe and South Africa (TEIXIDOR DE OTTO et al. 1980; MANTEL and BUTENANDT 1986; MU et al. 1990; LINEGAR et al. 1992), whereas sunflower and watermelon seeds are more common in the Middle East (FARKASH et al. 1982; ELHASSANI 1988; OGUZ et al. 2000; PASAOGLU et al. 1991). Due to their high protein concentration, most organic foreign bodies absorb water from bronchial secretions and tend to increase in size. Candies have been reported to have a similar effect due to their high sugar concentration (MEARNS and ENGLAND 1975). Oil, salt and vegetable proteins in cooked food irritate the mucosa, causing edema and formation of granulation tissue with resultant narrowing of the bronchial lumen. Hence, an organic foreign body can grow to be larger than the original diameter of the bronchus, and what was initially a partial obstruction can progress to become a complete obstruction (AYTAC et al. 1977; CATANEO et al. 1997).

Grass inhalation is not uncommon and has some

unique characteristics. The literature contains reports describing aspiration of several types of grass heads, all with the same structure of side spurs along the main stem. When inhaled stump-first, the spikes carry the grass heads distally into the bronchial tree and lung parenchyma. Being resistant to organic decay, they can remain in the chest for a long time and can cause unusual infections, as well as other complications (SPENCER et al. 1981; MAAYAN et al. 1993; DINDAR et al. 1994; BASOK et al. 1997; NEWSON et al. 1998).

Non-organic objects comprise 5%–9% of the foreign bodies aspirated by children (FARKASH et al. 1982). Of these, coins are the most common (REILLY and WALTER 1992), followed by plastic toy pieces and sharp objects such as pencils and pull-tabs from aluminum cans (ROGERS and IGINI 1975; BURRINGTON 1976; BLAZER et al. 1980; STRICKLAND et al. 1987). Inert foreign bodies have little effect on the bronchial mucosa and, unless they cause an obstruction by virtue of their size, can remain undiagnosed for long periods of time. Aspiration of pacifiers is not uncommon among toddlers (JAIN et al. 1986; BARRETT and DEBELLE 1995). Partially inflated balloons are particularly hazardous (ANAS and PERKIN 1983; ABDEL-RAHMAN 2000).

A tooth can be aspirated by a sleeping child at the age of permanent tooth eruption. This happened to a 10-year-old girl who had a loose deciduous tooth when she fell asleep at night. When she woke up the next morning the tooth had disappeared from her mouth. The episode was forgotten; 10 days later she developed symptoms of left lower lobe pneumonia, with no response to antibiotic therapy over several months. When she was admitted to the hospital, the missing tooth was evident in the left lower lobe bronchus on a chest radiograph, with atelectasis of most of the basal segments (Fig. 10.2). The tooth was removed by bronchoscopy; 2 months later residual bronchiectatic changes could still be seen in the left lower lobe.

Aspiration of tooth and dental fillings can also occur during anesthesia, dental treatment (STEELMAN et al. 1997), and intubation or resuscitation procedures, especially in victims of road traffic accidents.

Aspiration of gravel, dirt or sand can happen during a traffic accident or in a cave-in (BERGESON et al. 1978; WALES et al. 1983; AVITAL et al. 1989; CHOY and IDOWU 1996). Airway obstruction has also been reported as a result of non-accidental trauma, when forcible introduction of a foreign body caused tracheal obstruction, with a resultant death reported in one case (NOLTE 1993; BARRETT and DEBELLE 1995).

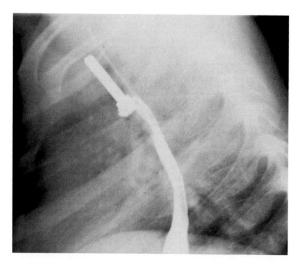

Fig. 10.1. Lateral view of a barium swallow shows a metallic bolt in the trachea of a 2-year-old boy

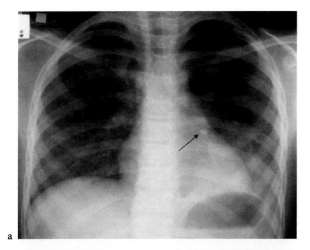

a

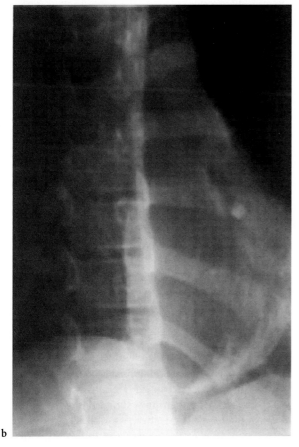

b

Fig. 10.2. Posteroanterior chest radiograph (**a**) of a 10-year-old girl and an oblique view (**b**) (obtained at fluoroscopy): A deciduous tooth (*arrow*) is present in the left lower lobe bronchus obstructing some of the basal segments and causing volume loss. Bronchiectasis, evident in the left lower lobe, is better demonstrated by the oblique projection

Aspiration of headscarf needles has been reported in adolescents in Islamic countries (UCAN et al. 1996; KAPTANOGLU et al. 1999).

10.3
Mechanisms of Airway Obstruction

A foreign body in the respiratory tract does not necessarily cause an obstruction, i.e. air can be inhaled and exhaled freely around the foreign body. This is known as a "two-way valve mechanism", and occurs when the foreign body, which is usually located in the trachea, is small in relation to the airway. A foreign body can cause complete obstruction when air entry is blocked during inspiration and the air cannot be exhaled during expiration. This is called a "no-way valve mechanism". A foreign body can allow air entry during inspiration but prevent the exit of air during expiration in a "one-way valve mechanism". This mechanism is explained by the larger diameter of the airway during inspiration due to higher intrathoracic negative pressure, and the smaller diameter during expiration.

Chest X-rays performed in cases of a non-obstructive tracheal or bronchial foreign body demonstrate uniform aeration bilaterally both in inspiration and expiration. In partial obstruction due to the one-way valve mechanism, the chest radiograph usually demonstrates air-trapping. Inspiratory films are often normal, and the air-trapping may become evident only in an expiratory study. In cases of complete airway obstruction (most commonly at the level of a bronchus), we often notice a combination of air-trapping in the non-dependent lobes with atelectasis of the dependent lobes. This is due to mucus plugging and the accumulation of secretions in the bronchial tree of the dependent segments (Fig. 10.3).

The incidence of right and left bronchial foreign bodies is almost equal in infants and children (MU et al. 1990; BLACK et al. 1994; BURTON et al. 1996; CATANEO et al. 1997; SENKAYA et al. 1997; METRANGELO et al. 1999; OGUZ et al. 2000), as opposed to predominance of the right bronchial tree in adults (BAHARLOO et al. 1999). The only slightly higher incidence of foreign bodies in the right bronchial tree in children is explained by the almost symmetrical tracheobronchial angle in this age group (CLEVELAND 1979). Migration of a small foreign body within the airways during different phases of the respiratory cycle, secondary to alterations of posture or following cough

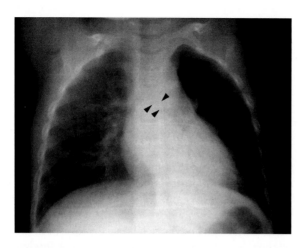

Fig. 10.3. A 3-year-old girl had cough and fever for 2 weeks. The history of an episode of choking on an almond was obtained from the mother following repeated questioning. Anteroposterior film using high kilovoltage copper filter technique demonstrates a segment in the left main bronchus deficient of air (*arrowheads*) and atelectasis of left lower lobe, with air-trapping in the left upper lobe. Notice air bronchogram in the atelectatic left lower lobe, in keeping with peripheral type of atelectasis. Bronchoscopy revealed a piece of almond in the proximal left main bronchus

is rare, but does occur, and can change the clinical and imaging findings (METRANGELO et al. 1999). The authors witnessed a case in which a foreign body that was located in the right main bronchus migrated to the right upper lobe bronchus when the father of the child turned her upside down in an attempt to expel the foreign body from the airway. Since in those days only rigid bronchoscopy was available, the foreign body could not be endoscopically removed and the patient required thoracotomy and lobectomy.

10.4
Clinical Findings and Differential Diagnosis

The clinical manifestations of aspirated foreign bodies vary according to the location and degree of obstruction.

Laryngeal and subglottic foreign bodies make up about 5% of foreign bodies in the airways (MANTEL and BUTENANDT 1986; ESCLAMADO and RICHARDSON 1987; COHEN et al. 1993; BLACK et al. 1994; BAHARLOO et al. 1999). When large enough, their presence in the major airway causes dyspnea, and when located adjacent to the vocal cords they may induce hoarseness, sudden loss of voice and inspiratory stridor

(BLAZER et al. 1980; HANUKOGLU et al. 1986; LAKS and BARZILAY 1988). Cyanosis may occur secondary to laryngeal spasm (HALVORSON et al. 1996; BAHARLOO et al. 1999). Similar symptoms can be induced by other processes such as a laryngeal web (CHEN et al. 1998), viral or bacterial croup, epiglottitis, papilloma or hemangioma, angioneurotic edema, or hypocalcemic tetany (GRAD and TAUSSIG 1990).

Tracheal foreign bodies constitute 4%–13% of foreign bodies in the airways (MU et al. 1990; BLACK et al. 1994; BURTON et al. 1996; METRANGELO et al. 1999). In one series, they represented 23% of the cases with early diagnosis and 7% of the cases with late diagnosis (OGUZ et al. 2000). In most patients there is a history of choking and dyspnea, yet they tend to be diagnosed later than bronchial foreign bodies, probably because they cause less severe respiratory symptoms (ESCLAMADO and RICHARDSON 1987). Inspiratory stridor and wheeze can also be caused by tracheomalacia or external compression on the trachea by a vascular structure (vascular ring, sling, etc.), bronchogenic cyst, enlarged lymph nodes (secondary to viral or bacterial infection or due to tuberculosis), mediastinal tumors (e.g., lymphoma), or an esophageal foreign body (Fig. 10.4).

The majority of aspirated foreign bodies (67%–80%) are found in the main bronchi (BLAZER et al. 1980; MANTEL and BUTENANDT 1986). A history of sudden choking is the most important clue for diagnosis (FARKASH et al. 1982; ESCLAMADO et al. 1987; SILVA et al. 1998; ZERELLA et al. 1998; METRANGELO et al. 1999; OGUZ et al. 2000). Such a history, however, was documented in only about one third of the cases in one series (OGUZ et al. 2000). The classical triad of a choking episode, cough and wheeze was found in over 90% of the patients in another series (BLAZER et al. 1980). Hemoptysis can be a presenting symptom (even in cases of a blunt foreign body) (SCULLY et al. 1983; MAAYAN et al. 1993; FABIAN and SMITHERINGALE 1996; CATANEO et al. 1997). Physical examination will reveal unequal chest expansion during inspiration, as well as decreased breath sounds over the obstructed lung (LAKS and BARZILAY 1988; OGUZ et al. 2000). Occasionally, a slapping sound of a loose foreign body can be heard (FELMAN 1982).

In cases of delayed diagnosis, pneumonia is a common presentation. The presence of an aspirated foreign body should be suspected in any patient with unexplained chronic pulmonary symptoms. Foreign body aspiration, however, is by no means the most common cause of recurrent pneumonia. Recurrent

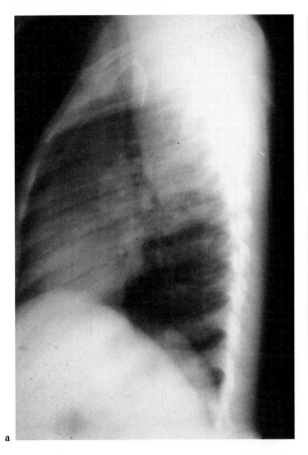

a

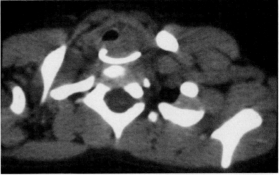

b

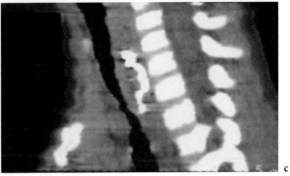

c

Fig. 10.4a–c. A 4-year-old child with stridor. Lateral chest radiograph (a), axial chest CT (b) and sagittal reconstructions (c) demonstrate a clam shell in the esophagus causing severe tracheal narrowing

pneumonia can also result from impaired clearance of secretions from the tracheo-bronchial tree as in asthma, ciliary dysmotility, cystic fibrosis, infected bronchiectasis or secondary to an immune deficiency. Tumors of the tracheo-bronchial tree are uncommon in children, but, when present, may cause a varying degree of airway obstruction.

Esophageal foreign bodies can mimic foreign bodies in any location of the airway due to external compression of the larynx, trachea or bronchi (Fig. 10.4). Such compression may cause laryngeal or tracheal spasm, resulting in respiratory distress, stridor or wheeze (SMITH et al. 1974). A tracheo-esophageal fistula may develop as a result of a decubitus ulcer caused by an esophageal foreign body of long-standing duration (SZOLD et al. 1991).

Nasal foreign bodies, when present for a long time, usually cause swelling of the nostrils or nasal discharge that may be foul smelling. They can ulcerate and damage the nasal septum or dislodge into the nasopharynx and be aspirated into the tracheo-bronchial tree (COHEN et al. 1993; FINI-STORCHI and NINU 1996).

10.5
Imaging Techniques

The plain chest X-ray remains the initial study in the evaluation of a suspected aspirated foreign body. Abnormal findings are found in 50%–65% of chest X-rays in children with proven foreign bodies (LAKS and BARZILAY 1988; MU et al. 1990; BLACK et al. 1994; OGUZ et al. 2000). These rates increase when using inspiratory–expiratory techniques (BLACK et al. 1984, 1994; LOSEK 1990). Opaque foreign bodies are easily identified, but most are radiolucent (see Figs. 10.1 and 10.3).

In cases of a non-opaque foreign body, inspiratory and expiratory films can provide important information. Comparison of the two hemithoraces is mandatory. The inspiratory film is often normal or near normal, while the expiratory film shows obvious airtrapping. The obstructed lung is of larger volume and more radiolucent. The decrease in ventilation of the obstructed lobe causes an increase in pCO_2. The higher pCO_2 leads to arterial vasoconstriction and therefore to reduced pulmonary perfusion. Thus,

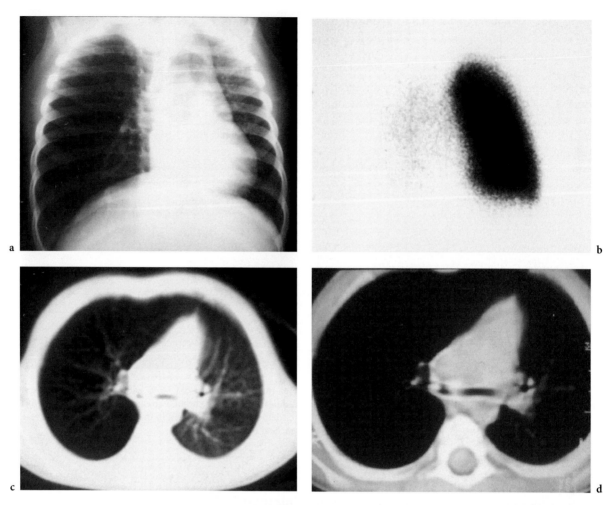

Fig. 10.5a–d. A 20-month-old boy had a choking episode. Initial chest radiograph (**a**) demonstrated obstructive emphysema of the right lung; bronchoscopy failed to reveal a foreign body. Lung scan (**b**) showed lack of perfusion to the right lung. Chest CT demonstrated obstructive emphysema of the right lung with contralateral mediastinal shift (**c**), as well as a foreign body in the right main bronchus (**d**). Repeat bronchoscopy identified a lentil

the vessels in the obstructed region become narrow and sparse. This finding, characteristic of obstructive emphysema, can be seen on both plain films and CT. There is usually a mediastinal shift to the opposite side in expiration, as well as a lower ipsilateral hemidiaphragm (Fig. 10.5a).

In young children, whose cooperation is not always optimal, two lateral decubitus films, one on each side, can replace the inspiratory–expiratory films (CAPITANIO and KIRKPATRICK 1972). An unobstructed dependent lung shows smaller volume and crowded vessels as a result of gravitational forces on the abdominal and mediastinal organs. In cases of partial obstruction, the dependent lung does not deflate as expected. The relative hyperinflation of the dependent lung thus indicates the presence of partial bronchial obstruction.

Alternatively, expiratory films can be obtained in non-cooperative patients by applying manual pressure on the upper abdomen using a lead glove during the examination (WESENBERG and BLUMHAGEN 1979). In infants this can also be done by inflating a blood-pressure cuff, wrapped around the abdomen. Careful monitoring must be performed to ascertain that at no time the pressure in the cuff exceeds the child's systolic blood pressure. Oblique projections enable better visualization of the trachea and main bronchi, and may demonstrate an otherwise "hidden" foreign body or discontinuation of the air column, depicted as an "absent segment" of the airway (Figs. 10.2b, 10.3, 10.6b).

The high kilovoltage (kV) copper filter technique increases the visibility of the major airways and of non-opaque foreign bodies (Figs. 10.6, 10.7). This technique combines the use of high kV with filters that absorb most of the low energy photons. As a result, the contrast between soft tissue and bone is reduced and the contrast between air and all other tissues is increased. Thus, the airway and its contents are sharply delineated over the background of the other tissues. Various filters have been used; however, the combination of 0.4 mm of tin, 0.5 mm of copper and 0.75 mm of aluminum is probably the most useful. The use of this technique enables improved visualization of the major airways with reduced radiation dose (JOSEPH et al. 1976).

The sensitivity, specificity and accuracy of chest radiographs for the detection and diagnosis of aspirated foreign bodies have been shown to be low when compared to bronchoscopy or to clinical signs in several retrospective studies (SVEDSTROM et al. 1989; HOEVE and ROMBOUT 1992; BARRIOS FONTOBA et al. 1997; SILVA et al. 1998; ZERELLA et al. 1998). In one series, up to 50% of chest X-rays obtained in children with proven foreign bodies were found to be normal when filmed in the early period (within 3 days) fol-

lowing aspiration; however, expiratory radiographs were not routinely obtained in this study (ZERELLA et al. 1998). Expiratory films have a high diagnostic value, but without clinical suspicion of foreign body aspiration, they will not be routinely performed. Therefore, it is mandatory that the clinician provide this sort of information to the radiologist in charge of the exam. Chest X-rays may also be normal in cases of bilateral bronchial foreign bodies (WISEMAN 1984; MUSEMECHE and KOSLOSKE 1986; LAKS and BARZILAY 1988).

Fluoroscopy used to be helpful in the investigation of foreign body aspiration. The proponents of this modality advocate its use because it is widely available, easy to use, and rapidly diagnostic in up to 90% of cases of a bronchial foreign body (BLAZER et al. 1980; ZERELLA et al. 1998). In our practice, fluoroscopy is seldom used. Nevertheless, the radiologist can optimally visualize the airways and detect obstruction or the presence of an opaque foreign body with fluoroscopy (see Fig. 10.2b), especially if a copper filter is used adjacent to the X-ray tube or close to the patient (W.E. Berdon, personal communication).

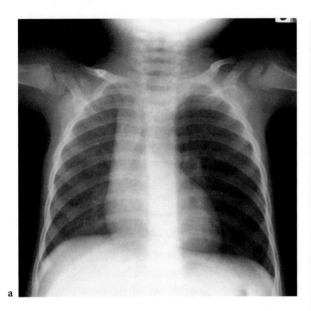

a

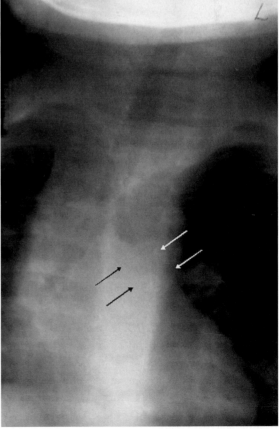

b

Fig. 10.6. Anteroposterior chest radiograph (**a**) and a high kilovoltage (kV) copper filter technique film (**b**) of the major airways of a 2-year-old girl. The chest radiograph demonstrates air-trapping in the left lung while the high kV copper filter technique demonstrates an "absent segment" (*arrows*) in the left main bronchus

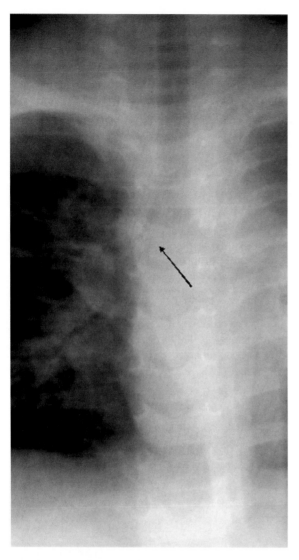

Fig. 10.7. High kilovoltage copper filter technique of the tracheobronchial tree of a 15-month-old girl. A non-opaque foreign body (*arrow*) surrounded by air is seen at the carina and in the right main bronchus . The inspiration and expiration films did not reveal air-trapping or any other pulmonary pathology

Mediastinal shift towards the obstructed side during inspiration and towards the contralateral side during expiration is easily recognized (THEANDER 1970; LAKS and BARZILAY 1988; MU et al. 1990). Unequal descent or ascent of the hemidiaphragms on inspiration and expiration can be seen in crying babies and in older children when requested to sniff rapidly. Diminished excursions of the diaphragmatic leaflets are invariably seen on the affected side, either with hyperinflation (in partial obstruction) or with volume loss (in complete obstruction) (THEANDER

1970). Use of any technique for assisted expiration, as described earlier, can facilitate demonstration of air-trapping.

Computed tomography (CT), due to its high contrast resolution, enables demonstration of foreign bodies that are frequently not visible on the chest X-ray. When foreign body aspiration is highly suspected and initial imaging studies or bronchoscopy are negative, CT may reveal the presence and location of a previously undiagnosed foreign body (BERGER et al. 1980; BERTOLANI et al. 1999). By varying window width and level, one can see not only the foreign body, but also the reaction of the tissue around and distal to it. One can also assess the presence and extent of complications such as air-trapping, atelectasis, pneumonia, empyema, bronchiectasis or chest wall involvement (Figs. 10.5, 10.8, 10.9, 10.10). Air-trapping is well demonstrated by decubitus scans (Fig. 10.11) (LUCAYA et al. 2000). Scanning in the semi-coronal plane can provide accurate localization of the obstructing foreign body (Figs. 10.9, 10.10) (BAR-ZIV and SOLOMON 1990). However, with current helical scanners using volumetric acquisition of data, a high pitch (1.5–2) and a short scanning time, accurate multi-planar reconstructions can be obtained, thereby replacing the semi-coronal scans. CT is a very sensitive modality for demonstrating small dense objects, such as thin fish or chicken bones, that may not be detected on plain films (BRAVERMAN et al. 1993; MIGNON et al. 1997).

We routinely use a helical technique with 5-mm collimation, 2.7-mm reconstructions and the smallest possible field of view. For infants and toddlers

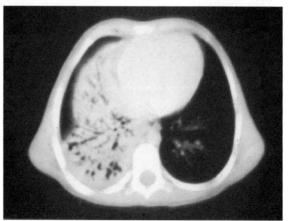

Fig. 10.8. Axial CT of the lower chest in a case of chronic foreign body aspiration into the right intermediate bronchus, causing collapse and bronchiectasis in the right middle lobe and right lower lobe

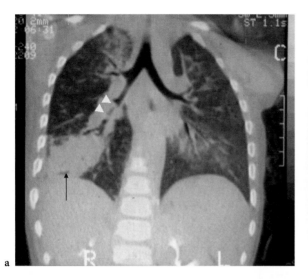

a

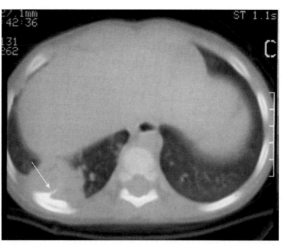

b

Fig. 10.9a,b. A 3-year-old boy aspirated a branch of Timothy grass. Semi-coronal (**a**) and axial (**b**) chest CT demonstrate narrowing and irregularity of the bronchus intermedius (*arrowheads*), distal atelectasis and abscess formation (*arrow*). Also note sclerosis of the adjacent rib representing osteomyelitis (*white arrow* in **b**)

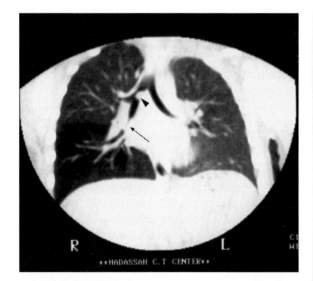

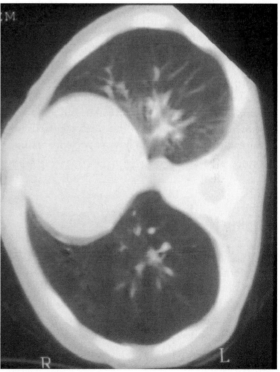

Fig. 10.10. A semi-coronal chest CT (lung settings) of a 2-year-old boy, obtained in expiration. Soft tissue density is demonstrated in the bronchus intermedius causing a partial obstruction (*arrow*). This is the equivalent of the "absent segment" sign that results from the presence of an obstructing foreign body and inflammatory changes in the adjacent bronchial wall. Note also the obvious air-trapping in the right lower lobe as compared to the normal-sized right upper lobe and left lung. Another partially obstructing foreign body is seen adjacent to the medial wall of the right main bronchus (*arrowhead*)

Fig. 10.11. Right lateral decubitus chest CT demonstrates air-trapping in the right (dependent) lung, following aspiration of a piece of an eraser

we may use 2.7-mm collimation with 1.3-mm reconstructions. Tube current can be reduced to as low as 50–60 mAs for such studies. Two- and three-dimensional reconstructions, including virtual bronchoscopy, can be helpful in detecting airway foreign bodies.

Nuclear medicine is not recommended for the diagnosis of a bronchial foreign body. When used, however, the lung scan can be helpful in defining regional decrease in ventilation and perfusion (see Fig. 10.5b), as well as air-trapping, and can thus guide endoscopy to the area of suspected obstruction (HOLLAND and TRUMBULL 1979; LULL et al. 1980). Magnetic resonance imaging (MRI) studies are also rarely used for investigating suspected foreign body aspiration, especially because at present the use of sedation is mandatory. Nevertheless, several reports have described the utility of MRI in the management of foreign body aspiration. Due to the multiplanar nature of this modality, MRI can accurately locate the foreign body prior to bronchoscopy, and can also reveal foreign bodies in multiple sites during the same study (IMAIZUMI et al. 1994; MORIJIRI et al. 1994). The high fat content of aspirated peanuts, as well as the high water content of most organic foreign bodies enable clear delineation of their size and site (O'UCHI et al. 1992; TASHITA et al. 1998). Ultrasound can be of value in defining the presence and extent of complications of foreign bodies, such as consolidation with an air bronchogram, pleural effusion or empyema, loculated pockets of fluid, chest wall abscess or rib osteomyelitis (SEIBERT et al. 1986; GIUDICELLI et al. 1996). Ultrasound can presumably demonstrate the foreign body within the collapsed lung; however the authors do not have experience in this.

10.6
Imaging Findings

Imaging findings in cases of foreign body aspiration are determined by the presence and the degree of airway obstruction, the site of the foreign body, its type and the time that has elapsed between aspiration and the performance of imaging studies.

A foreign body can be present in the airway without causing obstruction. This situation almost always involves an oblong foreign body in the trachea, small enough to have been aspirated yet not large enough to block the (relatively) larger airway. In such a case the chest X-ray and fluoroscopy will usually be negative,

although pneumonia might be present (ESCLAMADO and RICHARDSON 1987; MU et al. 1990; CATANEO et al. 1997). A high kV soft tissue technique with a copper filter may reveal the foreign body (see Figs. 10.6, 10.7). CT (GUPTA and BERRY 1991; MALIS and HAYES 1995; BERTOLANI et al. 1999) and MR imaging (O'UCHI et al. 1992; IMAIZUMI et al. 1994; MORIJIRI et al. 1994; TASHITA et al. 1998) can demonstrate the presence and often the nature of such a foreign body when the initial imaging is negative.

Obstruction of the airway can vary in severity and occur at different levels of the tracheo-bronchial tree. Laryngeal or sub-glottic foreign bodies tend to be thinner and are often arranged in an anteroposterior direction in the region of the vocal cords, as opposed to esophageal foreign bodies, which lie in a transverse direction. If the foreign body is a thin, rounded object (e.g., a coin or an egg shell), it will be seen as a thin line on the anteroposterior chest X-ray when located between the vocal cords, and as a rounded shadow when located in the esophagus. Tracheal foreign bodies usually cause no obstruction or incomplete obstruction. The imaging findings, when present, are often bilateral: either bilateral volume loss or bilateral hyperinflation. In the latter case, the diaphragms are flattened and in a low position. When small enough, the foreign body may move in the tracheobronchial tree during the different phases of the respiratory cycle or as a result of coughing, with consequent changes in the clinical and imaging findings (METRANGELO et al. 1999).

About three quarters of airway foreign bodies are found in the main bronchi (BLAZER et al. 1980; MANTEL and BUTENANDT 1986), where they cause partial or complete obstruction. Plain films and fluoroscopy seldom demonstrate a nonopaque foreign body. An oblique projection obtained with these modalities, placing the upper airway over the mediastinal soft tissues, creates better contrast and enhances demonstration of the foreign body (see Fig. 10.2). This technique may also indirectly reveal the presence of a foreign body by virtue of focal absence of the air column in the obstructed bronchus, the so-called "absent segment" or the "interrupted bronchus" sign (see Fig. 10.3) (GRUNEBAUM et al. 1979; LIMDUNHAM and YOUSEFZADEH 1999). Partial obstruction results in localized air-trapping distal to the site of the foreign body, with resultant widening of the intercostal spaces, and flattening of the ribs and diaphragms, and blunting of the costo-phrenic angles (LAKS and BARZILAY 1988; MU et al. 1990; BLACK et al. 1994; ERNST and MAHMUD 1994; OGUZ et al. 2000).

Pulmonary hyperexpansion with sparse vascularity or displacement of the mediastinum to the contralateral side on expiration indicates the presence of obstructive emphysema (see Figs. 10.5a, 10.6a) (Mu et al. 1990). Complete obstruction also causes segmental or lobar atelectasis (see Figs. 10.2a, 10.3), or even total collapse of the ipsilateral lung. The collapsed area may initially be homogeneously opaque, due to the absence of air in the alveoli and bronchi. Collateral diffusion of air to the bronchioles distal to the obstructing foreign body may result in a faint air bronchogram. In cases with lobar atelectasis, compensatory emphysema of the ipsilateral respected lobes and of the contralateral lung is often present (THEANDER 1970). In contrast to obstructive emphysema, pulmonary vessels are prominent in compensatory emphysema.

The presence of lobar collapse with localized pneumothorax should suggest the diagnosis of acute bronchial obstruction of any etiology (BERDON et al. 1984; NIMKIN et al. 1995) (Fig. 10.12). The combination of increased pressure and the presence of a sharp object in the bronchi can result in a broncho-pleural fistula. This complication, as well as pneumonia secondary to focal obstruction, may give rise to pleural effusion or empyema (DOGAN et al. 1999). Pleural effusion as the only imaging sign of foreign body aspiration has also been reported (AUERBACK 1990). In prolonged cases, localized or multi-focal bronchiectasis may develop and be evident on the plain radiograph (see Fig 10.2) or on CT (see Fig. 10.8.); these are best evaluated by high-resolution CT with thin section collimation (KUHN 1993). Subacute or chronic infection and inflammatory response may form a parenchymal abscess adjacent or distal to the foreign body, or a chest wall abscess and rib osteomyelitis (Figs. 10.9, 10.13).

10.7
Complications

Complications of foreign body aspiration can be immediate or long term. A foreign body can cause fatal asphyxia when there is complete obstruction of the major airways (BUNTAIN et al. 1979; BLACK et al. 1984, 1994; BYARD 1994). This occurrence is rare, although it was described in 7.5% of foreign body aspiration cases in one report (MENENDEZ et al. 1991). This high incidence has not been observed in the author's experience and is not corroborated in other reports. Asphyxia and hypoxemia can result in hypoxic-ischemic encephalopathy, convulsions, severe neurologic deterioration and death within several days (NORTHCOTE 1983).

Atelectasis is reported by some as the most common complication of foreign body aspiration (MU et al. 1990; CATANEO et al. 1997; OGUZ et al. 2000), and is seen in half of the patients who are diagnosed 24 h or more after the suspected aspiration event (WISEMAN 1984). Though atelectasis usually develops gradually, collapse of the entire lung may occur within an hour. When this happens on the right side, kinking of the superior vena cava may cause a sudden decrease of venous return to the heart and lead to loss of consciousness. Elevation of jugular venous pressure should alert the examining physician to the possibility of such a complication.

Pneumonia appears in about one third to one half of patients with an aspirated foreign body diagnosed 3 days or later consequent to the aspiration event (CATANEO et al. 1997; OGUZ et al. 2000). The pneumonia in these cases is usually located in the lower lobes, does not resolve following antibiotic therapy and is frequently associated with a pleural effusion. Pneumonia may at times be due to uncommon pathogens (CAVENS et al. 1973; BAETHGE et al. 1990). Dirt or shallow water aspiration can lead to diffuse pneumonitis (MANGGE et al. 1993).

A sudden increase in alveolar pressure due to proximal obstruction can cause an air leak into the inter-

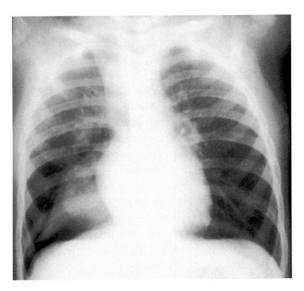

Fig. 10.12. Collapsed right lower lobe with localized pneumothorax due to acute foreign body aspiration

stitial space, leading to interstitial emphysema, pneumomediastinum (HANUKOGLU et al. 1980; BURTON et al. 1989; RAMADAN et al. 1992; BRATTON and O'ROURKE 1993), pneumothorax (see Fig. 10.12) (BERDON et al. 1984; NIMKIN et al. 1995; ESCLAMADO and RICHARDSON 1987; RAMADAN et al. 1992; CATANEO et al. 1997; NEWSON et al. 1998) or pneumopericardium (TJHEN et al. 1978; BRO and THAMSEN 1989). The abrupt onset of an air leak in a child under 2 years of age, without a history of chest trauma or asthma, should raise the suspicion of an aspirated foreign body (CATANEO et al. 1997).

The incidence and severity of long-term complications are directly related to the length of time that has passed between the actual event of aspiration and establishment of the diagnosis (AUERBACK 1990; MU et al. 1990; LINEGAR et al. 1992; SCHMIDT and MANEGOLD 2000). Positive radiological findings are more common in cases diagnosed 24 h or later consequent to the suspected aspiration (ESCLAMADO and RICHARDSON 1987; MU et al. 1990); the longer the delay in diagnosis, the higher the rate of complications (LEVY et al. 1983; MU et al. 1990). In most cases of delayed diagnosis the original episode passed unnoticed and the parents or physician do not relate recent, recurrent signs and symptoms as being linked to such an episode or to each other (MANTEL and BUTENANDT 1986). In such cases the presentation can be that of recurrent events of hyper-reactive airway disease, with incomplete response to treatment, or of recurrent pneumonia, with or without pleural effusion or empyema (AUERBACK 1990; BURTON et al. 1989; DOGAN et al. 1999; HANUKOGLU et al. 1980).

Chronic bronchitis and bronchiectasis (see Fig. 10.8) secondary to long-standing foreign body aspiration constitute approximately 5% of chronic suppurative lung disease. The presence of a bronchial foreign body of long duration causes atelectasis that can become infected and lead to the development of bronchiectasis. This can become so severe that surgical treatment may eventually be required (SPENCER et al. 1981; GATCH et al. 1987; MAAYAN et al. 1993; NIKOLAIZIK and WARMER 1994; CATANEO et al. 1997; SCULLY et al. 1998).

Grass heads of different types have been reported to cause a unique sequence of complications. If they have spikes that are soft and close together, as is the case of Timothy grass, they will soften with moisture following aspiration and will not penetrate into the lung periphery. The grass head may lodge in the bronchial tree and occlude it causing obstructive emphysema, collapse, pneumonia and lung abscess. If the spikes are stiff and do not become soft when

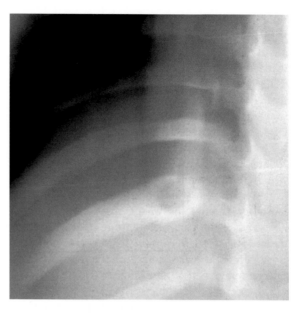

Fig. 10.13. A 2-year-old girl had repeated episodes of right lower lobe pneumonia for several months following an episode of choking around Christmas. Chest radiograph showed an osteolytic lesion with thickening and sclerosis in a rib at the right lower chest. At surgery, a pine tree needle was found in the rib, with osteomyelitis

moistened, or when inhaled stump-first, respiratory actions and cough can cause them to advance. Being carried by the spikes distally into the bronchial tree, they can penetrate the lung tissue and ultimately even extrude spontaneously through the chest wall (HILLMAN et al. 1980). During this process they can cause lung abscess (see Fig. 10.9), broncho-cutaneous fistula (CAVENS et al. 1973; BAETHGE et al. 1990; MAAYAN et al. 1993; DINDAR et al. 1994), rib osteomyelitis (see Figs. 10.9, 10.13), chest wall abscess or pneumocutaneous fistula (CHENG et al. 1991). Among several of our patients who suffered such a complication, one was a 3-year-old boy who had aspirated a branch of Timothy grass. Subsequently, the child developed cough and fever. A chest radiograph obtained several weeks later showed consolidation and volume loss in the right lower lobe. A semi-coronal chest CT study revealed irregularity and narrowing of the right lower lobe bronchus, partial consolidation and atelectasis of the right lower lobe with abscess formation. Thickening, sclerosis and irregularity of the inner border of the adjacent rib were also noted (see Fig. 10.9). Pathology of the resected right lower lobe revealed the presence of Timothy grass within the bronchus of the lateral basal segment with bronchiectasis and abscess formation.

Brain abscesses have been reported in association with foreign body aspiration, presumably due to faulty pulmonary capillary filter mechanisms (SPENCER et al. 1981; SANE et al. 1999).

Prolonged presence of a tracheal or an esophageal foreign body can result in a decubitus ulcer that can progress to a tracheo-esophageal fistula (Fig. 10.14) with possible mediastinitis, which might require surgery (SZOLD et al. 1991).

Pulmonary edema may occur subsequent to relief of an upper airway obstruction, regardless of the etiology. The pathophysiology of the pulmonary edema in these cases is not fully understood. It is thought that pulmonary congestion develops during obstruction as a result of raised pleural negative pressure, which increases venous return to the heart, in the presence of decreased left ventricular function. The hypoxia causes pulmonary hypertension and increased capillary permeability. This combination leads to greater pulmonary vascular volume, which may be radiographically difficult to detect because of associated air-trapping. Once the obstruction is relieved and lung aeration returns to normal, the pulmonary edema becomes apparent (SOFER et al. 1984a,b, 1985).

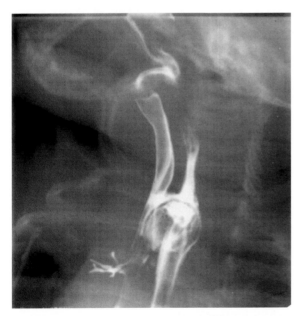

Fig. 10.14. A 6-week-old baby girl had suffered from respiratory symptoms since the age of 2 weeks. Tube esophagogram demonstrated a filling defect in the upper esophagus and a tracheo-esophageal fistula. A pistachio nutshell was surgically removed and the fistula excised

10.8
Conclusion

A wide variety of opaque or non-opaque foreign bodies can be aspirated by infants and young children. The history of choking is the most reliable clue for the diagnosis of foreign body aspiration, but many patients reach medical attention because of various non-specific clinical symptoms. The role of the radiologist in these cases is crucial. Knowledge of the imaging features of a foreign body in the respiratory tract is essential for diagnosis. Many clinical and imaging findings are the result of a one-way obstruction mechanism, most commonly affecting one of the main bronchi. A normal inspiratory chest radiograph does not rule out an endotracheo-bronchial foreign body. Hence, expiratory films are extremely important to demonstrate air-trapping. Alternatively, lateral decubitus or assisted expiration films can be used. The high kV copper filter technique is valuable for demonstrating the foreign body, and for indirectly showing an area of deficient aeration in the tracheobronchial tree, the "absent segment" sign.

Fluoroscopy can be very useful, but unfortunately the art of fluoroscopy is now almost lost. CT has become more valuable by virtue of its wide availability and high resolution. CT can establish the diagnosis of a foreign body, indicate its exact location and often show its composition, as well as any associated complications. Other imaging modalities can be used, though their role is not as well established. Nuclear scans are of some value only in cases of obstructive endobronchial foreign body. MRI has great potential and may be used extensively in the future. Currently, however, it is not widely available and usually requires sedation of the child. US is being used to demonstrate complications such as pleural effusion or chest wall abscesses.

An understanding of the mechanisms of obstruction and their resultant clinical and imaging manifestations, especially when foreign body aspiration is highly suspected, can lead to earlier diagnosis and lower the complication rate.

Acknowledgements. The authors thank Prof. B.S. Slasky for reviewing the manuscript; Prof. P. Mogle for his comments and for the contribution of the case described in Fig. 10.14; Prof. J. Strife for the case described in Fig. 10.13; and Mr. E. Koplewitz and Mrs. B. Koplewitz for their editorial comments and their continuous support.

References

Abdel-Rahman HA (2000) Fatal suffocation by rubber balloons in children: mechanism and prevention. Forensic Sci Int 108:97–105

Anas NG, Perkin RM (1983) Aspiration of a balloon by a 3-month-old infant. JAMA 250:385–386

Auerback ML (1990) Pleural effusion due to unsuspected aspiration of vegetable matter in a three-year-old boy. N Engl J Med 322:1238

Avital A, Springer C, Mogle P et al (1989) Successful treatment after 'drowning' in sand. Arch Dis Child 64:615–616

Aytac A, Yurdakul Y, Ikizler C et al (1977) Inhalation of foreign bodies in children. Report of 500 cases. J Thorac Cardiovasc Surg 74:145–151

Baethge BA, Eggerstedt JM, Olash FA Jr (1990) Group F streptococcal empyema from aspiration of a grass inflorescence. Ann Thoac Surg 49:319–320

Baharloo F, Veyckemans F, Francis C et al (1999) Tracheobronchial foreign bodies: presentation and management in children and adults. Chest 115:1357–1362

Bar-Ziv J, Solomon A (1990) Direct coronal CT scanning of tracheo-bronchial, pulmonary and thoraco-abdominal lesions in children. Pediatr Radiol 20:245–248

Barrios Fontoba JE, Gutierrez C, Lluna J (1977) Bronchial foreign body: should bronchoscopy be performed in all patients with a choking crisis? Pediatr Surg Int 12:118–120

Barrett TG, Debelle GD (1995) Near-fatal aspiration of a child's dummy: design fault or deliberate injury? J Accid Emerg Med 12:154–155

Basok O, Yaldiz S, Kilincer L (1997) Bronchiectasis resulting from aspirated grass inflorescences. Scand Cardiovasc J 31:157–159

Berdon WE, Dee GJ, Abramson SJ et al (1984) Localized pneumothorax adjacent to a collapsed lobe: a sign of bronchial obstruction. Radiology 150:691–694

Berger PE, Kuhn JP, Kuhn LR (1980) Computed tomography and the occult trecheobronchial foreign body. Radiology 134:133–135

Bergeson PS HW, Crawford RF, Sorenson MJ, Trump DS (1978) Asphyxia secondary to massive dirt aspiration. J Pediatr 92:506–507

Bertolani MF, Marotti F, Bergamini BM et al (1999) Extraction of a rubber bullet from a bronchus after 1 year: complete resolution of chronic pulmonary damage. Chest 115:1210–1213

Black RE, Choi KJ, Syme WC et al (1984) Bronchoscopic removal of aspirated foreign bodies in children. Am J Surg 148:778–781

Black RE, Johnson DG, Matlak MEB (1994) Bronchoscopic removal of aspirated foreign bodies in children. J Pediatr Surg 29:682–684

Blazer S, Naveh Y, Friedman A (1980) Foreign body in the airway. A review of 200 cases. Am J Dis Child 134:68–71

Bratton SL, O'Rourke PP (1993) Spontaneous pneumomediastinum. J Emerg Med 11:525–529

Braverman I, Gomori JM, Polv O et al (1993) The role of CT imaging in the evaluation of cervical esophageal foreign bodies. J Otolaryngol 22:311–314

Bro H, Thamsen H (1989) Pneumopericardium after aspiration of a pea into the respiratory tract. Ugeskr Laeger 151:2733

Buntain WL, Benton JW, Gutierrez JF (1979) Christmas bow tragedies. South Med J 72:1471–1472

Burrington DJ (1976) Aluminum "pop tops". A hazard to child health. JAMA 235:2614–2617

Burton EM, Riggs W Jr, Kaufman RA et al (1989) Pneumomediastinum caused by foreign body aspiration in children. Pediatr Radiol 20:45–47

Burton EM, Brick WG, Hall JD et al (1996) Tracheobronchial foreign body aspiration in children. South Med J 89:195–198

Byard RW (1994) Unexpected death due to acute airway obstruction in daycare centers. Pediatrics 94:113–114

Capitanio MA, Kirkpatrick JA (1972) The lateral decubitus film: an aid in determining air-trapping in children. Radiology 103:460–462

Cataneo AJ, Reibscheid SM, Ruiz Junior RL et al (1997) Foreign body in the tracheobronchial tree. Clin Pediatr (Phila) 36:701–706

Cavens TR, McGee MD, Miller RR et al (1973) Pneumocutaneous fistula secondary to aspiration of grass. J Pediatr 82:737–738

Chen YT, Singh R, Brett RH (1998) Diagnostic red herring in an infant with stridor. Singapore Med J 39:471–472

Cheng T, Herman G, Coulter K (1991) A tale of two diseases: Pneumonia and chest wall abscess. Pediatr Infect Dis J 10:414–418

Choy IO, Idowu O (1996) Sand aspiration: a case report. J Pediatr Surg 31:1448–1450

Cleveland RH (1979) Symmetry of bronchial angles in children. Radiology 133:89–93

Cohen HA, Goldberg E, Horev Z (1993) Removal of nasal foreign bodies in children (letter). Clin Pediatr (Phila) 32:192

Dindar H, Konkan R, Cakmak M et al (1994) A bronchopleurocutaneous fistula caused by an unusual foreign body aspiration simulating acute abdomen. Eur J Pediatr 153:136–137

Dogan K, Kaptanoglu M, Onen A et al (1999) Unusual sites of uncommon endobronchial foreign bodies. Reports of four cases. Scand Cardiovasc J 33:309–311

Elhassani NB (1988) Tracheobronchial foreign bodies in the Middle East. A Baghdad study. J Thorac Cardiovasc Surg 96:621–625

Ernst KD, Mahmud F (1994) Reversible cystic dilatation of distal airways due to foreign body. South Med J 87:404–406

Esclamado RM, Richardson MA (1987) Laryngotracheal foreign bodies in children: a comparison with bronchial foreign bodies. Am J Dis Child 141:259–262

Fabian MC, Smitheringale A (1996) Hemoptysis in children: the hospital for sick children experience. J Otolaryngol 25:44–45

Farkash J, Liberman A, Bar-Ziv J et al (1982) Respiratory tract foreign bodies in children. Harefuah 10:383–387

Felman AH (1982) The pediatric chest. Thomas, Springfield, Ill, pp 411–423

Fini-Storchi I, Ninu MB (1996) Atypical intranasal foreign body. Ear Nose Throat J 75:796–799

Fitzpatrick PC, Guarisco JL (1998) Pediatric airway foreign bodies. J LA State Med Soc 150:138–141

Friedman E (2000) Tracheobronchial foreign bodies. Otolaryngol Clin North Am 33:179–185

Garcia-Pena P, Lucaya J (1999) Chest CT in children: main applications and advantages. Pediatr Pulmonol S18:56–59

Gatch G, Myre L, Black RE (1987) Foreign body aspiration in children. Causes, diagnosis, and prevention. AORN J 46:850–861

Giudicelli J, Chapelon C, Louis D et al (1996) Intrabronchial inhaled seed migration. Value of ultrasonography in the diagnosis of pleural-cutaneous fistula. Rev Mal Respir 13:428–429

Grad R, Taussig LM (1990.Acute infections producing uper airway obstruction. In: Chenick V, Kendig EL (eds) Disorders of the respiratory tract in children, Saunders, Philadelphia, pp 336–348

Grunebaum M, Adler S, Varsano I (1979) The paradoxial movement of the mediastinum. A diagnostic sign of foreign-body aspiration during childhood. Pediatr Radiol 8:213–218

Gupta AK, Berry M (1991) Detection of a radiolucent bronchial foreign body by computed tomography. Pediatr Radiol 21:307–308

Halvorson DJ, Merritt RM, Mann C et al (1996) Management of subglottic foreign bodies. Ann Otol Rhinol Laryngol 105:141–144

Hanukoglu A, Fried D, Hadas E (1980) Pneumomediastinum and subcutaneous emphysema following foreign body aspiration. Harefuah 98:262–264

Hanukoglu A, Fried D, Segal S (1986) Loss of voice as sole symptom of subglottic foreign-body aspiration. Am J Dis Child 140:973

Hillman BC, Kurtzweg FT, McCook WW et al (1980) Foreign body aspiration of grass inflorescences as a cause of hemoptysis. Chest 78: 306–309

Hoeve LJ, Rombout J (1992) Pediatric laryngobronchoscopy. 1332 procedures stored in a data base. Int J Pediatr Otorhinolaryngol 24:73–82

Holland NJ, Trumbull HR (1979) Chronic foreign body aspiration diagnosed by lung scan. Clin Pediatr (Phila) 18:497–500

Imaizumi H, Kaneko M, Nara S et al (1994) Definitive diagnosis and location of peanuts in the airways using magnetic resonance imaging techniques. Ann Emerg Med 23:1379–1382

Jain L, Sivieri E, Bhutani VK (1986) Aspiration of pacifiers. Pediatrics 78:955–956

Joseph PM, Berdon WE, Baker DH et al (1976) Upper airway obstruction in infants and small children: improved radiographic diagnosis by combining filtration, high kilovoltage and magnification. Radiology 121:143–148

Kaptanoglu M, Dogan K, Onen A et al (1999) Turban pin aspiration; a potential risk for young Islamic girls. Int J Pediatr Otorhinolaryngol 48:131–135

Keith FM, Charrette EJ, Lynn RB et al (1980) Inhalation of foreign bodies by children: A continuing challege in management. Can Med Assoc J 122:55–57

Kuhn JP (1993) High-resolution computed tomography of pediatric pulmonary parenchymal disorders. Radiol Clin North Am 31:533–551

Laks Y, Barzilay Z (1988) Foreign body aspiration in childhood. Pediatr Emerg Care 4:102–106

Levy M, Glick B, Springer C et al (1983) Bronchoscopy and bronchography in children. Experience with 110 investigations. Am J Dis Child 137:14–16

Lim-Dunham JE, Yousefzadeh DK (1999) The interrupted bronchus:a fluoroscopic sign of bronchial foreign body ininfants and children. AJR Am J Roentgenol 173:969–972

Linegar AG, von Oppell UO, Hegemann S et al (1992) Tracheobronchial foreign bodies. Experience at Red Cross Children's Hospital 1985–1990. S Afr Med J 82:84–87

Losek JD (1990; Diagnostic difficulties of foreign body aspiration in children. Am J Emerg Med 8:348–350

Lucaya J, Garcia-Pena P, Herrera L et al (2000) Expiratory chest CT in children. AJR Am J Roentgenol 174:235–241

Lull RJ, Anderson JH, Telepak RJ et al (1980) Radionuclide imaging in the assessment of lung injury. Semin Nucl Med 10 :302–310

Maayan C, Avital A, Elpeleg ON et al (1993) Complications following oat head aspiration. Pediatr Pulmonol 15:52–54

Mangge H, Plecko B, Grubbauer HM et al (1993) Late-onset miliary pneumonitis after near drowning. Pediatr Pulmonol 15:122–124

Malis DJ, Hayes DK (1995) Retained bronchial foreign bodies: is there a role for high-resolution computed tomography scan? Otolaryngol Head Neck Surg 112:341–346

Mantel K, Butenandt I (1986) Tracheobronchial foreign body aspiration in childhood. A report on 224 cases. Eur J Pediatr 145:211–216

Mearns AJ, England JM (1975) Dissolving foreign bodies in the trachea and bronchus. Thorax 30:461–463

Menendez AA, Gotay Cruz F, Seda FJ et al (1991) Foreign body aspiration: experience at the University Pediatric Hospital. P R Health Sci J 10:127–133

Metrangelo S, Monetti C, Meneghini L et al (1999) Eight years' experience with foreign-body aspiration in children: what is really important for a timely diagnosis? J Pediatr Surg 34:1229–1231

Mignon F, Mesurolle B, Chambellan A et al (1997) Foreign body granuloma mimicking bronchial tumor. Aspects in x-ray computed tomography with views by virtual endoscopy. J Radiol 78:1181–1184

Morijiri M, Seto H, Kageyama M et al (1994) Assessment of peanut aspiration by MRI and lung perfusion scintigram. J Comput Assist Tomogr 18:836–838

Mu LC, Sun DQ, He P (1990) Radiological diagnosis of aspirated foreign bodies in children: review of 343 cases. J Laryngol Otol 104:778–782

Musemeche CA, Kosloske AM (1986) Normal radiographic findings after foreign body aspiration. When the history counts. Clin Pediatr (Phil) 25:624–625

Newson TP, Parshuram CS, Berkowitz RG et al (1998) Tension pneumothorax secondary to grass head aspiration. Pediatr Emerg Care 14:287–289

Nikolaizik WH, Warmer JO (1994) Aetiology of chronic suppurative lung disease. Arch Dis Child 70:141–142

Nimkin K, Kleinman PK, Zwerdling RG et al (1995) Localized pneumothorax with lobar collapse and diffuse obstructive airway disease. Pediatr Radiol 25:449–451

Nolte KB (1993) Esophageal foreign bodies as child abuse. Potential fatal mechanisms. Am J Forensic Med Pathol 14:323–326

Northcote RJ (1983) Pulmonary aspiration presenting with generalised convulsions. Scott Med J 28:368–370

Oguz F, Citak A, Unuvar E et al (2000) Airway foreign bodies in childhood. Int J Pediatr Otorhinolaryngol 52:11–16

O'Uchi T, Tokumaru A, Mikami I et al (1992) Value of MR imaging in detecting a peanut causing bronchial obstruction. AJR Am J Roentgenol 159:481–482

Pasaoglu I, Dogan R, Demircin M et al (1991) Bronchoscopic removal of foreign bodies in children: retrospective analysis of 822 cases. Thorac Cardiovasc Surg 39:95–98

Piepsz A (1988) Late sequelae of foreign body inhalation. A multicentric scintigraphic study. Eur J Nucl Med 13:578–581

Ramadan HH, Bu-Saba N, Baraka A et al (1992) Management of an unusual presentation of foreign body aspiration. J Laryngol Otol 106:751–752

Reilly JS, Walter MA (1992) Consumer product aspiration and ingestion in children: analysis of emergency room reports to the National Electronic Injury Surveillance System. Ann Otol Rhinol Laryngol 101:739–741

Rogers LF, Igini JP (1975) Beverage can pull-tabs. Inadvertent ingestion or aspiration. JAMA 233:345–348

Sane SM, Faerber EN, Belani KK (1999) Respiratory foreign bodies and *Eikenella corrodens* brain abscess in two children. Pediatr Radiol 29:327–330

Schmidt H, Manegold BC (2000) Foreign body aspiration in children. Surg Endosc 14:644–648

Scully RE, Mark EJ, McNeely BU (1983) Case recorrds of the Massachusets General Hospital: case 48–1983. N Engl J Med 309:1374–1381

Scully RE, Mark EJ, McNeely BU (1998) Case recorrds of the Massachusets General Hospital: case 31–1998. N Engl J Med 339:1144–1151

Seibert RW, Seibert JJ, Williamson SL (1986) The opaque chest: when to suspect a bronchial foreign body. Pediatr Radiol 16:193–196

Senkaya I, Sagdic K, Gebitekin C et al (1997) Management of foreign body aspiration in infancy and childhood. A life-threatening problem. Turk J Pediatr 39:353–362

Silva AB, Muntz HR, Clary R (1998) Utility of conventional radiography in the diagnosis and management of pediatric airway foreign bodies. Ann Otol Rhinol Laryngol 107 (10/1):834–838

Smith PC, Swischuk LE, Fagan CJ (1974) An elusive and often unsuspected cause of stridor or pneumonia (the esophageal foreign body). Am J Roentgenol Radium Ther Nucl Med 122:80–89

Sofer S, Bar-Ziv J, Scharf SM (1984a) Pulmonary edema following relief of upper airway obstruction. Chest 86:401–403

Sofer S, Baer R, Gussarsky Y et al (1984b) Pulmonary edema secondary to chronic upper airway obstruction. Hemodynamic study in a child. Intensive Care Med 10:317–319

Sofer S, Bar-Ziv J, Mogle P (1985) Pulmonary oedema following choking: report of two cases. Eur J Pediatr 143:295–296

Spencer MJ, Millet VE, Dudley JP et al (1981) Grassheads in the tracheobronchial tree: two different outcomes. Ann Otol Rhinol Laryngol 90:406–408

Steen KH, Zimmermann T (1990) Tracheobronchial aspiration of foreign bodies in children: a study of 94 cases. Laryngoscope 100:525–530

Steelman R, Millman E, Steiner M et al (1997) Aspiration of a primary tooth in a patient with a tracheostomy. Spec Care Dentist 17:97–99

Strickland AL, Elhassani SB, Stowe DG (1987) Aspiration of metallic foil by children: report of two cases. J S C Med Assoc 83:49–51

Svedstrom E, Puhakka H, Kero P (1989) How accurate is chest radiography in the diagnosis of tracheobronchial foreign bodies in children? Pediatr Radiol 19:520–522

Svensson G (1985) Foreign bodies in the tracheobronchial tree. Special references to experience in 97 children. Int J Pediatr Otorhinolaryngol 8:243–251

Szold A, Udassin R, Seror D et al (1991) Acquired tracheo-esophageal fistula in infancy and childhood. J Pediatr Surg 26:672–675

Tashita H, Inoue R, Goto E et al (1998) Magnetic resonance imaging for early detection of bronchial foreign bodies. Eur J Pediatr 157:442

Teixidor de Otto J, Negro F, Gutierrez C (1980) Removal of foreign bodies from the upper airways and the bronchial tree of small children. Z Kinderchir Grenzgeb 30:137–140

Theander G (1970) Motility of diaphragm in children with bronchial foreign bodies. Acta Radiol (Diagn) 10:113–129

Tjhen KY, Schmaltz AA, Ibrahim Z et al (1978) Pneumopericardium as a complication of foreign body aspiration. Pediatr Radiol 7:121–123

Ucan ES, Tahaoglu K, Mogolkoc N et al (1996) Turban pin aspiration syndrome: a new form of foreign body aspiration. Respir Med 90:427–428

Wales J, Jackimczyk K, Rosen P (1983) Aspiration following a cave-in. Ann Emerg Med 12:99–101

Wesenberg RL, Blumhagen JD (1979) Assisted expiratory chest radiography: an effective technique for the diagnosis of foreign-body aspiration. Radiology 130:538–539

Wiseman NE (1984) The diagnosis of foreign body aspiration in childhood. J Pediatr Surg 19:531–535

Witt WJ (1985) The role of rigid endoscopy in foreign body management. Ear Nose Throat J 64:70–74

Zerella JT, Dimler M, McGill LC et al (1998) Foreign body aspiration in children: value of radiography and complications of bronchoscopy. J Pediatr Surg 33:1651–1654

11 Imaging Evaluation of the Thymus and Thymic Disorders in Children

Donald P. Frush

11.1 Introduction

An understanding of the embryology and normal development, anatomy and histology, and the various pediatric disorders that can involve the thymus is important for radiologists for a number of reasons. Firstly, familiarity with the spectrum of appearances, including size and location (i.e., aberrancy or ectopia) of the normal thymus in infants and children minimizes the potential for diagnostic errors. In addition, the normal gross and microscopic constitution of the thymus gland determines the imaging appearances of the normal thymus gland. Each of the noninvasive imaging modalities including radiography, sonography, computed tomography (CT),

magnetic resonance imaging (MRI), and nuclear scintigraphy can provide a unique, often complimentary, role in the evaluation of thymic diseases. By understanding the benefits and limitations of each of these modalities with respect to thymic disorders, the radiologist is better able to design and implement an effective and expeditious imaging algorithm.

To this end, this chapter is divided into the following sections: historical perspective; thymic embryology, normal anatomy, and thymic function; imaging modalities and normal imaging appearances; and a pattern-oriented approach to imaging in thymic disorders. This pattern-oriented approach has been selected as it provides a familiar and practical method for the radiologist in the recognition and classification of thymic disease based on imaging features such as thymic masses (Table 11.1), diffuse thymic infiltration, or thymic calcification or fat (Table 11.2).

Table 11.1. Pediatric thymic masses

Non-neoplastic masses
Thymic cyst
Vascular malformation
Castleman's disease
Neoplastic masses
Epithelial tumors
Thymoma (invasive, noninvasive)
Thymic carcinoma
Lymphoid tumors
Hodgkin's lymphoma
Non-Hodgkin's lymphoma
Lymphoblastic
Large cell
Germ cell tumors
Stromal tumors
Thymolipoma
Neuroendocrine tumors
Carcinoid
Hemangioma
Metastasis
Neuroblastoma

Donald P. Frush, MD

Box 3808, Division of Pediatric Radiology, 1905 McGovern-Davison Children's Health Center, Department of Radiology, Duke University Medical Center, Erwin Road, Durham, North Carolina 27710, USA

Table 11.2. Specific thymic imaging features

Thymic cysts and cystic conditions
   True thymic cysts (unilocular, multilocular)
   Germ cell tumors
   Langerhans' cell histiocytosis
   Lymphatic malformation (e.g. cystic hygroma)
   Lymphoma
   Treated lymphoma
   Thymic dysplasia of HIV infection
   Thymoma
   Thymic carcinoma

Thymic calcification
   Germ cell tumor
   Langerhans' cell histiocytosis
   Lymphoma
   Thymic cysts

Fat containing thymic masses
   Thymolipoma
   Germ cell tumor (usually mature teratoma)
   Vascular malformations

11.2
Thymic Imaging: Historical Perspective

The history of the thymus gland is long, and is punctuated by a great deal of misunderstanding. This history was recently reviewed in greater detail (JACOBS et al. 1999). However, a brief summary of the historical perspective on the thymus gland is worthwhile, with particular emphasis on the relationship of the thymus to the origin and development of the subspecialty of pediatric radiology.

The name *thymus* is Latin and derived from the Greek *thymos* meaning "warty excrescence", a descriptor similar to the appearance of another namesake, the thyme plant. One of the earliest descriptions of the thymus dates back to circa 200 AD where the function of the thymus was said to be purification of the nervous system. It is interesting that the thymus gland was called at this time the "organ of mystery", a name which is appropriate even to this day. The first scientific treatise on the thymus was published in 1777; in 1832, SIR ASTLEY COOPER published *The Anatomy of the Thymus Gland* in which he noted a tremendous variability in size and appearance of the normal gland (COOPER 1832) (Fig. 11.1). While he offered no better explanation, COOPER did not believe the tenant of the time that the thymus gland simply occupied a space in the anterior mediastinum.

In the latter half of the nineteenth century, the thymus gland was implicated in two factitious conditions: thymic asthma and status thymicolymphaticus. Thymic asthma (also known as Kopp's asthma) was a disorder where the "enlarged" thymus caused sudden death. It is not hard to realize that those infants with sudden death (i.e., sudden infant death syndrome) likely had normal sized thymic glands, while those succumbing to more chronic illnesses would have had thymic atrophy.

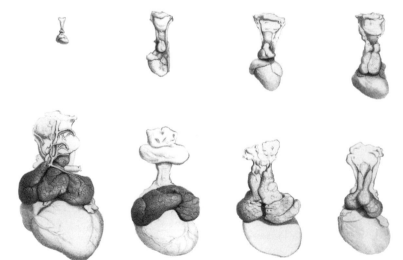

Fig. 11.1. Plate illustrating early work on the stages of thymic development. Each illustration, moving in a clockwise direction, represents the fetal thymus at monthly stages of development from 2 months (*left upper illustration*), to 9 months (*left lower illustration*). COOPER recognized the large normal thymic size (COOPER 1832)

In 1889, a constitutional disorder known as status thymicolymphaticus was proposed as another disorder of the thymus responsible for sudden death (PALTAUF 1889). This disorder was often implicated in the death of children during anesthesia. In fact, thymectomy was often advocated in children prior to anesthesia. About this time, the discovery of X-rays provided an important diagnostic opportunity to help clarify the appearance of the thymus gland in children; however, this discovery also provided an unfortunate therapeutic option for both thymicolymphaticus and thymic asthma (POHLE 1950) (Figs. 11.2, 11.3).

In 1907, the first treatment of thymic enlargement, associated with substantial respiratory distress, was reported, and recently reviewed by OESTREICH (1995). This treatment provided a total dose of 75–200 rad (0.75–2.0 Gy) to the affected infant. Despite the connection between radiation-induced cancer and radiation over the next 2–3 decades, thymic irradiation was still a requested therapy even until the 1960s (JACOBS et al. 1999).

Dr. JOHN CAFFEY, a pioneer in pediatric radiology, was instrumental in preventing further thymic misunderstanding and abuse. His description of the tremendous variability of the normal pediatric thymus gland is found in the earliest edition of his textbook (CAFFEY 1945). In addition, he considered that "destroying the thymus myth" (thymic asthma and status thymicolymphaticus) was one of his most important contributions to medicine (JACOBS et al. 1999).

Despite the tremendous advances in understanding the appearance and nature of the thymus gland, there are still many mysteries left to be solved from an imaging standpoint. Work is still needed to clarify contemporary issues with the thymus gland. These include whether there is recurrent or residual thymic involvement by lymphoma, the functional activity of normal thymic gland with positron emission tomography (PET), and the imaging manifestations of the thymus following immune constitution, such as thymic transplant for DiGeorge syndrome, and bone marrow transplant for severe combined immune deficiency.

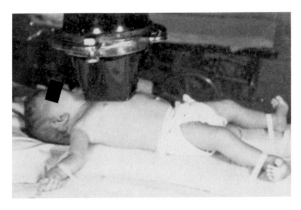

Fig. 11.2. The technique of thymic irradiation for status thymicolymphaticus or thymic asthma. (Reprinted with permission, POHLE 1950)

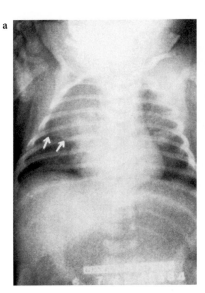
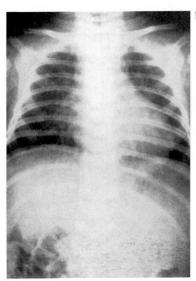

Fig. 11.3a,b. Effect of thymic irradiation on thymic size in an 8-week-old infant with "symptoms of thymic enlargement". **a** The opacity in the right upper lung was thought to be due to "atelectasis" secondary to thymic enlargement (*arrows*). **b** Following irradiation, frontal radiograph shows resolution of the opacity which likely represented normal thymic tissue. In the original text, it was noted that the child was "... now enjoying perfect health". (Reprinted with permission, POHLE 1950)

11.3
Thymic Development

A basic knowledge of the embryology and anatomy of the thymus is critical in understanding the variations in thymic anatomy and location. The thymus originates from the third pharyngeal pouch; a smaller contribution by the fourth pouch can also occur (KORNSTEIN 1995; SLOVIS et al. 1992). During fetal development, the thymus elongates with the development of the thymopharyngeal duct. This elongation begins in the neck, and the gland descends behind the thyroid and the sternocleidomastoid muscles. The two lobes fuse at the level of the transverse aorta (SLOVIS et al. 1992) beginning at about 8 weeks of gestational age. While the superior origin of the thymus gland usually atrophies, gross or microscopic rests of thymic tissue can persist from the origin of the gland, along the course of the thymopharyngeal duct. Thymopharyngeal duct remnants are the basis for thymic cysts.

Aberrant and ectopic locations of thymic tissue can be found with or without a coexistent normally located mediastinal thymus. While technically aberrancy is tissue along the normal embryologic course, and ectopia indicates tissue outside this course, the terms are often used interchangeably. These aberrant or ectopic locations include the neck, and the thorax including retrocaval and posterior mediastinal locations simulating mediastinal or apical masses (BACH et al. 1991; BAYSAL et al. 1999; KORNSTEIN 1995; SLOVIS et al. 1992; SWISCHUK and JOHN 1996).

Ectopic and aberrant thymic tissue does not usually cause symptoms. Reviews have noted that two-thirds of cases are seen in children under 10 years of age (CURE et al. 1995; KACKER et al. 1999; MARRA et al. 1995). In one review of imaging literature, 13 cases of posterior mediastinal thymus were identified (SLOVIS et al. 1992). In the five cases in which thymic ectopia was isolated, the gland was always located on the right. Most cervical ectopic or aberrant thymic tissue is lateral in location. In the mediastinum, retrocaval extension of the thymic gland has been noted in up to 10% of children (KUHN et al. 1993) (Fig. 11.4).

Both CT and MRI are well suited to the evaluation of abnormalities in a thymic location. The thymic tissue, which can be cystic or solid, is well circumscribed. When cystic, the mass can be multilocular with septations (CURE et al. 1995).

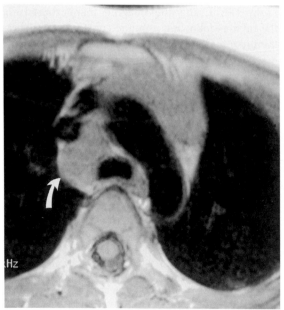
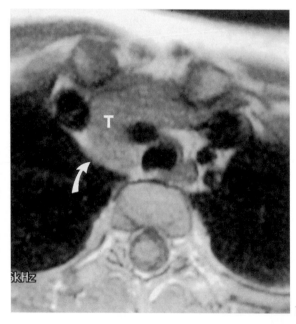

a   b

Fig. 11.4a,b. An 11-year-old male with retrocaval extension of normal thymus. **a** Axial T1-weighted (TR/TE 689/17; cardiac gated) magnetic resonance (MR) image at the level of the transverse thoracic aorta shows extension of the thymus (*curved arrow*) behind the superior vena cava. **b** MR image obtained at the level of the clavicular heads from the same sequence as in (**a**) shows the connection of the posteriorly extending thymus (*curved arrow*) to the thymus gland (*T*) in the typical anterior location. The MRI examination was obtained to evaluate for a mediastinal mass seen on echocardiography. The mass was the posterior extension of the thymus

11.4
Thymic Structure and Function

The normal thymus descends into the anterior mediastinum. The typical thymus gland begins just at or below the level of the left brachiocephalic vein, and is bordered anteriorly by the sternum and more lateral anterior chest wall, posteriorly by the aortic arch and branch vessels, and inferiorly by either the pulmonary outflow tract, the anterior heart, or the anteromedial hemidiaphragms (depending on the level of extent). In infancy and young childhood, the thymus takes on a quadrilateral configuration, with a triangular appearance typical of older children and adolescents. This configuration is best depicted with coronal imaging (Figs. 11.5, 11.6).

Arterial and venous structures for the thymus are variable. In general, the arterial supply rises from the internal thoracic, and superior and inferior thyroidal arteries. The arteries penetrate the gland laterally and superiorly; posterior penetration is less common (KORNSTEIN 1995). In this case, origin of the vessels can be from the common carotid or brachiocephalic arteries. Accessory thymic arteries can also occur. In addition, there may be asymmetry in vascular supply between the two lobes of the thymus in a child. Venous drainage is into the left brachiocephalic, internal thoracic, and inferior thyroidal vein. The thymic veins leave the gland through the medial aspect of both lobes. Occasionally, venous drainage can be into the superior vena cava or right brachiocephalic vein. While the vascular anatomy in the thymus gland has not received attention in imaging literature, these vessels can be identified particularly with the cross-sectional imaging modalities. With faster imaging times of helical and multislice CT,

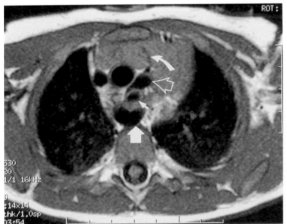

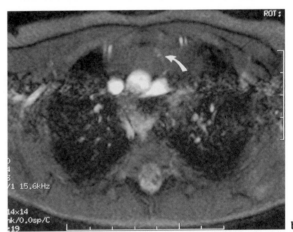

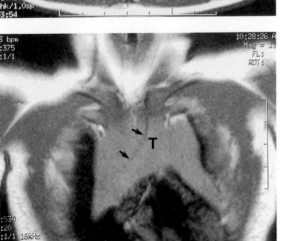

Fig. 11.5a–c. Normal thymus and demonstration of superior thymic vein. Magnetic resonance imaging was obtained to evaluate for an aberrant left subclavian artery arising from a right-sided aortic arch (not shown) in a child with obstructive airway symptoms. **a** Axial T1-weighted (TR/TE 530/20, cardiac-gated) axial image near the carina demonstrates a normal thymus with signal intensity slightly greater than that of skeletal muscle. A linear signal void is seen in the middle of the thymus (*curved arrow*) representing the superior thymic vein which originates from the brachiocephalic vein (*open arrow*). In this child, the course of the brachiocephalic vein was unusual in that it traveled in a retroesophageal course to the superior vena cava (not shown). Note also the diverticulum (*large arrow*) from the right-sided arch from which the aberrant subclavian artery originated, as well as mild tracheal narrowing (*small arrow*). **b** Gradient recall sequence (TR/TE 34/13; 33° flip angle) axial image identical to the level in (**a**) demonstrates high signal intensity representing flowing blood in the superior thymic vein (*curved arrow*). **c** Coronal T1-weighted (TR/TE 530/20, cardiac-gated) image of the anterior chest shows the quadrilateral configuration and the homogenous signal intensity of the thymus (*T*). The superior thymic vein (*small arrows*) that originates from the brachiocephalic vein is also evident

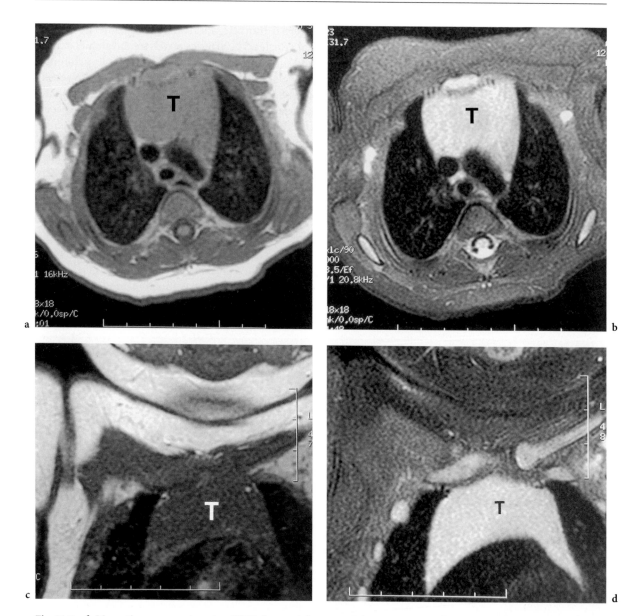

Fig. 11.6a–d. Magnetic resonance imaging (MRI) features of a normal thymus (*T*) in a 4-month-old male evaluated for Erb's palsy. **a** Axial T1-weighted (TR/TE 416/14) MR image at the level of the transverse thoracic aorta shows the homogeneous signal intensity which is isointense to skeletal muscle. **b** T2-weighted (TR/TE 4000/68; fast spin echo, fat saturated) MR image at the same level as in (**a**) demonstrates the homogeneous high signal intensity of the thymus. **c,d** Coronal T1-weighted (TR/TE 516/8) (**c**), and T2-weighted (TR/ 4000/65; fast spin echo, fat saturated) (**d**) MR images through the anterior mediastinum demonstrate the homogeneous signal intensity and quadrilateral configuration of the normal infant thymus

vascular opacification is improved and thymic vessels can be distinguished (Fig. 11.7). Using gradient recall sequences (or conceivably, intravenous contrast material), vascular structures are also identified and can be distinguished from other similar appearing structures such as fibrous septa (see Fig. 11.5).

Thymic size is highly variable even among children of the same age group. The size is either dis-cussed in terms of weight (grams) or dimension (centimeters); the latter description is typical for imaging literature. The normal variations and abnormalities in thymus size will be discussed below.

Grossly, the thymus is tan-yellow in color in children, being somewhat more pink in infancy. Because of fat, the adult gland becomes more yellow. Histolog-ically, the thymus contains a collection of cells which

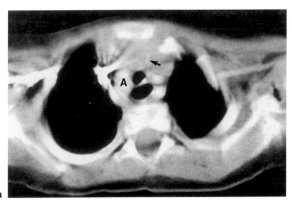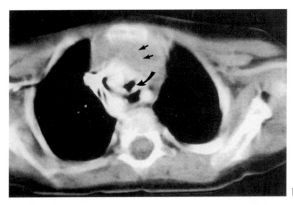

a   b

Fig. 11.7a,b. An 11-month-old male with normal thymus and thymic artery. Computed tomography (CT) angiography was performed to evaluate for a vascular ring. **a** IV contrast-enhanced CT examination is performed during dense arterial enhancement and demonstrates the superior thymic artery (*arrow*) at the level of the right-sided transverse thoracic aorta (*A*) in (**a**). **b** CT angiographic image obtained slightly more inferiorly shows thymic arteries (*arrows*). Note mild narrowing of the trachea (*curved arrow*) due to this vascular ring, completed by a small patent ductus arteriosis found at thoracotomy

are integral in the development of cellular immunity. It is these same cell types which contribute to the variety of thymic masses, including epithelial, stromal, and lymphoid tumors. The thymic gland contains cortical and medullary regions. Epithelial cells are found in either location. Those located in the medulla, which contain keratin and mucin, are slightly different to those in the cortex. These medullary epithelial cells are known more familiarly as Hassall's corpuses. The thymic gland also contains lympho-

cytes in various stages of maturation, macrophages and other mononuclear cells in addition to several other rarer cellular elements.

Thymic involution begins to occur in puberty. This process involves replacement of the septa with fat and enlargement of the perivascular spaces (KORNSTEIN 1995; HAYNES and HALE 1999) (Fig. 11.8). In addition, there is an overall decrease in cellular density and cystic degeneration of cell populations. These age-related changes result in the fatty replaced

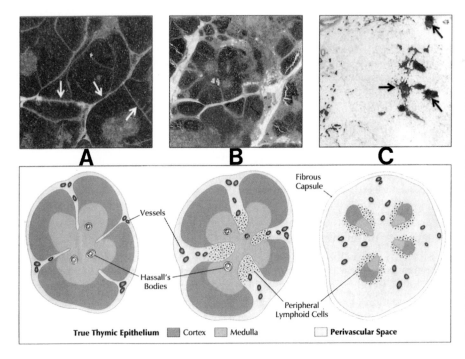

Fig. 11.8. Histologic and schematic representation of thymic structure at different ages. At 6 days of life (*A*), epithelial cells predominate. The perivascular compartment (*white arrows*) is small. At 15 years of age (*B*), the size of the perivascular space is increasing. At 65 years of age (*C*), the perivascular space contains fatty tissue, and surrounds small islands of true thymus (*white arrows*) (original histological preparations courtesy of Laura Hale, MD, Duke Medical Center; complete figure reprinted with permission, HAYNES and HALE 1999)

thymus characteristic in adults; the overall gland size, given fatty replacement, changes little if at all (HAYNES and HALE 1999). Age-related changes in thymic CT density have also been reported in children (SKLAIR-LEVY et al. 2000). Based on the image features, these investigators conclude that this cellular involution and fatty replacement is at least in part responsible for the decrease in CT density seen with advancing age in children.

The thymus gland is an integral component in the development and maintenance of immunocompetency. The primary function of the gland is differentiation and maturation of T (thymic)-cells which are key regulators in cellular immunity, as well as normal B-cell (humoral) immunity (HASSELBALCH et al. 1997). In disorders where the thymus gland fails to develop normally (i.e., severe combined immunodeficiency, DiGeorge syndrome), the deficiency in thymic size seen by imaging can be part of the clinical establishment of these disorders (YIN et al. 2000).

11.5
Imaging Appearance of the Normal Thymus Gland

The normal thymus gland can have a variety of appearances (e.g., size, location, homogeneity) for an individual imaging modality. The modalities that are useful for thymic imaging consist of radiography, sonography, CT, MRI, and nuclear medicine. While we still have yet to fully understand the variety of morphologic and functional imaging appearances of the thymus gland in children, a great deal of valuable information has been obtained in the last 2–3 decades with the advent of several imaging modalities. For this reason, the contribution of these relatively more recent modalities will be emphasized. As a basis for this more contemporary imaging approach, a brief discussion of the more traditional radiographic features (i.e., thymic size) will be provided, since this also applies to the more contemporary modalities.

As stated earlier in the chapter, the thymus gland has been historically misunderstood. Part of this reflects the past uncertainty concerning thymic function. However, thymic size itself is also implicated in misconception. Briefly, the thymus can vary greatly in size during infancy and childhood. In infancy, the thymus makes up the greatest proportion of overall bodyweight compared to any other time in life. This relationship changes over time. The consensus has

been that thymic size itself increases until puberty at which time the gland achieves its greatest gram weight. After this time, involution occurs. However, there is some disagreement about this; a recent review of this issue presented investigations that argued that thymic size actually varies little throughout childhood, ranging from 5–50 g from infancy to puberty (KORNSTEIN 1995).

Radiographically, the variations in thymus gland size can virtually always be identified based on location in the anterior mediastinum, homogeneous density, undulation of the lateral margins due to the subjacent ribs, and lack of mass effect on adjacent structures (Fig. 11.9). Most of these features, especially the homogeneity of the gland, transcend imaging modalities and provide a set of criteria which are important in determining whether the thymus is abnormal for other modalities as well.

Sonographically, the thymus has an echo texture similar to the liver (BEN-AMI et al. 1993; HASSELBALCH et al. 1997; KIM et al. 2000), but less than muscle (BEN-AMI et al. 1993), with punctate echoes and occasional echogenic lines (Fig. 11.10). Thymic size as determined using a thymic index (transverse and sagittal dimensions) has been reported to be variable in infants, but does correlate with birth weight (HASSELBALCH et al. 1997; ISCAN et al. 2000). Real time evaluation demonstrates the malleable appearance of the thymus during the respiratory cycle respiration that can help in separating normal tissue from a large mass.

The gland is easily identified in infants under about 1 year of age due to incomplete ossification of the sternum and manubrium (KIM et al. 2000). Routine thymic sonography includes transverse, and sagittal midline and parasternal images.

Sonography can be useful in thymic imaging, particularly given the lack of ionizing radiation, low cost, and relative availability. Indications include determining if an anterior mediastinal mass is normal thymus (KIM et al. 2000). In the setting of a mass, the presence of various features, including cysts, areas of calcification, or heterogeneous architecture, can suggest thymic pathology (KIM et al. 2000; BEN-AMI et al. 1993). Sonography should also be considered for biopsies or aspirations of thymic masses (Fig. 11.11). Recognition of variations in thymic position (e.g., retrocaval extension) during sonographic evaluation may also prevent additional and unnecessary imaging evaluation (KOUMANIDOU et al. 1998; LINDE et al. 1991) (see Fig. 11.4).

CT is an excellent modality for thymic evaluation. While ionizing radiation, the use of intravenous con-

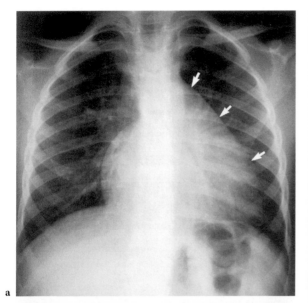

a

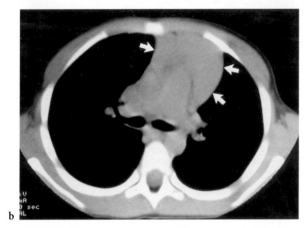

b

Fig. 11.9a,b. Normal thymic prominence in a 3-year-old boy referred for evaluation of a possible anterior mediastinal mass. a Posteroanterior chest radiograph demonstrates convex opacity that does not silhouette the main pulmonary artery (*arrows*). There is no displacement of the trachea or other mediastinal structures. b Axial non-contrast-enhanced computed tomography examination at the level of the main pulmonary artery demonstrates a normal thymus which is characterized by homogeneous soft tissue (isodense to skeletal muscle) in the anterior mediastinum with no displacement of intrathoracic structures

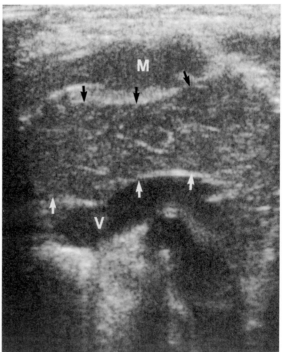

a

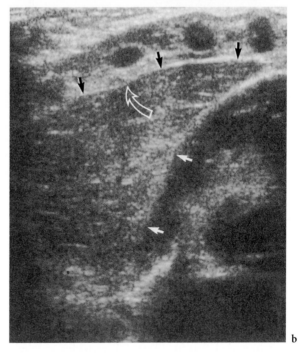

b

Fig. 11.10a,b. Normal thymic sonography in a 3-month-old male. a Transverse sonogram at the level of the brachiocephalic vein (*V*) shows hypoechoic thymic tissue (*arrows*) with punctate and linear echos. Note how the manubrium (*M*) is not completely ossified. b Parasternal sagittal view of the thymus (*arrows*) shows the anterior undulation of the gland (*curved arrow*) due to the rib; this feature of the thymus gland is well recognized with radiography

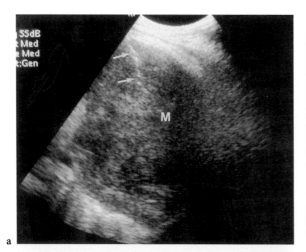

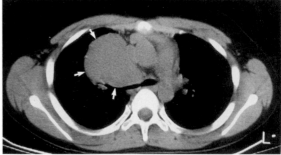

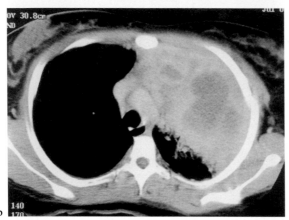

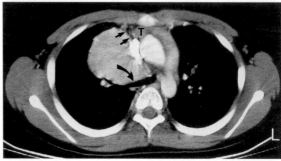

Fig. 11.12a,b. Distinguishing thymic from extrathymic disease: Castleman's disease of the anterior mediastinum in an 11-year-old boy. **a** Non-contrast-enhanced, axial computed tomography image just below the level of the transverse aorta arch demonstrates a mass in the anterior mediastinum (*arrows*). **b** Following administration of IV contrast material, there is greater enhancement than adjacent thymus. Note fat plane (*arrows*) separating nodal mass and thymus (*arrows*). The right main bronchus is also mildly narrowed (*curved arrow*)

Fig. 11.11a,b. An 18-year-old female with Hodgkin's lymphoma involving the anterior mediastinum and thymus gland. **a** Initial attempt at sonographically-guided percutaneous biopsy was unsuccessful given the high degree of fibrosis and necrotic tissue which was eventually determined after sternotomy and biopsy. Note that needle track (*arrows*) is well seen in the mass (*M*). **b** Axial IV contrast-enhanced computed tomography examination at the level of the transverse arch reveals a heterogeneous mass in the anterior mediastinum. Low attenuation regions represent areas of necrosis

trast material, and relatively greater cost are disadvantages compared with sonography, low dose scanning can minimize radiation risk. In addition, IV contrast reactions are actually quite rare in children (COHEN and SMITH 1994). CT provides excellent information on the thymus itself and the effect of thymic disorders on adjacent structures. CT helps to determine whether a mass is thymic in origin (Fig. 11.12), and can be used as a problem solving tool in cases of uncertain radiographic findings (Fig. 11.13). Abnormalities such as calcification, fat, cysts, and soft tissue heterogeneity are well depicted (Fig. 11.14). In

addition, an evaluation of the lung and airways and other adjacent structures are best evaluated by CT compared with sonography, MRI, and nuclear medicine.

The CT appearance of the normal thymus has been previously well described (ST. AMOUR et al. 1987). The thymus gland has homogenous soft tissue attenuation (see Fig. 11.9) with little variation in size in children aged 0–5 years (1.6+4.5 cm) to teenagers aged 16–19 years of age (1.8+4.2 cm) (ST. AMOUR et al. 1987). The left lobe is often slightly more prominent than the right lobe. The lateral edges of both the lobes are straight or slightly convex (infants and young children), or slightly concave (older children). Recently, age-related changes in thymic density have been reported in children (SKLAIR-LEVY et al. 2000). Thymic density was greatest during infancy with a mean attenuation of 80.8 HU with a gradual decrease in attenuation to 56 HU in teenage years probably due to fatty infiltration beginning in childhood (SKLAIR-

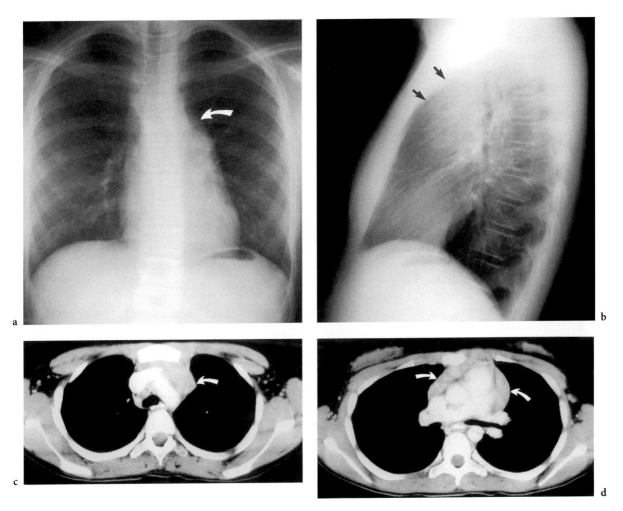

Fig. 11.13a–d. Unusual prominence of the thymus in a 12-year-old female who presented with substernal chest pain. **a** Posteroanterior view demonstrates soft tissue in the projection of the main pulmonary artery (*curved arrow*). **b** On the lateral radiograph there is increased opacity in the retrosternal region (*arrows*). **c,d** Axial IV contrast-enhanced chest computed tomography examination at the level of the aortic arch (**c**) and at the pulmonary artery bifurcation (**d**) show a homogeneous convex opacity (*curved arrows*) in both regions. While the enhancement was homogenous and normal thymus was a consideration, it was elected to perform a thymic biopsy because of chest pain rather than perform follow-up imaging. The biopsy confirmed normal thymic tissue

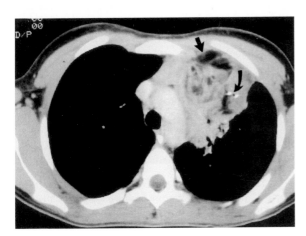

Fig. 11.14. A 12-year-old-female with a mature teratoma of the anterior mediastinum, involving the thymus. Axial IV contrast-enhanced computed tomography examination at the level of the transverse aorta shows a mixed attenuation mass of the left lobe of the thymus, involving the prevesicular region. Note soft tissue components, fat (*arrow*), and punctate calcification (*curved arrow*)

LEVY et al. 2000). Enhancement of the gland is homogenous, although the degree of enhancement in children has not been reported. With the advent of more rapid imaging provided by helical and, most recently, multislice CT, thymic vessels have been more evident. The cross sectional imaging appearance of thymic vessels has not yet been reported.

Routine chest CT techniques which have been previously described (ZEMAN et al. 1998) are usually adequate for dedicated thymic imaging. If depiction of calcification is important, then low dose (40–80 mA), and relatively thicker collimation (7–10 mm) images can be obtained to minimize additional radiation exposure prior to administration of contrast.

As with CT, the MRI appearance of the normal thymus has been well described (BOOTHROYD et al. 1992; SIEGEL et al. 1989; MOLINA et al. 1990). The multiplanar imaging sequences of MRI demonstrate the triangular or, in children generally under 5 years of age (SIEGEL et al. 1989), quadrilateral shape of the gland in the coronal plane (see Figs. 11.5, 11.6). MRI measurements of thymic dimensions support the contention that thymic size actually may vary little during childhood. In one report, dimensions of the lobes were not significantly different from infancy (3.0 cm width, 1.6 cm thickness) to 15–18 years of age (2.8 cm width, 1.5 cm thickness) (SIEGEL et al. 1989). With T1-weighting, the signal intensity is homogeneous and equal to, or slightly greater than, skeletal muscle. With T2-weighting, the signal intensity of the gland increases and is similar to fat; fat saturation does not decrease the high signal intensity of the thymus (Figs. 11.5, 11.6). As with CT, normal thymic arteries and veins can be depicted with the use of relatively high-resolution techniques, sequences, and coils.

The MRI technique for thymic evaluation is similar to techniques used with chest and mediastinal imaging (BOOTHROYD et al. 1992). Coil selection should be appropriate for age. A quadrature knee coil can be used in small infants. A head coil is appropriate for infants or small children. There are several torso coils designed for pediatric patients which provide excellent images. Typical thymic evaluation consists of T1- and T2-weighted axial, and either coronal or sagittal (or both) sequences. Cardiac gating is usually not necessary.

Nuclear scintigraphy is generally used as an imaging modality in staging and follow-up of lymphoma. There is only a limited role for focused evaluation of the thymus (LARAR et al. 1993). Gallium, thallium, and, more recently, ^{18}F-fluorodeoxyglucose positron emission tomography (PET) have been useful in the evaluation of the anterior mediastinum. Unfortunately, gallium and thallium uptake in rebound hyperplasia limits the usefulness of these agents in the setting of thymic lymphoma (LARAR et al. 1993; ROEBUCK et al. 1998). Increasing use of functional thymic imaging with fluorodeoxyglucose PET has provided helpful information in terms of lymphoma staging (O'HARA et al. 1999) (Fig. 11.15). However, it is not clear at this time what metabolic activity the normal thymus displays (O'HARA et al. 1996).

11.6
Thymic Disorders: Pattern-Oriented Classification

11.6.1
Abnormalities in Thymic size, Shape, or Location

The terms used to describe a small thymus include involution, hypoplasia, aplasia, and atrophy. Involution is a normal process of age-related decrease in gland size previously discussed. Thymic atrophy implies a previously normal thymus which has decreased in size most often due to some substantial systemic stress such as sepsis, major operative procedure, or agents such as steroids or a variety of chemotherapeutic agents. In these settings, thymic atrophy is easily recognized and transient and the thymus returns to normal size with resolution of the insult.

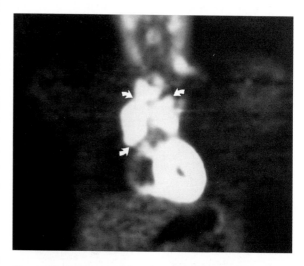

Fig. 11.15. A 15-year old male with Hodgkin's lymphoma. Coronal ^{18}F-fluorodeoxyglucose positron emission tomogram shows marked increase tracer activity in the anterior mediastinum (*small curved arrows*) as well as the left neck

Thymic aplasia and hypoplasia are other descriptors of a small (or absent) thymus. These are associated with T-cell related immune function. These terms are most familiar with DiGeorge syndrome. DiGeorge syndrome is due to abnormal development of the third and fourth pharyngeal pouch. Because of this, the syndrome is characterized by variable T-cell deficiency, and hypocalcemic seizures form parathyroid impairment. Great vessel, septal abnormalities and facial dysmorphology are also typical of DiGeorge syndrome. Thymic aplasia and hypoplasia are used interchangeably with partial (approximately 80% of cases) and complete DiGeorge syndrome, respectively. With partial DiGeorge syndrome, children can have a relatively intact immune system. This is in contradistinction to complete DiGeorge syndrome (thymic aplasia) where the immune dysfunction is severe, similar in type and degree to severe combined immunodeficiency (YIN et al. 2000). CT and MRI are of little use in thymic evaluation of immune disorders involving the thymus; however, in the setting of DiGeorge syndrome, these modalities can be useful in defining cardiovascular abnormalities when echocardiography may be inconclusive. Thymic epithelial transplants or bone marrow transplant are only recommended in cases of complete DiGeorge syndrome (MARKERT et al. 1999).

The thymus can also be absent or dysplastic in other immunodeficiencies with T-cell abnormalities such as ataxia-telangiectasia, or severe combined immune deficiency (SCID) syndrome (BUCKLEY et al. 1997; YIN et al. 2000). Perhaps the most familiar of these is SCID syndrome, which is characterized by an absence of normal thymic tissue in all cases (YIN et al. 2000) (Fig. 11.16). This lack of thymus can be an important observation in an infant in the first few months of life presenting with recurrent or severe infections; in this setting, the radiologist may be the first to suggest the diagnosis of an immunodeficiency (YIN et al., in press).

The thymus may be apparently absent due to an ectopic location. Most ectopic thymus glands have been reported to reside in the neck (90%), are lateral, and cystic in nature (KACKER et al. 1999). The imaging appearance depends on whether the ectopic tissue is solid or cystic. Solid ectopic glands have features of normal thymic tissue. The differential conditions for the solid gland include other masses in the neck such as lymphadenopathy or lymphadenitis, vascular malformations, hemangiomas, abnormal thyroid tissue, and sarcomas. Cystic considerations include cystic adenopathy, branchial cleft cysts, vas-

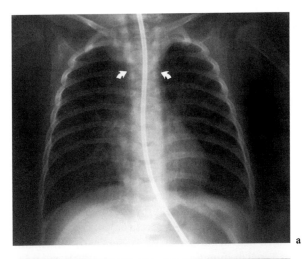

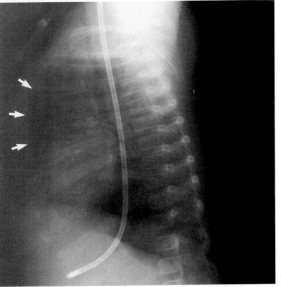

Fig. 11.16a,b. A 6-month-old female infant with severe combined immune deficiency syndrome. **a** Posteroanterior chest radiograph demonstrates absence of thymus (*curved arrows*). **b** On the lateral radiograph, there is increased lucency in the retrosternal region due to absent thymus. Hyperinflation is also present secondary to reactive airways disease due to past history of viral pneumonitis

cular malformations (i.e., lymphatic malformation or "cystic hygroma"), thyroglossal duct cysts, and dermoids or epidermoids.

One area of continued contention reminiscent of the historical association of the thymus with significant airway distress is that of the cervical thymus and its relationship to airway compression. While it has been noted that cervical herniation of the thymus is associated with innominate compression of the trachea due to crowding (MANDELL et al. 1994), similar anatomic relationships have been noted in children with no symptoms, or in children in whom the extent of tracheal narrowing is greater than that associated with a cervical thymus. In these children, investigators argue that the respiratory symptoms are due to an intrinsic problem with the trachea (MAHBOUBI et al. 1996).

Diffuse, homogeneous enlargement of the thymus gland is called hyperplasia (LINEGAR et al. 1993). The gland is hyperplastic if it is greater than about 50 g in weight. The hyperplastic thymus maintains the normal architecture and cellular components. Hyperplasia can be due to a provocation with rebound (also known as "true" hyperplasia), or it can be associated with syndromes such as Beckwith Widemann or T-cell dysfunction (WOYSODT et al. 1999), or endocrine or other disorders (usually only in adults) such as Grave's disease or myasthenia gravis, or be idiopathic, including the rare entity of giant thymic hyperplasia. Because of the association in adults with endocrine disorders, endocrine dysregulation is implicated as a possible mechanism; however, the etiology is unknown (WOYSODT et al. 1999). The most familiar condition in pediatric radiology is the true hyperplasia found following treatment for cancer. This is usually well recognized.

Massive thymic hyperplasia is an extreme of hyperplasia where there is no known provocation, and weights of up to 1260 g, with diameters of 17 cm, have been reported (LINEGAR et al. 1993; WOYSODT et al. 1999). Just over 70% of cases occur in children under 10 years of age, and virtually all cases are diagnosed during childhood, or before the third decade (DIMITRIOU et al. 2000; LINEGAR et al. 1993). Other than a massive enlargement, the imaging appearance is that of a normal thymus gland.

11.6.2
Focal Thymic Disorders

A variety of disorders can manifest with focal thymic disease in children (see Table 11.1). While focal thymic disorders include non-neoplastic conditions including abscesses and hemorrhage, these conditions, with the exception of thymic cysts, are sufficiently rare and clinically evident that the following discussion will focus on thymic neoplasms.

Thymic cysts are true epithelial lined fluids containing masses. Of all mediastinal cysts, only 3%–5% are of thymic origin (DAVIS et al. 1987). Thymic cysts represent less than 1% of all mediastinal masses in

children. Most thymic cysts are found in individuals of 20–50 years of age and are discovered incidentally.

Ectopic locations of thymic cysts have already been discussed. Those arising from the normally located thymus can vary in size from 1 to 18 cm (SUSTER and ROSAI 1991). The radiographic appearance is indistinguishable from a mediastinal mass or cardiac disease, including a pericardial effusion. Most cysts have fluid characteristics on CT or MRI, but the appearance of the fluid may be heterogeneous if there is associated hemorrhage (SUSTER and ROSAI 1991) (Fig. 11.17).

Tumors of thymus, excluding lymphoma, are rare causes of mediastinal masses in children (DEHNER et al. 1977). Benign pediatric neoplasms include thymolipoma and thymoma, and very rarely, hemangioma (NIEDZWIEDKI and WOOD 1990). Malignant tumors can be divided into primary and secondary tumors. Primary thymic malignancies include invasive thymoma, thymic carcinoma, and lymphoid tumors (ROSAI 1999). Thymic metastatic disease is rare in children; in a pediatric oncology textbook, the only primary tumor reference with thymic metastases was neuroblastoma (COHEN 1992). Thymic neoplasms can also be classified based on the cell type of origin. The most common are epithelial tumors (i.e., thymoma), germ cell tumors, stromal tumors (i.e., thymolipoma).

A thymolipoma is a tumor arising from thymic stroma. Most thymolipoma occur in children and young adults aged between 10 and 30 years. About one-third occur in individuals under 20 years of age, and half of these in the first decade (GREGORY et al. 1997; MORAN et al. 1995). The tumor has been reported in children as young as 2 years of age (MORAN et al. 1995). In two recent reviews it was noted that less than 10% of all thymic masses and 2%–9% of all thymic tumors were thymolipomas (GREGORY et al. 1997; MATSUDAIRA et al. 1994). Thymolipomas are asymptomatic in over 50% of cases (GREGORY et al. 1997; MORAN et al. 1995).

The appearance of a thymolipoma is fairly unique. This benign hamartoma is encapsulated with variable contributions of fat and thymic tissue. The location is anteromedial in 80% of cases. Because of the contribution of fat, either CT or MRI is an excellent imaging option (MORAN et al. 1995) (Fig. 11.18). The cross sectional imaging appearance is one of whorls of fatty tissue or soft tissue nodules interspersed in fat. These features are seen as low attenuation on CT and as high T1 and T2 signal intensity with MRI

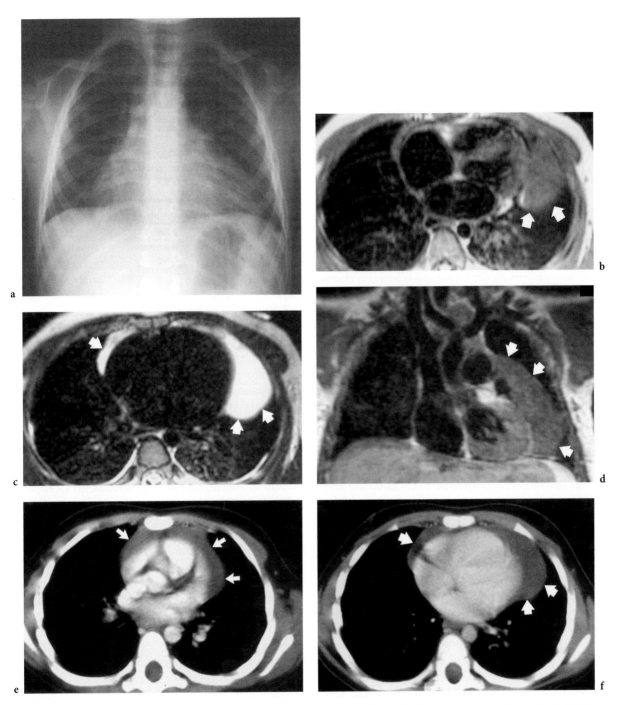

Fig. 11.17a–f. Thymic cyst in a 2-year-old-male. **a** Posteroanterior chest radiograph shows apparent cardiomegaly. Axial T1-weighted (TR/TE 540/20, cardiac gated) (**b**) and T2-weighted (TR/TE 5,000/144 fast spin echo) (**c**) magnetic resonance (MR) images obtained near the cardiac apex show a well-defined mass with T1-weighted signal intensity similar to skeletal muscle and T2-weighted signal intensity greater than fat. The mass is adjacent to both the left and right cardiac margin. **d** Coronal T1-weighted (TR/TE 555/20; cardiac gated) MR image at the level of the superior vena cava demonstrates the superior and inferior extent of the abnormality. Because there was concern about slightly heterogeneous signal intensity of this mass on MR imaging at some levels (not shown), a CT examination was performed. Axial IV contrast-enhanced CT examination at the level of the main pulmonary artery (**e**) and more inferiorly (**f**) demonstrate a homogenous fluid-attenuation mass which was confirmed at thoracotomy to be a thymic cyst (*arrows*). This was resected without complication. The heterogeneous signal intensity was due to hemorrhage within the cyst

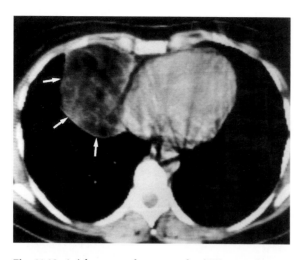

Fig. 11.18. Axial computed tomography (CT) scan shows a thymolipoma (*arrows*) with heterogeneous but predominately low (fatty) attenuation adjacent to the right atrium. (Original CT image courtesy of Daniel Melkus, MD, Herrin, Illinois; figure reprinted with permission, American College of Radiology)

(MATSUDAIRA et al. 1994; MOLINA et al. 1990; MORAN et al. 1995). Calcification and cystic spaces are not imaging features. Size can range up to 36 cm (MORAN et al. 1995). When this neoplasm also contains collagen, the mass is called a thymofibrolipoma (MORAN et al. 1994). Other than a teratoma, or a fat-containing vascular malformation, fatty masses of the thymus (e.g., lipoma) are extremely rare (CICCIARELLI et al. 1964).

Thymomas are either benign or invasive epithelial tumors of the thymus. The mean age for thymoma is 40–50 years (GRIPP et al. 1998). In total, 13% of thymomas occur between the ages of 10 and 29 years (GRIPP et al. 1998), and approximately 2% occur in the first decade. The tumor has been reported in infancy (DEHNER et al. 1977). Unlike in adults where there is a strong association with myasthenia gravis (30%–55%) (GAWRYCHOWSKI et al. 2000; GRIPP et al. 1998), thymomas in children are most often an isolated occurrence. There is an association in children with red cell aplasia and hypogammaglobulinemia (KORNSTEIN 1995). Histologically, thymomas are encapsulated and are characterized by epithelial proliferation. Cysts may be present histologically in up to 20% of tumors. The determination of invasion can be difficult and is based on evidence of either microscopic or gross evidence of capsular disruption, or distant metastases (KORNSTEIN 1995).

The appearance of a thymoma on CT and MRI is non-specific and based on only a few reports. The tumor presents as a focal mass, which may be lobulated (ST. AMOUR et al. 1987). Heterogeneous signal intensity with MRI has been noted, in addition to central hemorrhage (SIEGEL et al. 1989).

Thymic carcinoma is also rare in children. Most tumors occur from between the ages of 40 and 60 years, but have been noted in children as young as 4 years of age in a recent review (KORNSTEIN 1995). Thymic carcinoma is histologically distinct from invasive thymoma. There is no capsule and the tumor consists of areas of necrosis and hemorrhage, rare cystic change, and malignant cytology including high nuclear-to-cytoplasmic ratio, mitotic figures, among others (KORNSTEIN 1995). Because of these histologic features, attenuation or signal intensity is heterogeneous but not specific (Fig. 11.19).

Other thymic malignancies include thymic sarcoma (IYER et al. 1998) and carcinoid (LASTORIA et al. 1998). These are very rare in children.

Germ cell tumors of the thymus in children include teratomas (mature and immature), germinoma, embryonal carcinoma, yolk sac tumor, choriocarcinoma, and mixed types (ROSAI 1999). Teratoma is the most common type, accounting for 80% of all primary mediastinal germ cell tumors (RODGERS and McGAHREN 1996). With the exception of a teratoma, where the presence of calcification (20%–43%) (KORNSTEIN 1995), fat, cystic and soft tissue is characteristic (see Fig. 11.14), the features of germ cell tumors of the thymus are not specific (IYER et al. 1998) (Fig. 11.20). Elevations of serum tumor markers of beta-human chorionic gonadotrophin (B-HCG) or alpha-fetoprotein (AFP) are useful in identifying and following malignant germ cell tumors. Again, it is often impossible to discriminate primary thymic sites of origin from invasion from extra thymic sites of origin. This distinction is not important clinically.

11.6.3
Diffuse or Multifocal Thymic Disorders

Diffuse involvement of the thymus can be found with lymphoma, Langerhans' cell histiocytosis, HIV associated cystic dysplasia, or involvement by large tumors of the thymus discussed above in Sect. 11.6.2.

Lymphoid processes of the thymus which present as a multifocal or diffuse involvement include Hodgkin's disease, non-Hodgkin's lymphomas (i.e., lymphoblastic and large cell lymphoma) and Castleman's disease. The presence of adenopathy is very helpful in

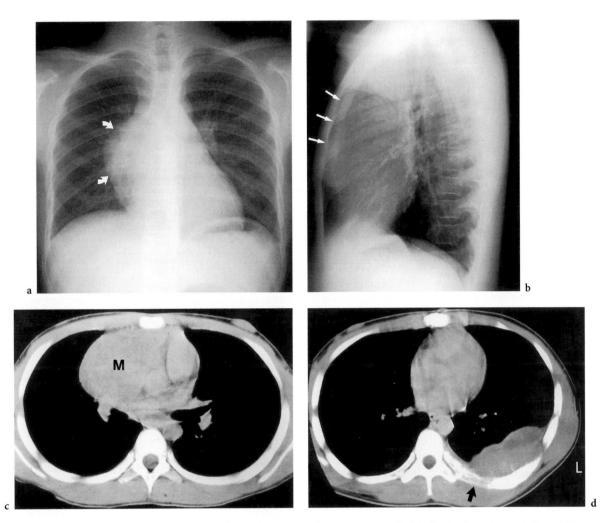

Fig. 11.19a–d. Thymic carcinoma in a teenage boy. **a** At 13 years of age, he presented with chest pain and an anterior medias-tinal mass (*small curved arrows*) evident predominately to the right on the posteroanterior chest radiograph. **b** On the lateral radiograph, there is dense opacification of the retrosternal region (*arrows*). **c** Axial non-contrast computed tomography (CT) performed at that time demonstrated a mass (*M*) with subtle heterogeneity in the anterior mediastinum. This was indistinguish-able from normal thymic tissue. Surgical findings and histology indicated that this was a thymoma. However, 18 months later he presented with pleural chest pain and a chest wall mass evident on a contrast-enhanced CT examination. **d** Note destruction of the adjacent rib (*arrow*). CT guided biopsy demonstrated that this was a carcinoma and the primary site was felt to be the previous thymic tumor

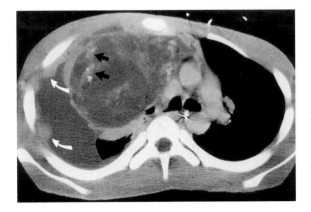

Fig. 11.20. A 14-year-old-male with a mixed germ cell tumor (seminoma and choriocarcinoma) involving the thymus. Axial IV contrast-enhanced computed tomography examination at the level of the carina shows a heterogeneous, prominently low attenuation mass with areas of calcification (*arrows*). Note also malignant pleura effusion and pleural metastases (*curved arrows*)

distinguishing lymphoma of the thymus from other masses (SIEGEL et al. 1989; SPIERS et al. 1997). For example, adenopathy was present in all children presenting with Hodgkin's lymphoma of the thymus in one report (SPIERS et al. 1997). In all patients with lymphoma, infiltration of the gland may be as much as 50% (SPIERS et al. 1997).

With lymphoma, the age of the child and presence of other regions of adenopathy can be helpful in prioritizing the histology (COHEN 1992). If the lymphoma is confined to thymus (or anterior mediastinum) in an older child or adolescent, a Hodgkin's-type lymphoma is likely. Hodgkin's disease is rare under 10 years of age; unlike with Hodgkin's lymphoma, non-Hodgkin's lymphoma can occur at any age. Large cell lymphoma occurs in older children.

The determination of whether or not residual thymic abnormalities represent residual disease is still problematic. In general, relapse is most often encountered in enlarged glands with heterogeneous signal intensity on MRI or attenuation with CT. On MRI, relapse is more likely if there are regions of T2-signal intensity greater than fat. T1-weighted signal intensity is not helpful; however, the presence of low heterogeneous signal intensity on T2-weighted sequences is reported to be seen only without relapse (SPIERS et al. 1997).

CT is recommended for initial evaluation of lymphoma. The appearance can be homogeneous or heterogeneous, due to areas of necrosis or fibrosis (see Fig. 11.11). It is important, as with any anterior mediastinal mass, to assess airway patency with radiography or CT. The MRI appearance of the thymus in lymphoma is variable. The gland can be diffusely enlarged, have asymmetric (lobar) enlargement, a lobular contour (Fig. 11.21), or have normal architecture. Areas of fibrosis are seen as relatively decreased T2-weighted signal intensity. Areas of hemorrhage and necrosis are seen as increased T2 signal intensity, greater than fat (SIEGEL et al. 1989).

T-cell lymphoblastic leukemia can also present as diffuse thymic disease (Fig. 11.22) with heterogeneous high signal on T2-weighted sequences (MOLINA et al. 1990). However, imaging of the thymus is not a routine evaluation for leukemia in children.

Langerhans' cell histiocytosis (LCH) is a solitary or multiorgan disorder characterized by infiltration of histiocytes of the Langerhans' cell type. Older nomenclatures for this disorder included eosinophilic granuloma. The incidence of thymic disease in LCH is unknown, but thymic involvement in up to 70% of children with multisystem disease has

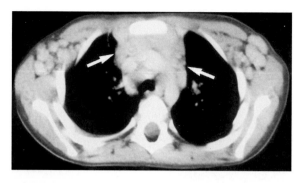

Fig. 11.21. A 3-year-old boy with T-cell non-Hodgkin's lymphoma. Axial IV contrast-enhanced computed tomography scan of the upper chest demonstrates anterior mediastinal adenopathy with lobular configuration of the thymus (*arrows*). Note also bilateral axillary adenopathy

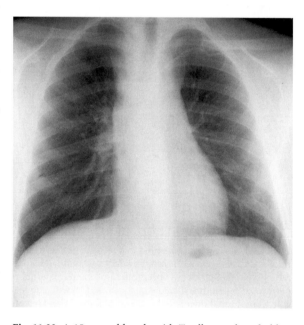

Fig. 11.22. A 15-year-old male with T-cell acute lymphoblastic leukemia. Posteroanterior chest radiograph shows anterior mediastinal widening which was due to thymic infiltration

been reported (HELLER et al. 1999; JUNEWICK and FITZGERALD 1999). In one small series of five children with thymic disease, cystic changes were evident in four, calcification in one, and thymic enlargement in all (JUNEWICK and FITZGERALD 1999). Diffuse heterogeneity with predominantly low attenuation with CT in systemic LCH with thymic involvement has also been reported (DONNELLY and FRUSH 2000) (Fig. 11.23).

Diffuse thymic disease can also be found in children with HIV infection. In a small series, including

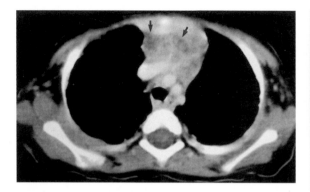

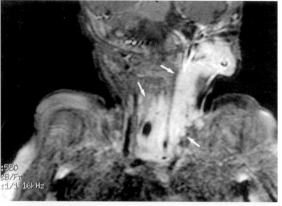

Fig. 11.23. A 20-month-old girl with thymic involvement by Langerhans' cell histiocytosis. Axial IV contrast-enhanced computed tomography of the upper chest shows diffuse, heterogeneous, predominately low, attenuation of the thymus gland (*arrows*)

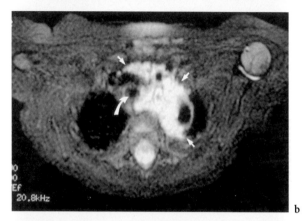

two children, the thymus was globally involved with cysts ranging in size from between 1 and 6 cm (LEON-IDAS et al. 1996) (Fig. 11.24). While some solid elements were evident, the abnormality was predominately cystic. Cystic thymic involvement, similar in appearance to that of the parotid glands with HIV, is felt to be associated with an accelerated lymphoid response with a relatively milder disease course (LEONIDAS et al. 1996).

Other diffuse or multifocal processes of the thymus include vascular malformations (Fig. 11.25).

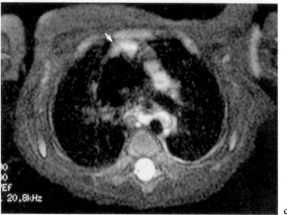

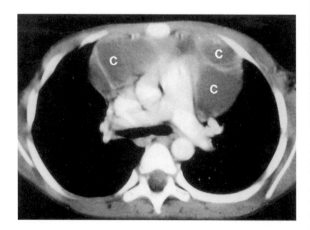

Fig. 11.24. HIV-associated cystic thymic dysplasia in an 8-year-old male. Axial IV contrast-enhanced computed tomography scan at the level of the pulmonary artery bifurcation shows variable-sized cystic spaces (*C*), with thin intervening septations, which replace the normal thymus gland

Fig. 11.25a–c. Thymic involvement by an extensive vascular malformation in a 3-month-old infant girl. **a** Coronal T1-weighted (TR/TE 550/8), contrast-enhanced magnetic resonance (MR) image shows the extensive involvement of the densely enhancing malformation (*arrows*) involving the left neck and mediastinum. **b** T2-weighted images (TR/TE 4000/96 fast spin echo; fat saturated) at the level of the brachiocephalic vein shows the infiltrating nature of the mass (*arrows*) and displacement of the trachea (*curved arrow*). **c** Axial MR image from the same sequence obtained at the level of the main pulmonary arteries demonstrates thymic involvement by the vascular malformation (*arrow*)

11.6.4
Specific Thymic Imaging Features: Calcification, Fat, Cysts

The identification of several imaging characteristics consisting of thymic calcification, fat, or cysts (Fig. 11.26) (Table 11.2) also proves to be useful in distinguishing between various thymic disorders. Rec-ognition of these features and familiarity with the individual imaging appearances on CT, sonography, and MRI is useful in the classification of disorders.

11.7
Conclusion

Imaging evaluation of the pediatric thymus gland can be challenging given the normal variation, as well as the wide variety of disorders that can involve the gland. It is important to be familiar with the spectrum of normal imaging appearances to prevent misdiagnosis of thymic disease. When the thymus is truly abnormal, classifying the pattern of involvement, as well as identifying certain imaging features, is useful in establishing the diagnosis or at least limiting the diagnostic possibilities. Understanding the advantages and disadvantages of the imaging options, especially sonography, CT and MRI, provides the radiologist with an opportunity for focused and successful thymic imaging strategies.

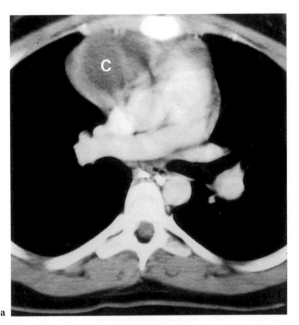

a

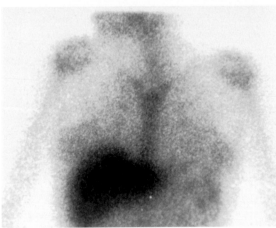

b

Fig. 11.26a,b. Thymic cyst in an 18-year-old female in remission for Hodgkin's lymphoma. **a** A thymic cyst (C) is shown on axial contrast-enhanced computed tomography examination at the level of the right pulmonary artery. High-density material in the region of the esophagus CT was due to previous lymphangiography. **b** At this time, a 67gallium-citrate study with images obtained at 72 h was negative for tracer activity in this region and the cyst gradually resolved during radiographic follow-up (not shown)

References

Bach AM, Hilfer CL, Holgersen (1991) Left-sided posterior mediastinal thymus-MRI findings. Pediatr Radiol 21:440–441

Baysal T, Kutlu R, Kutlu O et al (1999) Ectopic thymic tissue: a cause of emphysema in infants. Clin Imaging 23:19–21

Ben-Ami TE, O'Donovan JC, Yousefzadeh DK (1993) Sonography of the chest in children. Radiol Clin North Am 31:517–531

Boothroyd AE, Hall-Craggs MA, Dicks-Mireaux C et al (1992) The magnetic resonance appearances of the normal thymus in children. Clin Radiol 45:378–381

Buckley RH, Schiff RI, Schiff SE et al (1997) Human severe combined immunodeficiency: genetic, phenotypic, and functional diversity in one hundred eight infants. J Pediatr 130:378–387

Caffey J (1945) The mediastinum. In: Caffey J (ed) Pediatric x-ray diagnosis. Year Book, Chicago, pp 344–345

Cicciarelli FE, Soule EH, McGoon DW (1964) Lipoma and liposarcoma of the mediastinum: a report of 14 tumors including one lipoma of the thymus. J Thorac Cardiovasc Surg 47:411–429

Cohen MD (1992) Imaging of children with cancer, 1st edn. Mosby-Year Book, St Louis, pp 89–122, 136

Cohen MD, Smith JA (1994) Intravenous use of ionic and nonionic contrast agents in children. Radiology 191:793–794

Cooper AP (1832) The anatomy of the thymus gland. Longmand, Rees, Orme, Green and Brown, London, pp 1–48

Cure JK, Tagge EP, Richardson MS et al (1995) MR of cystic aberrant cervical thymus. AJNR 16:1124–1127

Davis RD, Oldham HN, Sabiston DC (1987) Primary cysts and neoplasms of the mediastinum: recent changes in clinical presentation, methods of diagnosis, management, and results. Ann Thorac Surg 44:229–237

Dehner LP, Martin SA, Sumner HW (1977) Thymus related tumors and tumor-like lesions in childhood with rapid clinical progression and death. Hum Pathol 8:53–66

Dimitriou G, Greenough A, Rafferty G et al (2000) Respiratory distress in a neonate with an enlarged thymus. Eur J Pediatr 159:237–238

Donnelly LF, Frush DP (2000) Langerhans' cell histiocytosis showing low-attenuation mediastinal mass and cystic lung disease. AJR 174:877–878

Gawrychowski J, Rokicki M, Gabriel A et al (2000) Thymoma – the usefulness of some prognostic factors for diagnosis and surgical treatment. Eur J Surg Oncol 26:203–208

Gregory AK, Connery CP, Resta-Flarer F et al (1997) A case of massive thymolipoma. J Pediatr Surg 32:1780–1782

Gripp S, Hilgers K, Wurm R et al (1998) Thymoma: prognostic factors and treatment outcomes. Cancer 83:1495–503

Hasselbalch H, Jeppesen DL, Ersboll AK et al (1997) Sonographic measurement of thymic size in healthy neonates. Relation to clinical variables. Acta Radiol 38:95–98

Haynes BF, Hale LP (1999) Thymic function, aging, and aids. Hospital Practice 34(3):59–87

Heller GD, Haller JO, Berdon WE, Sane S, Kleinman PK (1999) Punctate thymic calcification in infants with untreated Langerhans' cell histiocytosis: report of four new cases. Pediatr Radiol 29:813–815

Iscan A, Tarhan S, Guven H et al (2000) Sonographic measurement of the thymus in newborns: close association between thymus size and birth weight. Eur J Pediatr 159:223–224

Iyer R, Jaffe N, Ayala AG et al (1998) Thymic sarcoma in childhood. Br J Radiol 71:81–83

Jacobs MT, Frush DP, Donnelly LF (1999) The right place at the wrong time: historical perspective of the relation of the thymus gland and pediatric radiology. Radiology 210:11–16

Junewick JJ, Fitzgerald NE (1999) The thymus in Langerhans' cell histiocytosis. Pediatr Radiol 29:904–907

Kacker A, April M, Markentel CB et al (1999) Ectopic thymus presenting as a solid submandibular neck mass in an infant: case report and review of literature. Int J Pediatr Otorhinolaryngol 20:241–245

Kim OH, Kim WS, Kim MJ et al (2000) US in the diagnosis of pediatric chest diseases. Radiographics 20:653–671

Kornstein MJ (1995) Pathology of the thymus and mediastinum, 1st edn. Saunders, Philadelphia, pp 1–172

Koumanidou C, Vakaki M, Theophanopoulou M et al (1998) Aberrant thymus in infants: sonographic evaluation. Pediatr Radiol 28:987–989

Kuhn JP, Slovis TL, Silverman FN et al (1993) Part II: the neck and respiratory system. In: Silverman FN, Kuhn JP (eds) Caffey's pediatric x-ray diagnosis, 9th edn. Year Book Medical Publishers, Chicago, pp 637–695

Larar GN, O'Tuama LA, Treves ST (1993) Nuclear medicine in the pediatric chest. Radiol Clin North Am 31:481–498

Lastoria S, Vergara E, Palmieri G et al (1998) In vivo detection of malignant thymic masses by indium-111-DTPA-D-Phe–octreotide scintigraphy. J Nucl Med 39:634–639

Leonidas JC, Berdon WE, Valderrama E et al (1996) Human immunodeficiency virus infection and multilocular thymic cysts. Radiology 198:377–379

Linde LM, Marcus B, Padua E (1991) Normal thymus simulating pericardial disease: diagnostic value of magnetic resonance imaging. Pediatrics 88:328–331

Linegar AG, Odell JA, Fennell WMP et al (1993) Massive thymic hyperplasia. Ann Thorac Surg 55:1197–1201

Mahboubi S, Harty MP, Hubbard AM et al (1996) Innominate artery compression of the trachea in infants. Int J Pediatr Otorhinolaryngol 35:197–205

Mandell GA, McNicholas KW, Padman R et al (1994) Innominate artery compression of the trachea: relationship to cervical herniation of the normal thymus. Radiology 190:131–135

Markert ML, Boeck A, Hale LP et al (1999) Transplantation of thymus tissue in complete DiGeorge syndrome. N Engl J Med 341:1180–1189

Marra S, Hotaling AJ, Raslan W (1995) Cervical thymic cyst. Otolaryngol Head Neck Surg 112:338–340

Matsudaira N, Hirano H, Itou S et al (1994) MR imaging of thymolipoma. Magn Reson Imaging 12:959–961

Molina PL, Siegel MJ, Glazer HS (1990) Thymic masses on MR imaging. AJR 155:495–500

Moran CA, Zeren H, Koss MN (1994) Thymofibrolipoma: a histologic variant of thymolipoma. Arch Pathol Lab Med 118:281–282

Moran CA, Rosado-de-Christenson M, Suster S (1995) Thymolipoma: clinicopathologic review of 33 cases. Mod Pathol 8:741–744

Niedzwiecki G, Wood BP (1990) Radiological cases of the month. Thymic Hemangioma. Am J Dis Child 144:1149–1150

Oestreich AE (1995) William H Crane of Cincinnati and the first irradiation of the pediatric thymus. AJR 165:1064–1065

O'Hara SM, Betts JB, Coleman RE (1996) F-18 FDG PET imaging of the thymus gland in pediatric patients: preliminary results (abstract). Radiology 201(P):376

O'Hara SM, Donnelly LF, Coleman RE (1999) Pediatric body applications of FDG PET. AJR 172:1019–1024

Paltauf A (1889) Über die Beziehung der Thymus zum plötzlichen Tod. Wien Klin Wochenschr 2:877–881

Pohle EA (1950) The thymus. In: Pohle EA (ed) Clinical radiation therapy. Lea and Febiger, Philadelphia, pp 676–684

Rodgers BM, McGahren ED (1996) Mediastinum and pleura. In: Oldham KT, Colombani PM, Foglia RP (eds) Surgery of infants and children. Lippincott-Raven, Philadelphia, p 928

Roebuck DJ, Nicholls WD, Bernard EJ et al (1998) Misleading leads thallium-201 uptake in rebound thymic hyperplasia. Med Pediatr Oncol 30:297–300

Rosai J (1999) Histological typing of tumours of the thymus, 2nd edn. Springer, Berlin Heidelberg New York, pp 9–23

Siegel MJ, Glazer HS, Wiener JI et al (1989) Normal and abnormal thymus in childhood: MR imaging. Radiology 172:367–371

Sklair-Levy M, Agid R, Sella T et al (2000) Age-related changes in CT attenuation of the thymus in children. Pediatr Radiol 30:566–569

Slovis TL, Meza M, Kuhn JP (1992) Aberrant thymus-MR assessment. Pediatr Radiol 22:490–492

Spiers ASD, Husband JES, MacVicar AD (1997) Treated thymic lymphoma: comparison of MR imaging with CT. Radiology 203:369–376

St Amour TE, Siegel MJ, Glazer HS et al (1987) CT appearances of the normal and abnormal thymus in childhhod. J Comput Assist Tomogr 11:645–650

Suster S, Rosai J (1991) Multilocular thymic cyst: an acquired reactive process. Am J Surg Pathol 15:388–398

Swischuk LE, John SD (1996) Case report – normal thymus extending between the right brachiocephalic vein and the innominate artery. AJR 166:1462–1464

Woysodt A, Verhaart S, Kiss A (1999) Case report – massive true thymic hyperplasia. Eur J Pediatr Surg 9:331–333

Yin E, Frush DP, Donnelly LF, Buckley RH (2000) Primary immunodeficiency disorders in children: clinical features and imaging findings. AJR (in press)

Zeman RK, Baron RL, Jeffrey RB Jr et al (1998) Helical body CT: evolution of scanning protocols. AJR 170:1427–1438

12 Lymphoma – Controversies in Imaging the Chest

Sue C. Kaste

CONTENTS

12.1
Introduction

In the United States each year, approximately three cases of pediatric Hodgkin's disease and four cases of pediatric non-Hodgkin's lymphoma occur per 100,000 members of the population (LEVENTHAL and DONALDSON 1993). In such cases, diagnostic imaging is an integral part of staging and monitoring disease progression. However, staging and assessing disease activity in the chest is particularly difficult in pediatric patients because of the presence of the thymus, the lack of mediastinal fat, and the small size of anatomic structures. Thymic rebound or regrowth

SUE C. KASTE, DO
Associate Member, Department of Diagnostic Imaging, St. Jude Children's Research Hospital, 332 N. Lauderdale St., Memphis, TN 38105, USA

further complicates disease assessment. This chapter addresses staging complications caused by thymic tissue, the distinction between lymphoma-related pulmonary nodules and those related to other processes, and methods of differentiating between recurrent active disease and residual quiescent disease. The strengths and weaknesses of available imaging techniques is incorporated into each section.

12.2
Imaging Techniques for Differentiating Normal from Abnormal Thymic Tissue

Abnormal thymic tissue varies in size, contour, imaging characteristics, and may even obscure a mediastinal mass (BOOTHROYD et al. 1992; LIANG and HUANG 1997). Thymic tissue may develop in unusual locations; when such unusual findings are accompanied by symptoms, clinical and imaging problems may arise (HEIBERG et al. 1982; LEMAITRE et al. 1987; ROLLINS and CURRARINO 1988; THOMAS and GUPTA 1988). On imaging studies, even normal thymic tissue can mimic a mediastinal mass, and this fact can lead to a false-positive diagnosis (ADAM and IGNOTUS 1993; CHOYKE et al. 1987; HAN et al. 1989; LEMAITRE et al. 1987; LIANG and HUANG 1997). In contrast, the thymus may be the only site of involvement by Hodgkin's disease in children (LUKER and SIEGEL 1993). Thus, familiarity with the imaging characteristics of normal thymic tissue can facilitate staging and the differentiation of normal thymic tissue from diseased tissue (COHEN et al. 1980).

12.2.1
Radiographs of the Chest

Plain radiography is the least sensitive method of detecting normal thymic tissue. Characteristically, on plain radiographs the thymus appears as an anterior mediastinal mass that may be indented in relationship to anterior ribs. Although normal thymic tissue is usually low in density and appears relatively lucent, concurrent mediastinal disease may still be present (COHEN et al. 1980).

12.2.2
Computed Tomographic Imaging of the Chest

Because computed tomography (CT) is highly sensitive in detecting mediastinal, pericardial, pulmonary, and pleural abnormalities, it is the primary imaging method used for complete and accurate staging and follow-up of childhood Hodgkin's disease and non-Hodgkin's lymphoma (CHOYKE et al. 1987; HAMRICK-TURNER et al. 1994).

On CT images, the normal thymus generally has smooth, wavy lateral margins. During the first decade of life, the thymus generally maintains mildly convex lateral borders and a homogeneous density (FRANCIS et al. 1985), although straight or biconcave contours with intermediate soft tissue density may also be seen (HEIBERG et al. 1982; LUKER and SIEGEL 1993). However, in older children and adolescents, the biconcave configuration is typical (HEIBERG et al. 1982). After puberty, the density of the thymus becomes inhomogeneous because of fatty infiltration, and the gland itself becomes triangular in configuration (FRANCIS et al. 1985). Nodularity of the thymus is not a normal finding for patients of any age (FRANCIS et al. 1985; MOORE et al. 1983).

One factor that may aid in differentiating normal thymic tissue from diseased tissue is that on CT images the normal thymus appears to mold around the heart, great vessels, and anterior mediastinum without deforming them. In contrast, diseased thymic tissue lacks this characteristic; it appears more nodular and lobulated and may distort the shape of normal structures (HEIBERG et al. 1982; LEMAITRE et al. 1987).

12.2.3
Ultrasonography of the Chest

Because ultrasonography is noninvasive, it is an attractive method for evaluating the mediastinum in children. However, the results of sonographic imaging can be compromised by the presence of dense cartilage of the anterior ribs and by the calcified sternum. Ultrasonography allows good visualization of the thymus in children younger than 2 years when the parasternal, transternal, or suprasternal approaches are used (LEMAITRE et al. 1987; LIANG and HUANG 1997). On ultrasonographic images, the normal thymus has a sharply defined smooth margin with homogeneously low echogenicity that is similar to that of liver (HAN et al. 1989; LEMAITRE et al. 1987; LIANG and HUANG 1997; SIEGEL et al. 1989). This normal pattern of echogenicity does not vary with the age of the patient. On transverse images, the thymus has a bilobar or trapezoidal configuration, whereas on longitudinal images a lunate contour is typical (LEMAITRE et al. 1987; LIANG and HUANG 1997). The thymus is wider and thicker in boys than in girls, and its width increases with increasing age (LIANG and HUANG 1997).

12.2.4
Magnetic Resonance Imaging of the Chest

Magnetic resonance (MR) imaging is useful for defining the mediastinal structures without the need for radiation or iodinated contrast agents. However, the use of sedation, which is often needed to complete the examination in children, is particularly problematic when a mediastinal mass is compressing the airway. Furthermore, detection of adenopathy by MR imaging can be compromised by the limits of spatial resolution (DALDRUP et al. 1998).

BOOTHROYD and colleagues used images obtained at a field strength of 1.5 Tesla (T) to study the thymus in 31 children aged between 2 weeks and 12 years (BOOTHROYD et al. 1992). They found that normal thymus had an angular shape with acute angles, particularly in the coronal plane (one thymus had a rounded margin); homogeneous signal intensity similar to that of liver and muscle on T1-weighted sequences; signal intensity greater than that of fat on T2-weighted spin echo and short t inversion recovery (STIR) sequences; and normally distended mediastinal veins (ABRAHAMSEN et al. 1994; BOOTHROYD et al. 1992). SIEGEL and coworkers further defined age-related MR imaging characteristics of normal thymus. In children younger than 5 years, the thymus was quadrilateral in shape with biconvex lateral margins; in older children and adolescents, it had a characteristic triangular configuration with straight margins (SIEGEL et al. 1989). Although normal thymic tissue can occur in unusual locations, its normality can often be documented noninvasively by the presence of a homogeneous signal with intensity between those of muscle and fat on T1-weighted images and moderate intensity on T2-weighted images (Rollins and Currarino 1988) (Fig. 12.1).

In contrast, abnormal thymus has the following MR imaging characteristics: focal signal changes; an enlarged rounded shape with obtuse angles; heterogeneous signal intensity; and distortion, encasement, and displacement of mediastinal veins. In children with a histologically proven diagnosis of lymphoma, the thymus was characterized by rounded or distorted contours, focal signal changes, and extrinsic compression of the superior vena cava (Boothroyd

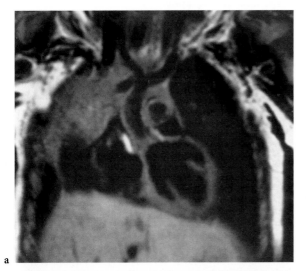

a

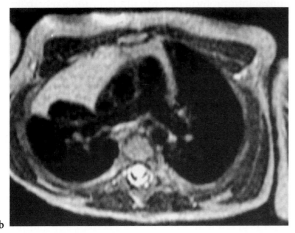

b

Fig. 12.1a,b. A 9-month-old girl undergoing evaluation for pulmonary hypoplasia. Coronal non-contrast T1-weighted (522/20) (**a**) and axial T2-weighted (2000/80) (**b**) magnetic resonance images of the chest show normal-appearing thymus gland occupying part of the right chests to compensate for right-sided pulmonary hypoplasia. Note homogeneous signal throughout the gland and distribution of the thymus molding around central structures. (Courtesy of Dr. Fred Hoffer)

et al. 1992; Siegel et al. 1989). When the thymus is involved by lymphoma, leukemia, or hyperplasia, inhomogeneous signal characteristics resulted from cystic degeneration, septations, fibrosis, calcifications, or hemorrhage. When hilar or mediastinal adenopathy occurs with these heterogeneous signal characteristics, lymphomatous involvement of the thymus is even more strongly suggested (Siegel et al. 1989) (Fig. 12.2).

12.2.5
Nuclear Imaging

12.2.5.1
⁶⁷Gallium Scintigraphy

Although gallium nuclear scintigraphy is variably sensitive in detecting tumor, it is the standard imaging modality for the staging of Hodgkin's disease and non-Hodgkin's lymphoma. In imaging non-Hodgkin's lymphoma, the sensitivity of this imaging method depends on the histologic subtype and grade of the disease (Hamrick-Turner et al. 1994). Gallium avidity in normal thymic tissue may complicate disease staging in children and adolescents. Hibi and colleagues found that gallium avidity occurred in 39% of cases of pediatric solid tumors and in 29% of thymus scans performed for cases of pediatric lymphoma. The incidence of gallium uptake by thymic tissue was greatest (90%) in children 1–2 years of age, regardless of tumor diagnoses, but including Hodgkin's disease and non-Hodgkin's lymphoma (Hibi et al. 1987). If gallium imaging is performed after therapy begins, false-negative findings may result. Furthermore, although ⁶⁷gallium scintigraphy is highly sensitive in detecting disease, its relative diagnostic accuracy is only 75%; when the findings are compared with those of other imaging modalities, false-positive findings occur in as many as 34% of cases (Cohen et al. 1986).

Single photon emission computed tomography (SPECT) can optimize the detection of avidity (Hamrick-Turner et al. 1994). This imaging method may be particularly helpful in conjunction with planar gallium imaging; because gallium is typically taken up by the normal skeleton, subtle areas of avidity may be obscured as the result of normal uptake of gallium by the bony thorax.

A study of 34 patients aged 8–49 years compared the sensitivity and specificity of ⁶⁷gallium scintig-

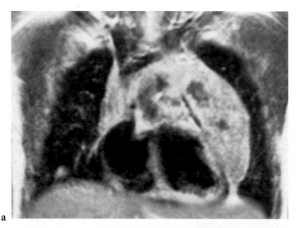

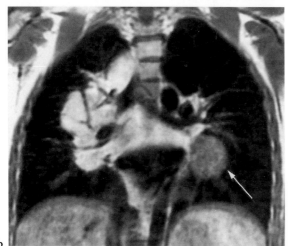

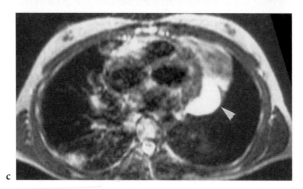

raphy and MR imaging in diagnosing disease. The results showed that [67]gallium scintigraphy was less sensitive but more specific than MR imaging in detecting disease (gallium sensitivity and specificity, 85.7% and 100%, respectively; MR imaging sensitivity and specificity, 92.8% and 80.6%, respectively). Furthermore, the positive predictive value of [67]gallium imaging was 100%, whereas that of MR imaging was 68.4%. Thus, the accuracy of [67]gallium imaging was 95.5%, whereas that of MR imaging was 84.4% (GASPARINI et al. 1993).

12.2.5.2
[201]Thallium Scintigraphy

A recent study of thallium avidity in mediastinal Hodgkin's disease and non-Hodgkin's lymphoma attempted to solve the problem of differentiating gallium-avidity in normal thymus from thymic involvement by tumor. FLETCHER and coworkers studied 33 pediatric patients with Hodgkin's disease and found that thallium scintigraphy is as accurate in predicting disease as either gallium scintigraphy or CT scanning. Thallium scintigraphy was 100% sensitive in detecting pediatric Hodgkin's disease; no false-positive findings occurred (FLETCHER et al. 1995). However, ROEBUCK and colleagues reported a single case of false-positive avidity in a 7-year-old girl with rebound thymic hyperplasia (ROEBUCK et al. 1998).

Thallium scintigraphy may be preferable to gallium scintigraphy because thallium is not taken up by normal bones, delivers a relatively lower whole-body radiation dose than gallium (TONAMI and HISADA 1977), and is not taken up by the normal mediastinum (NADEL 1993). In addition, thallium scintigraphy can be completed in one appointment, whereas gallium scintigraphy typically requires 2–3 days for completion (FLETCHER et al. 1995). Thallium uptake may indicate tumor grade, because low-grade Hodgkin's disease is characterized by greater thallium uptake than intermediate or high-grade disease (NADEL 1993). Although thallium is not taken up by normal bones, its intensity may be attenuated by overlying soft tissues. Thus, SPECT imaging may be helpful in conjunction with planar thallium scintigraphy in detecting disease.

12.2.5.3
FDG-PET Imaging

Positron emission tomography (PET) with 18-fluorodeoxyglucose (FDG) provides characterization of

Fig. 12.2a–c. This 16-year-old girl was undergoing staging evaluation for Hodgkin's disease. **a** Coronal contrast-enhanced T1-weighted (750/20) magnetic resonance (MR) image of the chest shows inhomogeneous signal characteristics of the enlarged thymus gland. **b** Coronal contrast-enhanced T1-weighted (750/20) MR image of the chest demonstrates extensive bilateral hilar and mediastinal adenopathy. The nonenhancing rounded structure in the left infrahilar region (*arrow*) is a cystic portion of thymic disease. **c** Axial T2-weighted MR image shows homogeneously increased signal in the cystic portion of the mediastinal mass. Also note associated right lower lobe pulmonary disease (*arrowhead*). (Courtesy of Dr. FRED HOFFER)

functional metabolic tissue regardless of morphology (ZINZANI et al. 1999). The role of FDG-PET in childhood lymphomas has not been fully defined. However, lymphomas demonstrate high FDG uptake that resolves after successful oncotherapy (SHULKIN 1997; SHULKIN et al. 1995). VALK and coworkers found that in 25% of untreated and 100% of treated patients with recurrent disease, PET identified sites of disease and correctly staged disease at a more advanced stage than CT, gallium scintigraphy, or lymphangiography (VALK et al. 1996). These findings prompted alteration of planned therapy in 12% of untreated patients and in half of those with recurrent disease (ZINZANI et al. 1999). Thus, PET is more accurate in diagnosing and staging recurrent Hodgkin's disease than are conventional imaging techniques (ZINZANI et al. 1999).

12.3
Lung Lesions: Differentiation Between Metastatic Sites and Benign Processes

12.3.1
Patterns of Pulmonary Lymphoma

The presence of pulmonary metastatic disease is a characteristic of stage IV Hodgkin's disease; this finding considerably alters therapy and prognosis. Thus, differentiating between benign and metastatic disease is imperative for proper staging of the disease status, for counseling the patient and the family about prognosis, and for designing proper therapy.

Disease metastasizes to the lungs by hematogeneous dissemination, lymphangitic spread, direct invasion, or a combination of the three. In non-Hodgkin's lymphoma and Hodgkin's disease, the mechanism of spread is typically hematogeneous or lymphangitic. Most hematogeneously disseminated pulmonary metastasis occurs through the pulmonary circulation. However, it has been suggested that the disease may also be disseminated through bronchial arteries. Hematogeneous dissemination of tumor emboli may occur along lymphatic channels, or lymphatic involvement may develop by retrograde proliferation along the lymphatic channels from mediastinal or hilar lymph nodes. Lymphangitic spread is less commonly caused by direct extension (SNYDER and PUGATCH 1998).

In patients with Hodgkin's disease, the pulmonary parenchyma is rarely involved at the time of diagnosis unless mediastinal or hilar adenopathy is present (AU and LEUNG 1997). Rare cases of primary pulmonary Hodgkin's disease have been reported in adults without hilar or disseminated disease (FRIEDLAND et al. 1982; NELSON et al. 1983; PIK et al. 1986). The incidence of pulmonary involvement by Hodgkin's disease in all patients is 5%–10% at the time of diagnosis (LEONE et al. 1990), increases to an overall incidence of 11%–40% (FRIEDLAND et al. 1982; NELSON et al. 1983; PIK et al. 1986; SHULKIN 1997; YOUSEM et al. 1986), is nearly 50% just before death (LEONE et al. 1990), and is more than 50% at the time of autopsy (SHAHAR et al. 1987; YOUSEM et al. 1986). In adults, pulmonary involvement is found in 50%–90% of cases of the nodular sclerosing subtype of Hodgkin's disease, but in only 5%–20% of cases of the other histologic subtypes (FRIEDLAND et al. 1982). Pulmonary involvement is twice as common in female patients; it is also more common among patients who are older at the time of diagnosis and those with B symptoms (YOUSEM et al. 1986), i.e., unexplained weight loss of at least 10% over the 6 months prior to diagnosis of Hodgkin's disease, unexplained fever for at least 3 consecutive days, and drenching night sweats (LEVENTHAL and DONALDSON 1993); these symptoms are usually associated with advanced-stage disease.

Pulmonary Hodgkin's disease is characterized by three patterns that can assist physicians in making an accurate diagnosis. Pulmonary involvement by Hodgkin's disease or non-Hodgkin's lymphoma is most commonly characterized by single or multiple pulmonary nodules of various sizes (AU and LEUNG 1997; LEONE et al. 1990) (Fig. 12.3). Whereas on CT images most pulmonary metastases originating from solid tumors are well-circumscribed solid nodules, pulmonary parenchymal tumors originating from the lymphomas may have somewhat irregular borders, may be cavitary, and may even mimic a pulmonary infiltrate (SHAHAR et al. 1987) (Figs. 12.4, 12.5).

In a study of 15 adults with primary pulmonary Hodgkin's disease, YOUSEM and colleagues found that histologic examination of all solitary pulmonary nodules showed central necrosis surrounded by a cellular border of lymphocytes, plasma cells, eosinophils, and Reed-Sternberg cells (YOUSEM et al. 1986). Alternatively, however, in the case of small bronchial obstructions, trapped air may lead to cavitation by a check-valve mechanism. The occurrence of cavitation after chemotherapy or radiation therapy is uncommon (SPIERS et al. 1997).

Unlike Hodgkin's disease, non-Hodgkin's lymphoma is associated with pulmonary involvement at

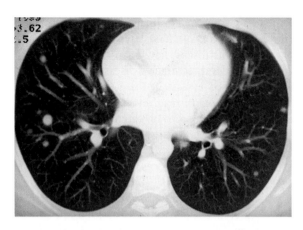

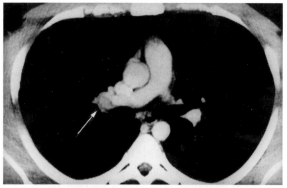

Fig. 12.3. This 19-year-old girl presented with multiple pulmonary nodules at the time of diagnosis of Hodgkin's disease as shown on this axial computed tomography image of through the chest, filmed with lung window

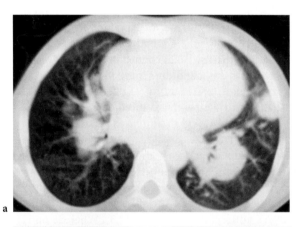

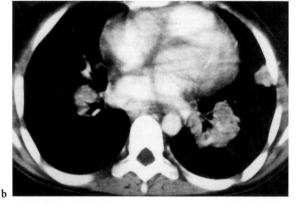

Fig. 12.5a,b. This 22-year-old man underwent routine off-therapy evaluation. Axial contrast-enhanced CT of the chest filmed with mediastinal (**a**) and lung windows (**b**), demonstrated right hilar adenopathy (*arrow*) and an irregular pleural-based pulmonary nodule (*arrowhead*). These findings were suspicious for pulmonary recurrence but serologic studies identified blastomycosis

Fig. 12.4a,b. This 12-year-old boy was diagnosed with nodular sclerosing Hodgkin's disease. Axial contrast-enhanced chest computed tomography filmed with lung window (**a**) and mediastinal window (**b**), demonstrate multiple pulmonary masses in concert with extensive bilateral hilar and mediastinal adenopathy. Note confluence and irregular margins of the pulmonary masses

the time of diagnosis in fewer than 5% of cases; lung involvement may occur without concurrent mediastinal or hilar disease (AU and LEUNG 1997). Like pulmonary parenchymal Hodgkin's disease, pulmonary parenchymal non-Hodgkin's lymphoma is most commonly manifested by multiple pulmonary nodules, but cavitation of nodules is rare at the time of diagnosis (AU and LEUNG 1997).

Pulmonary Hodgkin's disease is characterized by three patterns on imaging studies. The first pattern is the presence of both pulmonary nodules and ipsilateral mediastinal adenopathy; when both factors are present, the probability that the nodules are caused by metastatic lymphoma is increased (AU and LEUNG 1997). However, because histoplasmosis may also be characterized by pulmonary nodules with mediastinal adenopathy, making an accurate imaging diagnosis is more difficult when patients live in an area in which this inflammatory disease is endemic. Nevertheless, because pulmonary lymphoma does not typically form calcifications, the presence of central calcifications in lung nodules with or without mediastinal adenopathy suggests an inflammatory process such as histoplasmosis (CHAI and PATZ 1994; GURNEY and CONCES 1996). The presence of splenic calcifications, mediastinal calcifications, or both supports a granulomatous process (Fig. 12.6).

The second pattern characteristic of pulmonary Hodgkin's disease is the reticular interstitial pattern that results from venous or lymphatic obstruction caused by hilar or mediastinal adenopathy, or occurring intrinsically from interstitial tumor deposits (AU and LEUNG 1997) (Fig. 12.7).

The third pattern characteristic of pulmonary Hodgkin's disease is lobar or segmental consolidation. This pattern also occurs in non-Hodgkin's lym-

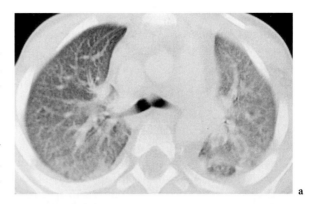

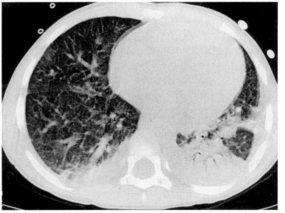

Fig. 12.7a,b. A 2-year-old boy presented in respiratory distress with anaplastic non-Hodgkin's lymphoma and biopsy proven pulmonary lymphoma. a Axial chest computed tomography, filmed with lung window, demonstrates diffuse bilateral interstitial pulmonary opacities associated with ground glass appearance of the lungs. b High resolution image of the chest, filmed with lung window shows to better advantage, the diffuse interstitial disease of pulmonary non-Hodgkin's lymphoma. Also note areas of consolidation with air bronchograms

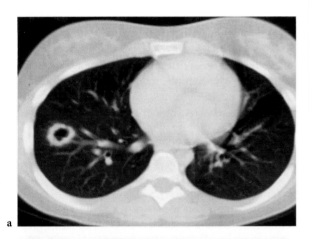

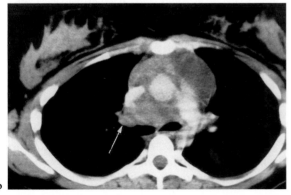

Fig. 12.6a,b. This 15-year-old girl was diagnosed with nodular sclerosing Hodgkin's disease. a Axial contrast-enhanced chest computed tomography filmed with lung window shows a cavitary right lower lobe pulmonary nodule with irregular margins. b Concurrent image filmed with mediastinal window shows extensive mediastinal and more subtle right hilar adenopathy (*arrow*)

phoma, and its appearance on radiographs may be confused with that of pneumonia (AU and LEUNG 1997). Primary extranodal pulmonary lymphoma with this pattern is thought to arise from bronchial lymphoid tissue and is usually a low-grade B-cell lymphoma (AU and LEUNG 1997).

Although imaging characteristics may suggest the correct diagnosis, a definitive diagnosis is possible only with biopsy. The results of percutaneous lung biopsy, which can be performed safely (WITTICH et al. 1992), are as accurate as those obtained by thoracotomy (DIEFENTHAL and TASHJIAN 1988; OGNIBENE et al. 1988). Alternatively, lung nodules may be adequately assessed by thoracoscopic biopsy with or without preoperative CT-directed localization.

12.3.2
Imaging Characteristics of Pulmonary Nodules

12.3.2.1
CT

The ability of CT to detect lung nodules has considerably improved tumor staging. Because CT can detect lung lesions as small as 2–3 mm in diameter, it is far more sensitive than chest radiography (ROSENFIELD et al. 1992). However, the radiographic appearance of pulmonary metastatic disease can mimic a wide spectrum of disease including infectious and non-infectious diseases, intrapulmonary lymph nodes, drug reactions, and septic emboli (SNYDER and PUGATCH 1998). In pediatric patients with primary malignancies, a tiny nodule may result from either benign or malignant disease, whereas in adults as many as 60% of nodules detected by CT may be benign (ROSENFIELD et al. 1992). Similarly, pulmonary nodules that develop in children undergoing treatment for cancer may be caused by metastatic disease, by infection, or by inflammation (HIDALGO et al. 1983; KASTE 2000; KASTE et al. 1999; ROSENFIELD et al. 1992). In adults, solitary malignant nodules are more likely than benign nodules to be less densely calcified and to have irregular margins as seen on CT images (SIEGELMAN et al. 1986). In other solid tumors, pulmonary nodules that enhance by at least 20 Housfield units are usually malignant (SWENSEN et al. 1992, 1995; YAMASHITA et al. 1995), but this finding has not been confirmed in the lymphomas. ROSENFIELD and colleagues have shown that these criteria used in adults are inadequate for differentiating benign from malignant lesions in children (ROSENFIELD et al. 1992). Thus, development of more sensitive and more specific imaging methods for distinguishing benign from malignant pulmonary nodules in pediatric patients is warranted.

12.3.2.2
Nuclear Imaging

12.3.2.2.1
67Gallium Imaging

Although gallium scintigraphy is a standard staging method for Hodgkin's disease and non-Hodgkin's lymphoma, it is nonspecific for malignancy (KASTE 2000; POSNIAK and OLSON 1996). Lung nodules resulting from Hodgkin's disease and non-Hodgkin's lymphoma can be gallium-avid but inflammatory lesions, such as infected pulmonary emboli from central venous access devices, and by focal pneumonia reactive processes, such as bronchiolitis obliterans-organizing pneumonia (BOOP) can also demonstrate gallium avidity (KASTE 2000; POSNIAK and OLSON 1996). In the case of inflammatory lesions, the absence of gallium avidity may nearly exclude a diagnosis of active tumor.

12.3.2.2.2
201Thallium

SPECT imaging with [201]thallium shows promise in detecting mediastinal and hilar lymph nodes and in differentiating benign from malignant lung lesions. ARBAB and coworkers compared the results of thallium SPECT of lung nodules and hilar lymphadenopathy with those of helical CT (ARBAB et al. 1998). They determined that the sensitivity of CT imaging in detecting lymph nodes was 83%, its specificity was 60%, and its negative predictive value was 90%. In contrast, the sensitivity of [201]thallium SPECT was 50%, its specificity was 80%, and its positive predictive value was 80%. Furthermore, these authors determined that even lymph nodes larger than 1 cm on CT images could be considered benign if they were not thallium-avid (ARBAB et al. 1998).

12.3.2.2.3
FDG-PET Imaging

Recent experience indicates that FDG-PET is a useful noninvasive method for estimating the risk that a pulmonary nodule is malignant (GUPTA et al. 1992, 1996; VALK et al. 1996; WORSLEY et al. 1997). PET scanning detects the increased glucose metabolism, thus exploiting the biochemical differences between benign and malignant cells. FDG-PET has a sensitivity of 93%, a specificity of 88%, and a positive predictive value of 92% in differentiating malignant from benign solitary pulmonary nodules (GUPTA et al. 1992, 1996). Negative results from a PET scan were associated with only a 4.7% likelihood of malignancy (GUPTA et al. 1996). Although PET imaging shows promise in determining whether pulmonary nodules are malignant, its routine use is hampered by its cost and its limited availability (ARBAB et al. 1998). However, in a study of cost-effectiveness of PET imaging, VALK and colleagues found that PET was more accurate than conventional imaging techniques in staging Hodgkin's disease and was more cost-effective than unnecessary surgical procedures in analyzing pulmonary nodules (VALK et al. 1996).

12.3.2.2.4
Somatostatin-Receptor Scintigraphy

Somatostatin receptors have been identified in both Hodgkin's disease and non-Hodgkin's lymphoma. However, few clinical trials have used somatostatin-receptor scintigraphy to identify disease (BANGERTER et al. 1996; BARES et al. 1993; KRENNING et al. 1993; VANHAGEN et al. 1993). BARES and colleagues found that ^{111}In-labeled octreotide scintigraphy was useful in detecting supradiaphragmatic disease, but that infradiaphragmatic disease was largely obscured by the superimposition of the tracer on bowel, spleen, kidneys, and liver (BANGERTER et al. 1996; BARES et al. 1993). However, using ^{111}In-labeled somatostatin analogs, VANHAGEN and coworkers identified additional sites of disease in ten patients (VANHAGEN et al. 1993). Thus, with further clinical development, ^{111}In-labeled octreotide scintigraphy may aid in differentiating malignant from benign disease.

12.3.2.2.5
Immunoscintigraphy

As is true for somatostatin-receptor scintigraphy, clinical experience with immunoscintigraphy for Hodgkin's disease is limited. Immunoscintigraphic agents demonstrate affinity for the CD-30-associated antigen that is present in Hodgkin's disease and anaplastic large cell lymphoma (DACOSTA et al. 1992; FALINI et al. 1992). FALINI and colleagues used a ^{131}I-labeled Ber-H$_2$ (CD30) monoclonal antibody to study six patients with advanced Hodgkin's disease. Unlike immunohistological studies, this method only detected half of the tumor sites (BANGERTER et al. 1996; FALINI et al. 1992). DACOSTA and coworkers found that ^{125}I-labeled HRS-3 Hodgkin-associated monoclonal antibody was highly specific in detecting disease in their study of 18 patients with Hodgkin's disease (DACOSTA et al. 1992). CARDE et al. (1990) had similar results using ^{123}I-labeled HRS-1 Hodgkin's associated monoclonal antibody.

12.4
Detecting Recurrent Disease in Residual Mediastinal Mass

Disease response is typically associated with a decrease in the size of the primary mass and a decrease in adenopathy (LUKER and SIEGEL 1993; NYMAN et al. 1989; RAHMOUNI et al. 1993). In children, residual mediastinal abnormality is common, usually benign (BRISSE et al. 1998; LUKER and SIEGEL 1993; PEYLAN-RAMU et al. 1989; THOMAS et al. 1988), and typically composed of necrosis, fibrosis, and inflammation (DURKIN and DURANT 1979). A residual mass may be present in as many as 88% of patients with Hodgkin's disease after the completion of therapy (JOCHELSON et al. 1985), and is most often associated with the nodular sclerosing subtype of Hodgkin's disease because of its large fibrotic component (MICHEL et al. 1995; NYMAN et al. 1989). Residual mediastinal widening may also occur with non-Hodgkin's lymphoma, even though this disease less commonly involves the mediastinum (SMITH et al. 1998). A decrease in the size of the mediastinal mass may continue for more than 8 months with therapy, and the size of the mass may not stabilize for as long as 20 months (LUKER and SIEGEL 1993). Thus, the significance of residual mediastinal abnormality must be determined by correlating its presence with the clinical information obtained in each case.

Residual mediastinal widening is managed in one of three ways: expectant watching, further evaluation by imaging or biopsy with action dictated by the results, and immediate therapeutic intervention for patients with high-risk disease (DJULBEGOVIC et al. 1992). Notably, consideration of residual active disease or delineation of recurrent disease warrants therapeutic modifications or reinstitution of chemotherapy or additional radiation therapy. In contrast, documentation of an inactive residual mediastinal mass obviates the need for more treatment (Fig. 12.8).

However, a recurrent mediastinal mass raises great concern about the tumor's response to therapy and about the possibility of unidentified recurrent disease. Although the mediastinum is the most common site of relapse of Hodgkin's disease, thymic rebound can occur as soon as 1 week after completion of therapy in as many as 25% of pediatric patients and can complicate evaluation (CHOYKE et al. 1987; FLETCHER et al. 1998; MICHEL et al. 1995; PEYLAN-RAMU et al. 1989). Thymic rebound is usually self-limiting and reversible, but increased [67]gallium avidity may persist in this tissue for 2–59 months (HARRIS et al. 1993; PEYLAN-RAMU et al. 1989). Differentiating between thymic rebound and residual or recurrent disease may require further imaging studies when clinical findings are inconclusive.

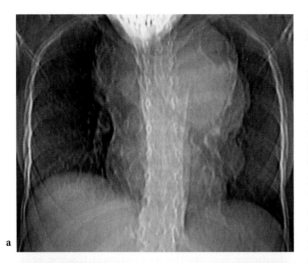

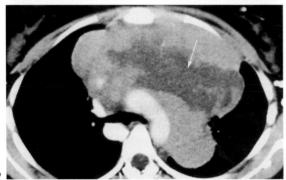

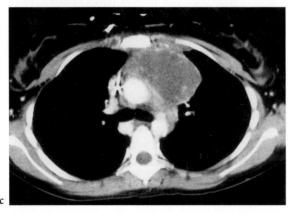

Fig. 12.8a–c. Chest computed tomography (CT) at diagnosis and follow-up of a 14-year-old girl with non-Hodgkin's lymphoma. Coronal CT topogram (a) and, B, axial contrast-enhanced chest CT image (b) at diagnosis show a large mediastinal mass extending bilaterally, involving the thymus, and encasing the great vessels. Note density inhomogeneity indicative of necrosis within the mass (*arrow*). The mass also demonstrated marked gallium-avidity (not shown). c Axial contrast-enhanced CT image after 4 months of therapy and with the patient in clinical remission demonstrates marked reduction in the size of the mediastinal mass in association with marked diffuse decrease in density indicative of tumor necrosis. The mass lacked gallium-avidity

12.4.1
Radiography of the Chest

As many as 88% of patients with mediastinal Hodgkin's disease have residual mediastinal abnormalities that are visible on chest radiographs and can persist for years after completion of therapy (JOCHELSON et al. 1985). Such changes include residual mediastinal widening, straightening of the aorticopulmonary window, and right paratracheal fullness. Patients with mediastinal disease that is larger than one-third the transthoracic ratio are more likely to have residual abnormalities; the treatment method – chemotherapy or radiation therapy – does not seem to affect the incidence of mediastinal abnormality (JOCHELSON et al. 1985). Furthermore, no difference was found in the incidence of relapse between patients with mild residual widening (<6 cm) and those with larger widening (JOCHELSON et al. 1985).

12.4.2
CT Imaging of the Chest

Studies of patients with advanced Hodgkin's disease treated with chemotherapy, radiation therapy, or both found residual mediastinal abnormalities in 38%–64% (ORLANDI et al. 1990; RADFORD et al. 1988). As was true for non-Hodgkin's lymphoma, the presence of mediastinal abnormality in association with Hodgkin's disease did not routinely predict relapse (RADFORD et al. 1988). However, in one series, the rate of isolated intrathoracic relapse was 11% for patients with no residual mass but 20.5% for those with residual widening (ORLANDI et al. 1990).

Residual mediastinal soft tissue abnormalities are less common in patients with non-Hodgkin's lymphoma than in those with Hodgkin's disease. In a large series of 252 adult and pediatric patients treated with chemotherapy for non-Hodgkin's lymphoma, TREDANIEL and coworkers found an 8% incidence of residual mediastinal mass (defined as an abnormality larger than 2 cm in diameter) that initially responded to chemotherapy, remained stable in size for at least 3 months, and was associated with complete resolution of all clinical and biologic signs of active lymphoma. The predominant histological pattern of such masses was diffuse large cell non-Hodgkin's lymphoma. The investigators found no difference in estimates of disease-free survival or overall survival for those patients with residual mediastinal masses and for those with complete disease remission (TREDANIEL et al. 1992). In contrast, a study of adults with mediastinal non-Hodgkin's lymphoma found that residual mediastinal disease at a volume of more than 100 ml predicted disease relapse (SMITH et al. 1998).

CT is sensitive in detecting residual or recurrent mediastinal masses, but its specificity is limited, particularly in light of the intensive treatment that is required for salvage therapy or bone marrow transplantation. ELKOWITZ and colleagues found that CT had a sensitivity of 100% in detecting residual mediastinal mass after therapy, a specificity of 27%, a positive predictive value of 17%, and a negative predictive value of 100% (ELKOWITZ et al. 1993). CT cannot differentiate between fibrous tissue and viable neoplasm (ELKOWITZ et al. 1993; LEWIS and MANOHARAN 1987; TREDANIEL et al. 1992); however, cystic changes suggest that the mass is benign (TREDANIEL et al. 1992).

Although recurrent mediastinal widening is cause for concerning regarding disease relapse, thymic regrowth commonly mimics disease recurrence, but other factors may also cause mediastinal widening. Gallium-avid thymic hyperplasia has been reported in association with thyrotoxicosis after successful completion of therapy for Hodgkin's disease (PENDLE-BURY et al. 1992). Thymic cysts typically appear on CT images as well-defined, low-density mediastinal masses and can occur during therapy for Hodgkin's disease, but are more common after completion of therapy (BORGNA-PIGNATTI 1994; EL-SHARKAWI and PATEL 1995; LEWIS and MANOHARAN 1987; MURRAY and PARKER 1984). They rarely occur after completion of therapy for non-Hodgkin's lymphoma and are probably degenerative in origin (BORGNA-PIGNATTI 1994; EL-SHARKAWI and PATEL 1995; LEWIS and MANOHARAN 1987; MURRAY and PARKER 1984).

12.4.3
MR Imaging

The sensitivity of MR imaging in detecting mediastinal masses may complement CT findings (TRE-DANIEL et al. 1992). However, motion significantly degrades mediastinal assessment. Thus, cardiac gating and sometimes respiratory gating are required for diagnostic MR imaging studies. Adenopathy and active tumor in a mediastinal mass are characterized by decreased signal on T1-weighted MR images and by increased signal on T2-weighted images. Inactive tumor is characterized by decreased signal both on

T1-weighted images and on T2-weighted sequences, and by a decrease in overall tumor volume (MICHEL et al. 1995; NYMAN et al. 1989; RAHMOUNI et al. 1993). The most striking change in the appearance of mediastinal disease on MR images occurs during the early part of treatment (NYMAN et al. 1989; RAHMOUNI et al. 1993).

Like CT, MR imaging has a sensitivity of 100% and a negative predictive value of 100% in detecting malignant mediastinal disease. However, the specificity of MR imaging (73%) and its positive predictive value (35%) are higher than those of CT. The improved specificity of MR imaging is largely due to detection of fibrotic changes in residual mediastinal mass as evidenced by decreased signal on T2-weighted images (ELKOWITZ et al. 1993). These signal changes may be due to tissue necrosis, active tumor, early fibrosis, or inflammation (BRISSE et al. 1998; ELKOWITZ et al. 1993; GASPARINI et al. 1993; RAHMOUNI et al. 1993). In the presence of clinical remission, inhomogeneous increase in signal within the mass may demonstrate fibrotic changes 3–5 months after documentation of remission. The persistent increase in signal on T2-weighted images may continue in some patients for more than 1 year even though clinical remission continues (ELKOWITZ et al. 1993).

In contrast, SPIERS and coworkers found that signal changes detected by MR imaging in large-volume residual masses were associated with disease relapse; the authors advocated close follow-up or biopsy (SPIERS et al. 1997). The inflammatory changes caused by oncotherapy can cause the changes on MR images to be less specific in detecting residual disease (RAH-MOUNI et al. 1993). Thus, the specificity of MR imaging is limited but exceeds that of CT. Signal changes indicative of fibrosis are useful for clinical decision making. However, when areas of increased signal on T2-weighted images persist in a residual mediastinal mass, MR imaging is no more specific than CT in identifying active disease (ELKOWITZ et al. 1993).

12.4.4
Nuclear Imaging

12.4.4.1
⁶⁷Gallium

Gallium scintigraphy has been used to assess tumor viability in the mediastinum. Absence of gallium avidity suggests a quiescent mass. In contrast, however, although the presence of gallium avidity strongly suggests active disease, false-positive results occur in as many as 43% of patients (BRISSE et al. 1998).

Whole-body [67]gallium imaging is 95% sensitive in detecting lymphoma and 98% sensitive in detecting its recurrence (FRONT et al. 1993). One study found that [67]gallium scintigraphy could detect disease recurrence approximately 7 months prior to development of clinical symptoms or before CT detected an abnormality (FRONT et al. 1993). The whole-body imaging technique is particularly useful for patients with lymphoma as disease recurrence may develop at sites other than that of the original disease (FRONT et al. 1993).

False-positive results of gallium scintigraphy may suggest disease recurrence when in fact gallium avidity may be due to localization in normal thymic tissue (BRISSE et al. 1998; FLETCHER et al. 1998; HARRIS et al. 1993; HIBI et al. 1987). Thus, a patient may undergo therapy and suffer its toxic effects (including death) even though no active disease was present if determination of active disease rested with gallium avidity alone (DJULBEGOVIC et al. 1992). Results of the study by DJULBEGOVIC and colleagues of determining the probability of disease in residual mediastinal mass after completion of multiagent chemotherapy indicated that if the probability of disease relapse exceeds 3%, then gallium imaging is warranted before retreatment is initiated (DJULBEGOVIC et al. 1992).

Gallium avidity in cases of thymic rebound tends to be more common in pediatric patients under the age of 15 years; it may or may not be associated with mediastinal widening (PEYLAN-RAMU et al. 1989). Clinical characteristics that can support a benign cause of [67]gallium avidity include the small non-cleaved cell histologic subtype of non-Hodgkin's lymphoma, the absence of disease elsewhere, the absence of mediastinal disease at the time of diagnosis, and the lack of disease progression over the course of serial studies (PEYLAN-RAMU et al. 1989).

A comparison of the sensitivity of [67]gallium SPECT and MR imaging for patients with Hodgkin's disease found that MR imaging had 90% specificity for predicting relapse but only 45% sensitivity. The sensitivity of [67]gallium SPECT was similar to that of MR imaging, but its specificity was lower (33%) (BANGERTER et al. 1996).

12.4.4.2
[201]Thallium

More recently, [201]thallium imaging of the mediastinum has shown strong promise in differentiating benign from malignant mediastinal masses.

As FLETCHER and colleagues showed, [201]thallium is 100% sensitive in detecting active mediastinal disease at the time of diagnosis of Hodgkin's disease and is also useful for detecting relapse in treated patients (FLETCHER et al. 1998). These investigators found that gallium scintigraphy has greater specificity (90%±5%) than thallium scintigraphy (85%±6%), but the specificity of thallium and gallium scintigraphy together (97%±2%) exceeds that of either modality independently (FLETCHER et al. 1998). Thus, for pediatric patients less than 18 years of age, thallium scintigraphy coupled with gallium scintigraphy may be advantageous in differentiating benign thymic regrowth from recurrent disease (FLETCHER et al. 1998; HARRIS et al. 1993). The absence of thallium uptake by residual or recurrent mediastinal mass suggests a quiescent process.

12.4.4.3
FDG-PET Imaging

FDG-PET imaging provides a metabolic road map of foci of increased glycolytic activity, which has been shown to be an indicator of increased metabolism in tumors. PET delineates active tumor mass rather than total tumor volume (ZINZANI et al. 1999). Thus, it is useful for predicting malignant histology of hilar and mediastinal lymphadenopathy (GUPTA et al. 1992, 1996), and can be particularly useful in differentiating active tumor from necrotic tumor when large masses remain after the completion of therapy (Fig. 12.9).

ZINZANI and coworkers (1999) compared the findings of FDG-PET and CT in 44 patients with Hodgkin's disease or non-Hodgkin's lymphoma and residual abdominal masses. They found that disease relapse occurred in 100% of patients with positive findings from both CT and FDG-PET, but in only 4% of patients with positive CT findings but negative FDG-PET findings. No relapses occurred in patients with negative findings on both studies (ZINZANI et al. 1999). Thus, it may be beneficial to use FDG-PET imaging to detect recurrent disease when CT scanning demonstrates residual mediastinal mass.

12.5
Summary

Pediatric Hodgkin's disease and non-Hodgkin's lymphoma present unique diagnostic challenges. Identifying active disease, differentiating quiescent resid-

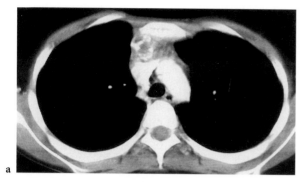

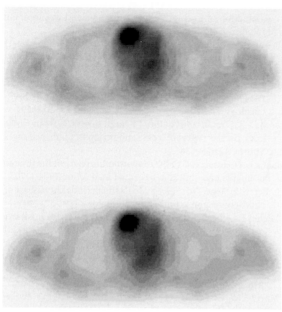

Fig. 12.9a,b. This 12-year-old girl underwent routine imaging after 4 months of therapy for mediastinal B-cell non-Hodgkin's lymphoma. **a** Axial contrast-enhanced chest computed tomography filmed with mediastinal windows shows a residual, partially calcified anterior mediastinal mass which had considerably decreased in size since diagnosis. **b** 18-Fluorodeoxyglucose positron emission tomography (FDG-PET) imaging demonstrates persistent avidity within the mass indicative of residual active disease. With additional therapy, FDG-PET avidity resolved. (Courtesy of Dr. BARRY SHULKIN)

ual mass from recurrent disease, and distinguishing findings related to lymphoma from those related to other causes are vital for proper disease staging and therapeutic planning. Contemporary imaging techniques do well at identifying anatomic abnormalities but are limited in determining disease activity. Established nuclear scintigraphic techniques, such as FDG-PET, and evolving immunoscintigraphic techniques herald the evolution of functional and metabolic techniques with great promise in solving the problems discussed in this chapter.

Acknowledgements. The author thanks Flo Witte for editorial assistance and Jean Littlejohn and Marcine Eddins for manuscript preparation.

References

Abrahamsen AF, Lien HH, Aas M et al (1994) Magnetic resonance imaging and [67]gallium scan in mediastinal malignant lymphoma: a prospective pilot study. Ann Oncol 5:433–436

Adam EJ, Ignotus PI (1993) Sonography of the thymus in healthy children: frequency of visualization, size, and appearance. AJR Am J Roentgenol 161:153–155

Arbab AS, Koizumi K, Toyama K et al (1998) Detection of lung lesions and lymph nodes with ^{201}Tl SPET. Nucl Med Commun 19:411–416

Au V, Leung AN (1997) Radiologic manifestations of lymphoma in the thorax. AJR Am J Roentgenol 168:93–98

Bangerter M, Griesshammer M, Binder T et al (1996) New diagnostic imaging procedures in Hodgkin's disease. Ann Oncol 7 [Suppl 4]:55–59

Bares R, Galonska P, Dempke W et al (1993) Somatostatin receptor scintigraphy in malignant lymphoma: first results and comparison with glucose metabolism measured by positron-emission tomography. Horm Metab Res Suppl 27:56–58

Boothroyd AE, Hall-Craggs MA, Dicks-Mireaux C et al (1992) The magnetic resonance appearances of the normal thymus in children. Clin Radiol 45:378–381

Borgna-Pignatti C, Andreis IB, Rugolotto S et al (1994) Thymic cyst appearing after treatment of mediastinal non-Hodgkin lymphoma. Med Pediatr Oncol 22:70–72

Brisse H, Pacquement H, Burdairon E et al (1998) Outcome of residual mediastinal masses of thoracic lymphomas in children: impact on management and radiological follow-up strategy. Pediatr Radiol 28:444–450

Carde P, DaCosta L, Manil L et al (1990) Immunoscintigraphy of Hodgkin's Disease: in vivo use of radiolabelled monoclonal antibodies derived from Hodgkin cell lines. Eur J Cancer 26:474–479

Chai JL, Patz EF Jr (1994) CT of the lung: patterns of calcification and other high-attenuation abnormalities. AJR Am J Roentgenol 162:1063–1066

Choyke PL, Zeman RK, Gootenberg JE et al (1987) Thymic atrophy and regrowth in response to chemotherapy: CT evaluation. AJR Am J Roentgenol 149:269–272

Cohen M, Hill CA, Cangir A et al (1980) Thymic rebound after treatment of childhood tumors. AJR Am J Roentgenol 135:151–156

Cohen MD, Siddiqui A, Weetman R et al (1986) Hodgkin disease and non-Hodgkin lymphomas in children: utilization of radiological modalities. Radiology 158:499–505

DaCosta L, Carde P, Lumbroso JD et al (1992) Immunoscintigraphy in Hodgkin's disease and anaplastic large cell lymphomas: results in 18 patients using the iodine radiolabeled monoclonal antibody HRS-3. Ann Oncol Suppl 4:53–57

Daldrup HE, Link TM, Wörtler K et al (1998) MR imaging of thoracic tumors in pediatric patients. AJR Am J Roentgenol 170:1639–1644

Diefenthal HC, Tashjian J (1988) The role of plain films, CT, tomography, ultrasound, and percutaneous needle aspiration in the diagnosis of inflammatory lung disease. Semin Respir Infect 3:83–105

Djulbegovic B, Hendler FJ, Hamm J et al (1992) Residual mediastinal mass after treatment of Hodgin's disease: a decision analysis. Med Hypotheses 38:166–175

Durkin W, Durant J (1979) Benign mass lesions after therapy for Hodgkin's disease. Arch Intern Med 139:333–336

Elkowitz SS, Leonidas JC, Lopez M et al (1993) Comparison of CT and MRI in the evaluation of therapeutic response in thoracic Hodgkin disease. Pediatr Radiol 23:301–304

El-Sharkawi AMM, Patel B (1995) Management of residual thymic cysts in patients treated for mediastinal Hodgkin's disease. Thorax 50:1118–1119

Falini B, Flenghi L, Fedeli L et al (1992) In vivo targeting of Hodgkin and Reed-Sternberg cells of Hodgkin's disease with monoclonal antibody Ber-H2 (CD-30): immunohistological evidence. Br J Haematol 82:38–45

Fletcher BD, Kauffman WM, Kaste SC et al (1995) Use of Tl-201 to detect untreated pediatric Hodgkin disease. Radiology 196:851–855

Fletcher BD, Xiong X, Kauffman WM et al (1998) Hodgkin disease: use of Tl-201 to monitor mediastinal involvement after treatment. Radiology 209:471–475

Francis IR, Glazer GM, Bookstein FL et al (1985) The thymus: re-examination of age-related changes in size and shape. AJR Am J Roentgenol 145:249–254

Friedland ML, Wittels EG, Deutsch A (1982) Hodgkin's disease with pulmonary cavitation. Postgrad Med J 58:794–796

Front D, Bar-Shalom R, Epelbaum R et al (1993) Early detection of lymphoma recurrence with gallium-67 scintigraphy. J Nucl Med 34:2101–2104

Gasparini MD, Balzarini L, Castellani MR et al (1993) Current role of gallium scan and magnetic resonance imaging in the management of mediastinal Hodgkin lymphoma. Cancer 72:577–582.

Gupta NC, Frank AR, Dewan NA et al (1992) Solitary pulmonary nodules: detection of malignancy with PET with 2-[F-18]-fluoro-2-deoxy-D-glucose. Radiology 184:441–444

Gupta NC, Maloof J, Gunel E (1996) Probability of malignancy in solitary pulmonary nodules using fluorine-18-FDG and PET. J Nucl Med 37:943–948

Gurney JW, Conces DJ (1996) Pulmonary histoplasmosis. Radiology 199:297–306

Hamrick-Turner JE, Saif MF, Powers CI et al (1994) Imaging of childhood non-Hodgkin lymphoma: assessment by histologic subtype. Radiographics 14:11–28

Han BK, Babcock DS, Oestreich AE (1989) Normal thymus in infancy: sonographic characteristics. Radiology 170:471–474

Harris EW, Rakow JI, Weiner M et al (1993) Thallium-201 scintigraphy for assessment of a gallium-67-avid mediastinal mass following therapy for Hodgkin's disease. J Nucl Med 34:1326–1330

Heiberg E, Wolverson MK, Sundaram M et al (1982) Normal thymus: CT characteristics in subjects under age 20. AJR Am J Roentgenol 138:491–494

Hibi S, Todo S, Imashuku (1987) Thymic localization of gallium-67 in pediatric patients with lymphoid and nonlymphoid tumors. J Nucl Med 28:293–297

Hidalgo H, Korobkin M, Kinney TR et al (1983) The problem of benign pulmonary nodules in children receiving cytotoxic chemotherapy. AJR Am J Roentgenol 140:21–24

Jochelson M, Mauch P, Balikian J et al (1985) The significance of the residual mediastinal mass in treated Hodgkin's Disease. J Clin Oncol 3:637–640

Kaste SC (2000) Infection imaging of children and adolescents undergoing cancer therapy: a review of modalities and an organ system approach. Semin Pediatr Infect Dis 11:122–141

Kaste SC, Pratt CB, Cain AM et al (1999) Metastases detected at the time of diagnosis of primary pediatric extremity osteosarcoma at diagnosis: imaging features. Cancer 86:1602–1608

Krenning EP, Kwekkeboom DJ, Reubi JC et al (1993) 111In-octreotide scintigraphy in oncology. Digestion 54 [Suppl 1]:84–87

Lemaitre L, Marconi V, Avni F et al (1987) The sonographic evaluation of normal thymus in infants and children. Eur J Radiol 7:130–136

Leone G, Castellana M, Rabitti C (1990) Escavative pulmonary Hodgkin's lymphoma: diagnosis by cutting needle biopsy. Eur J Haematol 44:139–141

Leventhal BG, Donaldson SS (1993) Hodgkin's disease. In: Pizzo PA, Poplack DG (eds) Principles and practice of pediatric oncology, 2nd edn. Lippincott, Philadelphia, pp 577–594

Lewis CR, Manoharan A (1987) Benign thymic cysts in Hodgkin's disease: report of a case and review of published cases. Thorax 42:633–634

Liang C-D, Huang S-C (1997) Sonographic study of the thymus in infants and children. J Formos Med Assoc 96:700–703

Luker GD, Siegel MJ (1993) Mediastinal Hodgkin disease in children: response to therapy. Radiology 189:737–740

Michel F, Gilbeau J-P, Six C et al (1995) Progressive mediastinal widening after therapy for Hodgkin's disease. Acta Clin Belg 50:282–287

Moore AV, Korobkin M, Olanow W et al (1983) Age-related changes in the thymus gland: CT-pathologic correlation. AJR Am J Roentgenol 141:241–246

Murray JA, Parker AC (1984) Mediastinal Hodgkin's disease and thymic cysts. Acta Haematol 71:282–284

Nadel HR (1993) Thallium-201 for oncologic imaging in children. Semin Nucl Med 23:243–254

Nelson S, Prince D, Terry P (1983) Primary Hodgkin's disease of the lung: case report. Thorax 38:310–311

Nyman RS, Rehn SM, Glimelius BLG et al (1989) Residual mediastinal masses in Hodgkin disease: prediction of size with MR imaging. Radiology 170:435–440

Ognibene FP, Pass HI, Roth JA et al (1988) Role of imaging and interventional techniques in the diagnosis of respiratory disease in the immunocompromised host. J Thorac Imaging 3:1–20

Orlandi E, Lazzarino M, Brusamolino E et al (1990) Residual mediastinal widening following therapy in Hodgkin's disease. Hematol Oncol 8:125–31

Peylan-Ramu N, Haddy TB, Jones E et al (1989) High frequency of benign mediastinal uptake of gallium-67 after completion of chemotherapy in children with high-grade non-Hodgkin's lymphoma. J Clin Oncol 7:1800–1806

Pendlebury SC, Boyages S, Koutts J et al (1992) Thymic hyperplasia associated with Hodgkin disease and thyrotoxicosis. Cancer 70:1985–1987

Pik A, Cohen N, Weissgarten J et al (1986) Primary pulmonary Hodgkin's disease with air bronchogram. Respiration 50:226–229

Posniak HV, Olson MC (1996) Correlative imaging of abdominal infection. In: Henkin RE, Boles MA, Dillehay GL et al (eds) Nuclear medicine, vol II. Mosby, St Louis, pp 1662–1685

Radford J, Cowan R, Flanagan M et al (1988) The significance of residual mediastinal abnormality on the chest radiograph following treatment for Hodgkin's disease. J Clin Oncol 6:940–946]

Rahmouni A, Tempany C, Jones R et al (1993) Lymphoma: monitoring tumor size and signal intensity with MR imaging. Radiology 188:445–451

Roebuck DJ, Nicholls WD, Bernard EJ et al (1998) Misleading leads. Thallium-201 uptake in rebound thymic hyperplasia. Med Pediatr Oncol 30:297–300

Rollins NK, Currarino G (1988) MR imaging of posterior mediastinal thymus. J Comput Assist Tomogr 12:518–520

Rosenfield NS, Keller MS, Markowitz RI (1992) CT differentiation of benign and malignant lung nodules in children. J Pediatr Surg 27:459–461

Shahar J, Angelillo VA, Katz D et al (1987) Recurrent cavitary nodules secondary to Hodgkin's disease. Chest 91:273–274

Shulkin BL (1997) PET applications in pediatrics. Q J Nucl Med 41:281–291

Shulkin BL, Mitchell DS, Ungar DR et al (1995) Neoplasms in a pediatric population:2-[F-18]-fluoro-2-deoxy-D-glucose PET studies. Radiology 194:495–500

Siegel MJ, Glazer HS, Wiener JI et al (1989) Normal and abnormal thymus in childhood: MR imaging. Radiology 172:367–371

Siegelman SS, Khouri NF, Leo FP et al (1986) Solitary pulmonary nodules: CT assessment. Radiology 160:307–312

Smith D, Shaffer K, Kirn D et al (1998) Mediastinal large cell lymphoma: prognostic significance of CT findings at presentation and after treatment. Oncology 55:284–288

Snyder BJ, Pugatch RD (1998) Imaging characteristics of metastatic disease to the chest. Chest Surg Clin North Am 8:29–48

Spiers ASD, Husband JES, MacVicar AD (1997) Treated thymic lymphoma: comparison of MR imaging with CT. Radiology 203:369–376

Swensen SJ, Morin RL, Schueler BA et al (1992) Solitary pulmonary nodule: CT evaluation of enhancement with iodinated contrast material– a preliminary report. Radiology 182:343–347

Swensen SJ, Brown LR, Colby TV et al (1995) Pulmonary nodules: CT evaluation of enhancement with iodinated contrast material. Radiology 194:393–398

Thomas NB, Gupta SC (1988) Unilobar enlargement of normal thymus gland causing mass effect. Br J Radiol 61:244–246

Thomas F, Cosset JM, Cheret P et al (1988) Thoracic CT-scanning follow-up of residual mediastinal masses after treatment of Hodgkin's disease. Radiother Oncol 11:119–122

Tonami N, Hisada K (1977) Clinical experience of tumor imaging with 201Tl-chloride. Clin Nucl Med 2:75–81

Tredaniel J, Brice P, Lepage E et al (1992) The significance of a residual mediastinal mass following treatment for aggressive non-Hodgkin's lymphomas. Eur Respir J 5:170–173

Valk PE, Pounds TR, Tesar RD et al (1996) Cost-effectiveness of PET imaging in clinical oncology. Nucl Med Biol 23:737–743

Vanhagen PM, Krenning EP, Reubi JC et al (1993) Somatostatin analogue scintigraphy of malignant lymphomas. Br J Haematol 83:75–79

Wittich GR, Nowels KW, Korn RL et al (1992) Coaxial transthoracic fine-needle biopsy in patients with a history of malignant lymphoma. Radiology 183:175–178

Worsley DF, Celler A, Adam MJ et al (1997) Pulmonary nodules: Differential diagnosis using ^{18}F-fluorodeoxyglucose single-photon emission computed tomography. AJR Am J Roentgenol 168:771–774

Yamashita K, Matsunobe S, Tsuda T et al (1995) Solitary pulmonary nodule: preliminary study of evaluation with incremental dynamic CT. Radiology 194:399–405

Yankelevitz DF, Henschke CI (1997) Does 2-year stability imply that pulmonary nodules are benign? AJR Am J Roentgenol 168:325–328

Yousem SA, Weiss LM, Colby TV (1986) Primary pulmonary Hodgkin's disease. A clinicopathologic study of 15 cases. Cancer 57:1217–1224

Zinzani PL, Magagnoli M, Chierichetti F et al (1999) The role of positron emission tomography (PET) in the management of lymphoma patients. Ann Oncol 10:1181–1184

13 Chest Tumours Other Than Lymphoma

Kieran McHugh

CONTENTS

13.1 Introduction

Thoracic tumours are generally arbitrarily classified, despite some inevitable overlap, as originating in three major compartments within the chest, namely the lung parenchyma, the mediastinum, and the chest wall. In the interests of simplicity and convention, that anatomical approach will be used in this chapter with an additional brief reference to diaphragmatic tumours. As the mediastinal tumours mentioned, other than lymphangioma, have varying degrees of malignancy depending on the exact histological sub-type, that section has not been divided into benign and malignant categories. Benign chest wall tumours are described in Chap. 15 and will not be mentioned here. The imaging at diagnosis for all lesions has been emphasised throughout. The subsequent fol-low-up radiology of benign conditions is governed by the clinical course, and that of malignant masses is largely determined thereafter by imaging proto-cols devised by the various international paediatric oncology co-operative groups and should take place in specialist paediatric centres.

13.2 Clinical Features

Most tumours occurring in the thorax in childhood, particularly those encountered in paediatric oncology centers, are pulmonary metastases. These will usually be found during staging of a known or new malig-nancy and the dominant clinical findings will be those of the primary lesion. Primary thoracic neoplasia is uncommon in childhood and seldom an early diag-nostic consideration, but a wide variety of tumours within the chest do occur and ideally should be recog-nised and imaged appropriately. It is noteworthy that there is essentially no major difference between the sexes in the incidence of the primary and secondary chest tumours described here. Tumours also essen-tially occur with equal frequency in either lung.

Similar to tumours elsewhere, primary chest neo-plasms largely manifest due to pressure effects sec-ondary to local compression of adjacent organs, systemic symptoms when there is disseminated malignancy or as an incidental finding. Paraneo-plastic syndromes are exceedingly rare. With airway obstruction or respiratory symptoms that do not respond to the usual medical treatment, computed tomography (CT) in particular can be very useful in excluding other pathology or documenting an unsus-pected lesion. Whilst the presenting symptomatology can vary enormously even within the same histolog-ical group, some generalisations with regard to the presentation of chest masses can be made.

In both benign and malignant lung tumours the most frequent presenting complaints are fever, cough

Kieran McHugh, FRCR, FRCPI, DCH
Radiology Department, Great Ormond Street Hospital for Children, London WC1N 3JH, UK

and pneumonitis (HANCOCK et al. 1993; HARTMAN and SHOCHAT 1983). Haemoptysis and respiratory distress are more common with malignant pulmonary lesions. In one large review series, 27.9% of benign tumours were asymptomatic as compared to 6.3% of malignant lung tumours (HANCOCK et al. 1993). A child who is truly asymptomatic is twice as likely to harbour a benign pulmonary tumour, and this likelihood is even greater in children over 4 years of age. Endobronchial masses typically result in lung collapse, persistent hyperinflation or wheezing which again fails to respond to conventional treatment and may be complicated by bronchiectasis. The endobronchial location of many such lesions is often only apparent after bronchoscopy. Occasionally CT may reveal an abnormality prior to bronchoscopy being performed or, albeit less likely, when bronchoscopy is negative or not considered feasible.

Some chest wall tumours come to attention because of a superficial chest mass. Thoracic neuroblastoma and more especially the benign ganglioneuroma are often found incidentally on chest X-rays (CXRs) performed for other reasons. The majority of chest wall and mediastinal tumours generally present, however, with non-specific respiratory symptoms such as airway obstruction, cough or fever due to a complicating pneumonia. In contrast to many pulmonary tumours the likely nature of the illness becomes apparent after a chest radiograph has been performed – if the film is interpreted correctly. The lung opacity is generally not typical for pneumonia with often clearly defined margins suggesting a pleural or chest wall component. Mediastinal shift or adenopathy may be seen and rib changes, in particular, should be sought as this latter finding virtually always indicates an extrapleural malignancy. In fact, the vast majority of mediastinal and chest wall tumours seen in children are malignant.

13.3
Imaging

Radiological studies should always begin with a frontal chest radiograph. When an unusual opacity is evident, a lateral film can be particularly helpful in assessing the trachea for compression and/or displacement, and in accurately defining the location of the abnormality, which aids greatly in differential diagnosis. For pulmonary lesions the next imaging study should be CT, as this remains the best modality to evaluate the lung parenchyma. A few limited low dose non-enhanced sections may be performed to assess for calcification, although calcification is usually easily discernible on post-contrast studies also. It is crucial that intravenous contrast is given to best delineate tumour extent and the relationship of a mass to the adjacent airway, major blood vessels or chest wall. A solely non-enhanced study of the thorax in this context is in essence a waste of time and such CT studies invariably need to be repeated. When bronchoscopy suggests an endobronchial lesion CT may be used with thin 2–5 mm sections to confirm these findings and assess the extrabronchial spread of disease. Despite meticulous technique in examining smaller endobronchial lesions associated with atelectasis, the atelectatic segment may obscure tumour resulting in a false negative CT study. Alternatively, bronchiectasis with atelectasis may be the dominant clinical finding and so prompt a high-resolution chest CT which, with 1–2 cm gaps between sections, could easily miss an underlying endobronchial mass.

In the routine screening for pulmonary metastases, contiguous 5-mm sections without intravenous contrast enhancement through the entire thorax are generally adequate in paediatric patients – many centres, including our own department, use 5-mm sections in children up to an arbitrary age, e.g. 5 years, with 8-mm sections in older children. A pitch of 1.5 on a spiral CT scanner seems a reasonable compromise between resolution and dose reduction. As has been well documented for high-resolution chest CT, the lung parenchyma because of its high inherent contrast can also be adequately examined for pulmonary nodules at relatively low tube current, e.g. 50 mA (DIEDERICH et al. 1999). Overlapping reconstructions are favoured by some to increase nodule detection and one paper described a maximum intensity projection (MIP) technique that may have improved sensitivity particularly for small, high-density pulmonary nodules (COAKLEY et al. 1998). In everyday practice, however, contiguous sections are adequate for nodule detection. Low dose techniques increase noise and render assessment of the mediastinum less reliable. When there is suspicion of mediastinal adenopathy, it is mandatory that intravenous contrast is given as the lack of mediastinal fat in children, unlike in adult patients, makes evaluation of the mediastinum difficult.

CT after intravenous contrast administration can accurately define mediastinal and chest wall masses and is sensitive in the detection of adjacent bony destruction. CT will also be necessary to evaluate the pulmonary parenchyma in patients with malignant tumours. Magnetic resonance imaging (MRI), however, where available, has become the optimal technique for examining the chest wall and mediastinum, mainly as a result of improved ECG- and respiratory-gating, cine modes and MR angiography, in addition to the usual advantages of better soft-tissue contrast, lack of radiation and multiplanar capability. Most tumours have intermediate T1 signal, are hyperintense to varying degrees on T2 and display variable contrast enhancement after gadolinium administration. Rather than actual signal characteristics, it is the pattern and site of tumour occurrence and the age of the patient that suggests the likely tumour in an individual case.

13.4
Pulmonary Tumours

Pulmonary masses are unusual in childhood. The absence of systemic upset or pyrexia generally excludes a round pneumonia or lung abscess, and so other diagnostic possibilities need to be considered. Low attenuating cystic appearances are common on CT with abscesses or bronchogenic cysts, for example, allowing correct diagnoses in most cases. Once the common causes of a pulmonary mass and a primary extra-thoracic malignancy with metastases have been excluded, primary tumours are the next major consideration in the differential diagnosis of pulmonary masses in childhood (Table 13.1) (MAS ESTELLES et al. 1995).

Table 13.1. Summary of primary pulmonary neoplasms in children. (Reprinted with permission, HANCOCK et al. 1993)

Tumour type	Number (%)
Benign (n=92)	
Inflammatory	48 (52)
Hamartoma	22 (24)
Neurogenic tumour	9 (10)
Leiomyoma	6 (7)
Mucous gland adenoma	3 (3)
Malignant (n=291)	
Bronchial 'adenoma'	118 (40)
Bronchogenic carcinoma	49 (17)
Pulmonary blastoma	45 (16)
Fibrosarcoma	28 (10)
Rhabdomyosarcoma	17 (6)
Leiomyosarcoma	11 (4)
Sarcoma	6 (2)
Haemangiopericytoma	4 (1)

13.4.1
Previous Cystic Lung Lesion

The vast majority of lung neoplasms are thought to occur de novo without pre-existing lung pathology. The association between prior cystic lung lesions and subsequent pulmonary tumours has been controversial. Nevertheless, 4.3% of benign tumours and 8.6% of malignant tumours reported by HANCOCK et al. (1993) were associated with previously documented cystic malformations. TAGGE et al. (1996) cite 16 reports noting a relationship in children between pulmonary cystic disease and pleuropulmonary blastoma and related tumours. Other tumours with known prior cysts have included hamartomas, bronchogenic carcinomas, rhabdomyosarcomas and other sarcomas. At least two reported cases of rhabdomyosarcoma have arisen in congenital cystic adenomatoid malformations. Some sarcomas, however, previously reported in association with prior lung cysts may in fact have been unrecognised pleuropulmonary blastomas (PRIEST et al. 1997). So-called lung cysts have even included alleged 'pneumatoceles' in some cases (TAGGE et al. 1996).

The correct approach to asymptomatic lung cysts is therefore uncertain. Follow-up may need to be life-long, e.g. two pulmonary adenocarcinomas developing in young adult non-smokers who had had large peripheral lung cysts of longstanding duration have been described (TAGGE et al. 1996). It has even been suggested that an asymptomatic pulmonary cyst in a child should be resected unless radiographic evidence can show it to be acquired, as there is a widespread assumption that congenital lung lesions are more likely to undergo malignant change (McHUGH and BOOTHROYD 1999). There are a large number of cystic lung pathologies, e.g. congenital cystic adenomatoid malformation, bronchogenic cyst, sequestration, parenchymal cysts and pneumatoceles. There is an increasing tendency to manage at least some of these lesions conservatively, particularly if small, an asymptomatic antenatal pick-up or an incidental finding. When a solid component is detected in any of these abnormalities on CT or ultrasound, surgical resection should be strongly considered (TAGGE et al. 1996). This topic is further alluded to in Sect. 13.4.3.2.

13.4.2
Benign Tumours

13.4.2.1
Inflammatory Pseudotumour

Inflammatory pseudotumour, originally termed plasma cell granuloma, has a variety of other synonyms, including inflammatory myofibroblastic tumour. Because the histological findings may vary greatly, there are some objections to using the term inflammatory pseudotumour, but the label is entrenched in the literature and does convey the benign nature of this process. It is an uncommon lesion characterised histologically by a localised proliferation of mononuclear inflammatory cells in the form of plasma cells, lymphocytes, eosinophils and mesenchymal cells comprising spindle cells and myofibroblasts (BROWN and SHAW 1995). It is the most common benign pulmonary 'tumour' in childhood and accounts for approximately half of all benign lesions. The aetiology of inflammatory pseudotumour is likely multifactorial and seems to be an unregulated reparative response of injured tissue. The important function of the myofibroblast in tissue repair is also consistent with the hypothesis that an aberrant response to tissue injury is the pathogenesis of these lesions.

There is seldom a history of trauma or of preceding infection at the site of involvement by the inflammatory pseudotumour, although up to one-fifth of older patients give a history of recent lower respiratory tract infection. A variety of unusual micro-organisms have been implicated in individual case reports, including *Mycobacterium avium intracellulare*, *Corynebacterium equi*, *Coxiella burnetii*, *Bacillus sphaericus* and, more recently, Epstein-Barr virus (HEDLUND et al. 1999).

The condition has been increasingly recognised in children and the lung is the most common site in the body (MAS ESTELLES et al. 1995). A history of systemic upset with fever, malaise and weight loss is generally present although up to 30% of children may be asymptomatic. An endobronchial lesion may manifest as an exacerbation of asthma and persistent hyperinflation (JAYNE et al. 1997). Unusual for pulmonary masses, pain at the site of the lesion is not uncommon. An association with hypertrophic pulmonary osteoarthropathy has been reported and this association may be more frequent than is generally believed (MAS ESTELLES et al. 1995). Although bronchi and vessels may be trapped within the pulmo-

nary masses and become narrowed distally or even obliterated, this seldom leads to radiologically obvious atelectasis. Focal collapse is evident in only 14% of paediatric patients (VERBEKE et al. 1999). Pleural effusion is found in less than 5%.

Most patients present with a solitary sharply circumscribed peripheral mass in a lower lobe (Fig. 13.1). The lesions are often around 3–4 cm in diameter with usually no invasion of adjacent structures. Masses that abut the pleura can be amenable to ultrasound evaluation and typically appear solid and homogeneous. CT, however, is the major modality used in the evaluation of these lesions in the chest. The masses are typically well circumscribed (AGRONS et al. 1998). Three distinct CT appearances have been reported (BROWN and SHAW 1995). The most common finding is of a large coin lesion that may contain areas of calcification (Fig. 13.1). In fact, calcification seems to be more a feature of inflammatory lung pseudotumours in young patients than in adults (AGRONS et al. 1998). A small non-calcified endobronchial mass that can mimic an endobronchial adenoma is another manifestation in up to 20% of cases. The least common appearance is that of a large spiculated mass that may show features of necrosis or cavitation. Varied enhancement is seen following intravenous contrast administration (AGRONS et al. 1998). Hilar lymphadenopathy and pleural effusion are not commonly associated and their presence should cast doubt on this diagnosis (MAS ESTELLES et al. 1995). The CT features of inflammatory pseudotumour are notoriously nonspecific, however. A few MRI studies have demonstrated signal characteristics of pulmonary masses that paralleled those of adjacent lung parenchyma, thus rendering the lesions difficult to visualise (VERBEKE et al. 1999).

Atypical thoracic manifestations of inflammatory pseudotumours also occur. Lesions arising solely in the oesophagus have been described. More locally aggressive masses are occasionally seen and these are probably detected late in the natural history of the disorder. More extensive lesions may encase bronchi or other mediastinal structures, present as a mediastinal mass, or invade the chest wall, vertebrae or diaphragm (HEDLUND et al. 1999; VERBEKE et al. 1999). Invasive inflammatory pseudotumours appear to be more common in children than in adults. CT and MRI are both useful in characterising the extent of these aggressive lesions in relation to the tracheobronchial tree, oesophagus, vascular structures and chest wall. Angioinvasion including cardiac involve-

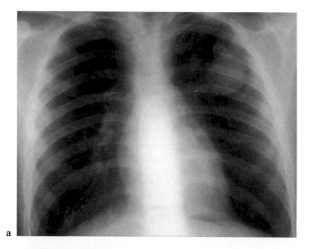

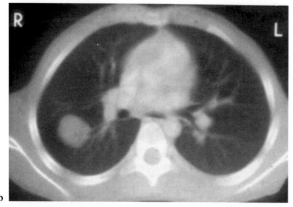

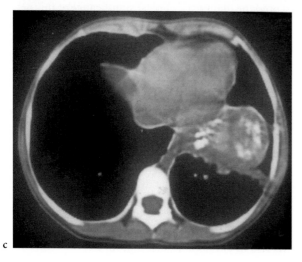

Fig. 13.1a–c. Inflammatory pseudotumour: varied appearances. **a** Chest radiograph revealing a rounded, well-circumscribed opacity in the left upper zone. Note absence of hilar adenopathy, pleural effusion and rib changes. **b** Axial CT showing a well-defined lesion in the right lower lobe. **c** A calcified inflammatory pseudotumour on unenhanced CT – the margins of this mass and its relationship to the pericardium and chest wall would be optimally evaluated after intravenous contrast administration

ment may be better demonstrated with MRI or echocardiography (HEDLUND et al. 1999). Barium studies are essential for characterising oesophageal involvement when suspected.

The relationship between inflammatory pseudotumour and malignancy is controversial and unclear. It has been suggested that inflammatory pseudotumour represents the benign end of a spectrum that also includes other fibrohistiocytic lesions with varying malignancy (AGRONS et al. 1998). Most investigators regard inflammatory pseudotumour, particularly the paediatric variety, as a distinct entity with no malignant potential. On presentation, these masses are often suspected to be primary thoracic malignancies and the diagnosis of inflammatory pseudotumour may not be entertained. In children without a known underlying malignancy a solitary peripheral pulmonary nodule or mass is more likely to represent an inflammatory pseudotumour than a neoplasm (AGRONS et al. 1998). A calcified lesion may suggest a hamartoma but hamartomas are less common in the paediatric population.

Although some cases have resolved without recourse to surgery, conservative pulmonary resection with removal of all gross evidence of disease is the mainstay of treatment and is generally curative. Locally aggressive lesions may require more radical surgery including pneumonectomy rather than the more usual segmental or lobar resection. Tumour recurrence following incomplete resection or sclerosing mediastinitis may rarely complicate the clinical course. Relapse or invasion of the mediastinum have occasionally been treated with immunosuppressive corticosteroid therapy and even multi-agent chemotherapy with good results (VERBEKE et al. 1999).

13.4.2.2
Hamartoma

Hamartomas account for approximately 20% of benign tumours that occur in the lung parenchyma in childhood (HANCOCK et al. 1993). Hamartomas are generally regarded as developmental anomalies and are composed of tissues native to the lung but present in an abnormal configuration. Some consider congenital cystic adenomatoid malformation (CCAM) to be a hamartomatous lesion but this lesion is dealt with in more detail in Chap. 5. Briefly, the fundamental pathological feature of CCAM is a proliferation of bronchioles that form cysts instead of normal alveoli and so they are clearly different from classic lung hamartomas (KIM et al. 1997). Most patients with CCAMs present in the first 6 months of life with respiratory distress, older children tend to come to attention due to recurrent chest infections, and CCAMs are also being increasingly recognised antenatally. They all manifest on plain radiographs and CT as multiple, thin-walled, air- or fluid-filled cysts expanding a lobe, in contrast to true hamartomas, which generally present as a solid mass lesion in older children.

Despite being regarded as developmental anomalies, the majority of pulmonary hamartomas are discovered in adults between the fourth and sixth decades. VAN DEN BOSCH et al. (1987) cited 30 adults among their cohort of 154 patients with pulmonary hamartomas who had had preceding normal chest radiographs, thereby lending credence to the belief that hamartomas are actually acquired lesions. Pulmonary hamartomas are frequently asymptomatic and often incidental findings (HARTMAN and SHOCHAT 1983). The characteristic radiological finding is a round opacity in the periphery of the lung parenchyma. Altogether, 10% of lesions show calcification, often with a curvilinear or speckled configuration, and sometimes this calcification has the classic 'popcorn' appearance. The frequency of calcification increases significantly with the size of the lesion. Occasionally a central fat density is seen on CT.

In contrast to adult patients, many of the reported cases of pulmonary hamartomas in younger children have fared poorly. Four lesions seen in the neonatal period were all fatal (HARTMAN and SHOCHAT 1983). Only a minority of the reported paediatric cases have been asymptomatic. At least three other childhood hamartomas occurred as part of a triad of lesions in young girls that also included an extraadrenal paraganglioma and a gastric smooth muscle tumour (HARTMAN and SHOCHAT 1983). Although pulmonary hamartomas manifest typically as isolated pulmonary nodules, in young children in particular these lesions may be quite large. Their true nature only becomes apparent at histological examination.

Endobronchial hamartomas, which are particularly uncommon in childhood, present with respiratory symptoms or infections due to airway obstruction. A few sporadic reports of tracheal hamartomas exist. One tracheal hamartoma with a large extraluminal component has also been described which manifested as a neck mass in a young girl (GROSS et al. 1996). Surgery for all hamartomas is curative although the less common endobronchial hamartoma may require lobectomy or even pneumonectomy.

13.4.2.3
Leiomyoma

The majority of leiomyomas are found in the lung parenchyma; fewer than one-third of cases manifest as endobronchial lesions. Most leiomyomas are seen in adult patients, with only one in three cases presenting before 20 years of age (KARNAK et al. 2000). HARTMAN and SHOCHAT (1983) reported four leiomyomas in children between the ages of 5 and 11 years, which were all cured by surgery. They also cited two reports in the literature of neonates who died from respiratory distress secondary to large pulmonary leiomyomas. Although quite rare, leiomyoma is also the most common benign tumour of the oesophagus. The involved oesophagus demonstrates marked circumferential wall thickening and there is an association with Alport syndrome (GUEST et al. 2000).

There is now a well documented association between the acquired immune deficiency syndrome (AIDS) and tumours of smooth muscle origin. Pulmonary leiomyomas have been seen in children with AIDS and it is likely that the incidence of these tumours will increase in paediatric practice (CHADWICK et al. 1990). DE CHADAREVIAN et al. (1997) reported two further patients with AIDS who presented with recent onset of wheezing due to bronchopulmonary leiomyomas. This, they believed, underscored the diagnostic clinical significance of this new symptom in young patients with AIDS, particularly when the wheezing is unilateral or does not respond to bronchodilators. Four centrally located leiomyomas were seen in one of their patients, and in their other patient a leiomyoma was evident on CT merely as severe narrowing of the left main bronchus with no direct evidence of a tumour. Similar tumours have been observed in patients with various immunocompromising conditions such as renal and hepatic transplants. Epstein-Barr virus has been detected in every AIDS-related soft tissue tumour and is assumed to play an active role in the development of these tumours (DE CHADAREVIAN et al. 1997). Prolonged survival in paediatric patients with AIDS may increase the risk of developing such tumours.

13.4.2.4
Laryngotracheal Papilloma

Laryngeal papilloma is the most common benign laryngeal epithelial tumour. It is caused by the human papillomavirus, mainly types 6 and 11. Papillomas spread inferiorly from the larynx by direct contiguous extension as far as the major bronchi but rarely beyond. Lung parenchymal nodules occur in approximately 1% of cases possibly exacerbated by treatment to the primary laryngeal lesions. It is hypothesised that fragments are detached during endoscopy and are carried down the airways during inspiration. Those that lodge proximal to the respiratory bronchioles may be expelled by mucociliary clearance (KRAMER et al. 1985). Those that travel more distally are not cleared and thus enlarge.

Airway papillomas may be localised or extensive. Conglomerate lesions typically manifest as endotracheal or endobronchial masses (Fig. 13.2). Papillomas have a classic fimbriated or 'salmon egg' appearance on endoscopy. They are predominantly endoluminal with usually little submucosal infiltration although this does occur with more extensive papillomas. Pulmonary parenchymal lesions typically have a nodular appearance. Parenchymal lesions may be widely scattered remote from the major bronchi and a subpleural location is not uncommon. The nodules may be small or large, thin or thick-walled and may cavitate (Fig. 13.2). Air-fluid levels can be seen in larger pulmonary lesions, and these may occur without superadded infection. Some lesions occasionally resemble dilated bronchi or bronchiectasis but close inspection shows no direct communication to more central bronchi. An intraluminal airway mass with concomitant solitary or multiple pulmonary nodules or cavities is very suggestive of laryngotracheal papillomatosis. There is usually a history of treated laryngeal papillomatosis. It is my experience and impression that asymptomatic lung nodules may be more frequent in this population than is generally believed but chest CT is not, of course, indicated in children who are symptom free. More significantly, severe lung damage may result from multiple destructive parenchymal lesions such that symptoms of restrictive lung disease are seen in addition to upper airway obstruction.

13.4.3
Malignant Tumours

13.4.3.1
Bronchial Adenoma

The term 'adenoma' is a misnomer implying benign disease but is in common usage to categorise all neoplasms of the tracheobronchial glands. The tumours grouped under the label bronchial adenoma are low grade malignant lesions with the capacity for dis-

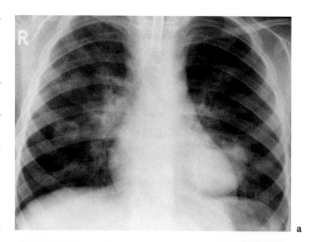

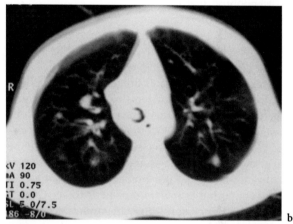

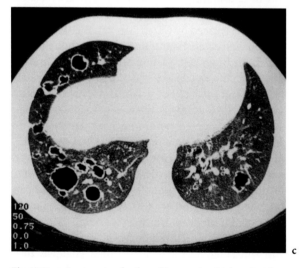

Fig. 13.2a–c. Laryngotracheal papillomatosis with lung involvement. **a** Frontal erect chest radiograph showing two cavitary lung nodules. The larger left-sided lesion has an air-fluid level but was not secondarily infected. Note the lower aspect of a tracheostomy tube. **b** Axial CT showing a relatively large endotracheal mass and parenchymal nodules in each lung. **c** Numerous cavitary nodules of varying size, many with irregular thick walls due to parenchymal spread of disease

semination with the exception of the extremely rare true mucinous adenoma. The other tumours comprising this group include the bronchial carcinoid, mucoepidermoid carcinoma and adenoid cystic carcinoma (cylindroma). Most tumours occur in the main bronchi and are unusual in the trachea.

In reality, bronchial adenomas are difficult to suspect in everyday paediatric practice as commoner causes of persistent lung collapse such as an aspirated foreign body lead to a low threshold for bronchoscopy which often makes the diagnosis. Endobronchial lesions should be included in the differential diagnoses in such cases, however, and the airway should be scrutinised closely on radiographs and CT. An endobronchial mass is generally evident on CT when eventually performed, although it should be stressed that 2–5 mm sections are best to depict an endobronchial lesion when suspected. Thicker sections may result in an indeterminate study – when there is doubt a repeat examination with narrower sections through the major airways should be performed. So-called three-dimensional (3D) CT virtual endoscopy may show endobronchial lesions elegantly, but bronchoscopic biopsy will ultimately be needed. Bronchography can demonstrate distinctive outward flaring of the bronchus proximal to an obstruction but is seldom now performed (CURTIS et al. 1998). Previously, bronchography was important in considering the extent of surgical resection when bronchiectasis was present, but this role has now been replaced by CT.

Bronchial *carcinoid* tumours account for up to one half of all bronchial adenomas. Carcinoid tumours arise from the Kulchitsky cell of the respiratory epithelium, and their cell of origin is part of the amine precursor uptake and decarboxylase (APUD) system. The actual carcinoid syndrome is extremely rare in childhood, having been reported in a large review in only one child who had metastatic disease (HANCOCK et al. 1993). Cushing's syndrome from ectopic adrenocorticotrophic hormone secretion has also been described but is similarly uncommon (WANG et al. 1993). Children with bronchial carcinoids are much more likely than their adult counterparts to present with wheezing, haemoptysis or lobar collapse. In a series of 25 young patients with bronchial carcinoid tumours, none was asymptomatic (WANG et al. 1993). An asymptomatic young patient is probably more likely to have a peripheral pulmonary lesion since any resultant area of atelectasis could be clinically silent (CURTIS et al. 1998). Endobronchial carcinoids (Fig. 13.3; see also Chap. 3, Fig. 3.15) have an intra-

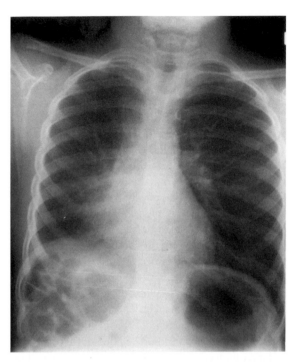

Fig. 13.3. Bronchial adenoma: carcinoid tumour. Persisting right middle and lower lobe collapse for over 6 months, proven at bronchoscopy to be due to an endobronchial carcinoid tumour in the bronchus intermedius

luminal, mural and extrabronchial component. They are vascular polypoid tumours and characteristically show prominent contrast enhancement at CT. The majority of carcinoid tumours, despite generally occurring in the central airways, are visible neither on chest radiography nor, often, on routine CT. Occasionally the mass external to the bronchus is larger than that in the lumen, and the extrabronchial component may consequently be visible as a hilar mass. The incidence of metastases with bronchial carcinoids, usually lymphatic metastases, has been reported in children to be between 5%–20% (WANG et al. 1993). Approximately one quarter of carcinoid tumours in adult patients are calcified, but the frequency of calcification appears to be much less in childhood.

Mucoepidermoid carcinoma accounts for approximately one third of bronchial adenomas. It is histologically similar to tumours described in the major salivary glands and is thought to originate from the minor salivary glands lining the tracheobronchial tree. As with other endobronchial lesions the history is usually that of respiratory infections or lobar collapse with or without air trapping. Calcification is seen in 50% of tumours. Contrast enhancement may be marked suggesting hypervascularity (Fig. 13.4).

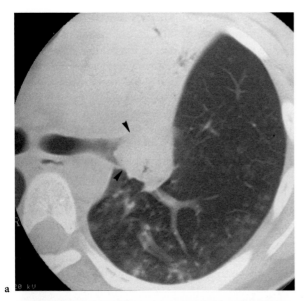

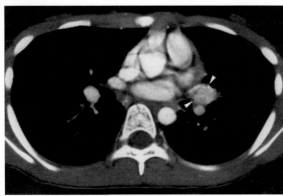

Fig. 13.4a, b. Bronchial adenoma: mucoepidermoid carcinomas. **a** CT showing an endobronchial mass (*arrowheads*) virtually occluding the left main bronchus close to the origin of the upper lobe bronchus with associated upper lobe collapse. **b** Enhanced CT scan in a different patient demonstrating an enhancing, hypervascular tumour (*arrowheads*) at the origin of the lingular bronchus. (Courtesy of Dr. H. Hara, Tokyo)

Mucoepidermoid carcinoma of the bronchus in children has low-grade malignant potential but complete resection should result in a good outcome.

Adenoid cystic carcinoma or *cylindroma* is a malignant lesion, characterised by slow growth and a potential for submucosal spread. In upper airway lesions, pathological examination reveals invasion beyond the wall of the trachea in virtually all cases (MAZIAK et al. 1996). Lung metastases may rarely be seen hence there is a need for both detailed fine sections through the tumour in addition to a CT study of the entire pulmonary parenchyma.

Mucous gland adenoma is the sole truly benign bronchial adenoma. It originates from the submucosal glands of the trachea and larger bronchi, and is extremely rare. Seven reported paediatric cases were reviewed by DICKSTEIN et al. (1993). A round opacity or merely lung hyperinflation or atelectasis may be evident on chest radiographs. Abundant mucous production may result in an apparent cystic mass on CT obscuring the endobronchial lesion.

13.4.3.2
Pleuropulmonary Blastoma

Pleuropulmonary blastoma is a rare lung tumour that occurs almost exclusively in children less than 6 years of age (WRIGHT 2000). It is now thought to represent an entity distinct from pulmonary blastoma, which is predominantly an adult tumour. It is exclusively mesenchymal, there is an absence of epithelial carcinomatous elements but rather a variably mixed blastematous and sarcomatous appearance. A recent hypothesis suggests pleuropulmonary blastoma may arise in a precursor lung developmental anomaly as in the relationship of nephrogenic rests and nephroblastomatosis to Wilms' tumour (PRIEST et al. 1997). Pleuropulmonary blastoma is regarded as a true dysembryonic neoplasm of thoracopulmonary mesenchyme in childhood. It is thus the pulmonary dysontogenetic analogue not only to Wilms' tumour but also to neuroblastoma in the adrenal gland and hepatoblastoma in the liver (PRIEST et al. 1997). A classification of pleuropulmonary blastomas into types I to III has been proposed (DEHNER et al. 1995). Predominantly cystic (type I), cystic and solid (type II) and mainly solid (type III) sub-types are described with increasing histological evidence of malignancy. There appears to be a significant difference in the age at presentation. In a review of 50 cases the median ages at diagnosis were 10 months for type I lesions, 34 months for type II, and 44 months of age in type III lesions (PRIEST et al. 1997).

There is a well documented association with prior cystic disease of the lung. In the Pleuropulmonary Blastoma Register cystic lung disease was present at diagnosis in almost 40% of patients (ROMEO et al. 1999). As the radiological follow-up of some of these preceding lung abnormalities appears to have been brief, it is not clear how often these allegedly innocuous 'cysts' were actually an early manifestation of the tumour in a more benign and less complex form. Nevertheless, some pleuropulmonary blastomas do seem to arise from pre-existing lung cysts. In addition, 25% of cases occur in a constitutional and familial setting in which the patients themselves or other family members have other dysplastic or neoplastic conditions. For example, in the Pleuropulmonary Blastoma Register, children with contralateral CCAM and bilateral cystic lung changes have been seen and another child had a sibling with CCAM (Priest et al. 1997). Moreover, any one of the three tumour types can be found in a familial setting. A thorough family history is therefore essential. Early surgical intervention is indicated for any cystic pulmonary abnormality in children from these families.

Although lesions may be intrapulmonary adjacent to the mediastinum, most pleuropulmonary blastomas arise in a subpleural location with over half of cases occurring in the lower lobes (Fig. 13.5). Like all thoracic mass lesions the clinical symptomatology

of pleuropulmonary blastomas is non-specific. Chest or abdominal pain, cough or pulmonary infections are the most frequent presenting complaints. A large pleural effusion may mimic an empyaema. Pneumothorax is an uncommon but well recognised presentation (Romeo et al. 1999). Pleuropulmonary blastomas manifest as mixed cystic and solid masses in the lung periphery adjacent to the pleura usually in the lower zones. Large lesions occupying virtually the entire hemithorax with mediastinal displacement may occur (Senac et al. 1991). A pulmonary cyst or complex mass lesion of uncertain aetiology is the usual indication for surgery (Fig. 13.5). The solid components of the mass lesion are seen to enhance with intravenous contrast administration on CT and MRI. Some lesions are sharply demarcated from adjacent lung parenchyma while others may be more

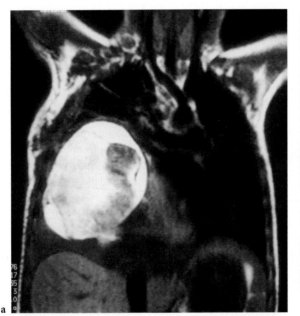

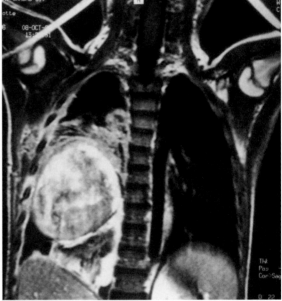

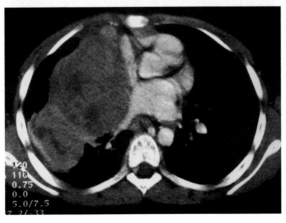

Fig. 13.5a–c. Pleuropulmonary blastomas. a Unenhanced coronal T1 W MRI showing a large hyperintense lesion in the region of the right middle lobe. This patient had had aspiration of haemorrhagic fluid on two occasions prior to this study and the hyperintense T1 appearance may be largely due to methaemoglobin. b Coronal T1 W MRI after gadolinium administration in the same patient showing diffuse pleural and lower lobe enhancement and upper lobe consolidation. Only haemorrhagic friable tissue was found at surgery and no discrete cyst could be identified. c Axial contrast-enhanced CT in another patient showing wide separation of the right pulmonary veins by a large heterogeneous intrapulmonary tumour. This 10-year-old boy had a right lung 'cyst' removed a few years previously and it is very unusual for a pleuropulmonary blastoma to occur at this age – the current lesion may well be a recurrence of the same tumour now in a more malignant form

infiltrative. Confident designation as to the site of origin i.e. lung or pleura, is often difficult to determine. Cross-sectional imaging should include the mediastinum as hilar metastases can occur. As with all chest masses, precise diagnosis depends on histological evaluation which in most cases takes place after attempted or successful surgical resection. It is actually quite common that these tumours are so friable intra-operatively, and this has been our experience also, that empyaema is still suspected during surgery. Thoracoscopic, open or percutaneous biopsy may be required for pre-operative diagnosis in more invasive, suspicious lesions as their peripheral location renders these tumours inaccessible to bronchoscopic biopsy.

Type I lesions, which comprise only 14% of all pleuropulmonary blastomas, have a better prognosis than the other sub-types. Large lesions (>5 cm) frequently recur or metastasise despite primary resection. Patients with pleural or mediastinal involvement fare significantly worse than those without such involvement. Actual metastatic disease is unusual at diagnosis but should be excluded. Metastases appear to occur exclusively in those with type II or III lesions. Pleuropulmonary blastomas have a particular tendency to metastasise to the central nervous system including the spinal cord – 44% of recurrences are in the CNS (PRIEST et al. 1997). All patients therefore merit craniospinal MRI for staging purposes and during follow-up. The second most common site for metastatic spread is the skeletal system. As there is little data on screening for skeletal metastases in children with pleuropulmonary blastoma, it seems advisable to perform both Tc99m-MDP radionuclide bone scanning and radiographic skeletal surveys in all patients with types II and III tumours. Responses to chemotherapy occur but the prognosis for other than type I lesions is not good. Five-year survival has been reported as 83% for type I, and 42% for types II and III (PRIEST et al. 1997).

13.4.3.3
Bronchogenic Carcinoma

Bronchogenic carcinoma is rare in childhood with approximately 50 cases reported in the world literature (KIM et al. 2000). Nevertheless, it accounts for 17% of malignant lung tumours in the paediatric age range. Undifferentiated tumours and adenocarcinomas account for 80% of lesions. There has been a notable scarcity of squamous cell tumours (12%) reported compared to an incidence in adults of between 40%–50% (HARTMAN and SHOCHAT 1983). Bronchogenic carcinoma in childhood is most common in adolescence. It is an aggressive malignancy with disseminated disease frequent at diagnosis and a mortality rate of around 90%. The common presenting complaints of cough, haemoptysis and weight loss are more likely to suggest pulmonary tuberculosis, particularly in endemic areas. As in adult patients, a central mass with endobronchial growth appears to be typical.

13.4.3.4
Pulmonary Metastases

The lungs are the predominant site of metastatic spread in the vast majority of solid extra-cranial malignancies. Disseminated neuroblastoma is an exception as it typically results in osseous secondaries and only rarely metastasises to the lung (Fig. 13.6).

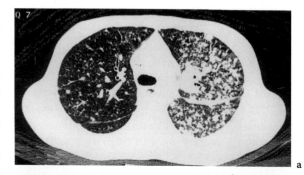

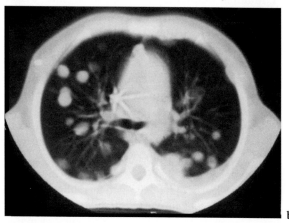

Fig. 13.6a, b. Pulmonary metastases. a Predominantly left-sided nodularity, pleural and interstitial thickening due to neuroblastoma metastases. An unusual lymphangitic pattern of tumour spread has occurred in this patient. b Numerous rounded opacities in a non-febrile 2-year-old child with a renal tumour – these lesions are undoubtedly metastases and were also visible on the chest radiograph at diagnosis

Pulmonary or pleural metastases in neuroblastoma are found in less than 1% of cases but this figure may well be an underestimate as chest CT is not routinely performed in these patients at diagnosis (COWIE et al. 1997). Common paediatric tumours which are associated with lung secondaries (with an approximate percentage incidence of pulmonary metastases at diagnosis) include Wilms' tumour (10%), rhabdomyosarcoma (10%), hepatoblastoma (10%), Ewing's (15%–20%) and osteosarcoma (15%–20%) (PAULUSSEN et al. 1998; KASTE et al. 1999). All of these primary neoplasms, and also other less common malignancies, merit routine chest CT for staging purposes at diagnosis.

CT is, of course, more sensitive than plain radiography in the detection of lung deposits. A successful response to chemotherapy should be accompanied by disappearance of the pulmonary secondaries. Occasionally larger metastases may respond with some shrinkage but not total disappearance – residual fibrosis is then assumed but ultimately proof of benignity rests on stable, unchanged appearances on follow-up, particularly off treatment in these so-called sterilised metastases. If the initial chest CT is negative for metastases, later follow-up is largely with chest radiography with CT reserved for suspected relapses or equivocal CXR findings. As up to 30%–40% of children with osteosarcoma eventually develop lung secondaries, more routine screening with CT of patients with osteosarcoma is justified.

Multiple pulmonary nodules in a child with a known solid tumour, particularly when some lesions are over 1 cm in diameter, are invariably metastases (Fig. 13.6). Diagnostic dilemmas arise when nodules are small (a few millimetres in diameter) and indistinct or only a solitary nodule is present. In one group of 52 children with a variety of solid malignancies who underwent 74 thoracotomies, over 80% of small (10 mm or less) nodules were metastatic lesions (CRISP et al. 1996). In 18 Wilms' tumour patients with nodules visible on CT but not CXR, 15 positive biopsies for metastatic disease were found (MEISEL et al. 1999). Clearly there exist patients, however, with solitary or small pulmonary nodules who may not have lung metastases. The true frequency of malignant nodules detected by CT in children with cancer is unknown. A solitary lesion or a few small equivocal lesions require either biopsy, which is often impractical, or close surveillance to reveal their true nature. A conservative approach to these equivocal lesions is generally adopted in most centres.

CONNOLLY et al. (1999) reported a series of core needle biopsies of small pulmonary nodules in children under CT guidance using a co-axial system. The rationale behind their use of a co-axial system was that it allowed multiple biopsies through a single pleural pass to be obtained which should reduce the potential for haemo- or pneumothorax. In their study attempted biopsy of 18 nodules resulted in adequate cores of tissue for diagnosis in 15. Nine nodules were positive for malignancy, five were benign and there was one false-negative result in whom later thoracoscopic biopsy revealed malignancy. No clinically significant pneumothorax was encountered (CONNOLLY et al. 1999). This type of interventional practice has not as yet gained widespread acceptance. Fine needle aspiration cytology is practised widely in adult patients with carcinoma and the yield is usually diagnostic. In children, however, sarcomas and lymphomas are relatively much more common. Differentiation from other cells can be extremely difficult on small cytological specimens and architectural information is lost such that aspiration cytology is generally regarded as unreliable for the diagnosis of childhood tumours.

Small nodules, particularly if ossified, in a patient with osteosarcoma are almost always significant and should be regarded as malignant until proven otherwise. Osteosarcoma may also metastasise to the mediastinal lymph nodes and pleura, which can also show ossified deposits. Innumerable tiny miliary metastases are a well-recognised manifestation of thyroid carcinoma. Cavitary metastases are unusual in childhood but are occasionally seen with sarcomatous tumours or rarely Wilms' tumour, or after chemotherapy or irradiation. There is some suggestion in adult patients that malignant lung nodules demonstrate contrast enhancement on CT and that absence of enhancement is predictive of benignity, but no studies corroborating this have been performed in children.

The differential diagnosis of a few or even multiple pulmonary nodules includes tuberculosis or histoplasmosis particularly in endemic areas. Other diagnostic considerations include septic emboli, previous varicella infection, Wegener's granulomatosis, Langerhans cell histiocytosis, laryngeal papillomatosis and a variety of opportunistic infections in an immunodeficient child. In an oncology child on parenteral nutrition, complications such as lipid or septic emboli or infarction can be difficult to differentiate from metastases. Although all these possibilities should be borne in mind, the clinical picture is usually straightforward.

Multiple lung nodules in a child with a malignancy, who is neither pyrexial nor tachypnoeic, are usually indicative of metastatic disease.

Controversy exists regarding the significance of pulmonary nodules detectable only on CT in patients with Wilms' tumour. Co-operative paediatric oncology groups in North America and Europe all suggest that positive findings for pulmonary nodules on CT (presumed metastases) can be ignored if no lesions are visible on the postero-anterior and lateral chest radiograph. Although the recommended imaging protocols state that lung CT is unnecessary when the CXR is normal, CT is performed routinely in most centres nevertheless! The rationale behind CT-positive, CXR-negative findings being classified according to the local abdominal stage, and not metastatic disease, rests on an unproven assumption, that patients with a small pulmonary metastatic volume may be treated with less chemotherapy because the tumour burden is smaller than in those patients with metastases evident on chest radiographs. This topic has been well reviewed by COHEN (1996). There is a widespread belief among paediatric oncologists that there is a continuum of pulmonary metastatic disease in Wilms' patients and possibly other childhood malignancies also (J. Pritchard, personal communication). Nodules visible on CXR represent the largest metastases, lesions only evident on CT are intermediate-sized deposits, but there may also be an unknown cohort of Wilms' patients with invisible 'micrometastases'. Thus only the largest metastases require local irradiation – systemic chemotherapy should eradicate all other deposits. There are conflicting reports as to whether those patients who are CT-positive but CXR-negative for metastases do in fact have an increased risk of later pulmonary relapse. There is also much confusion as some of these patients are treated as metastatic stage 4 disease by some oncologists while others, adhering to protocol, treat these patients as non-metastatic disease with less intensive chemotherapy (MEISEL et al. 1999). Pulmonary nodules, whether on CXR or CT, are frequently significant in these patients and it is known that at the time of relapse in Wilms' patients, 47% have pulmonary metastases. Finally, the situation whereby findings on one imaging modality are ignored i.e. abnormal CT but normal CXR, is unusual within paediatric oncology practice as staging is conventionally dependent on disease distribution rather than on the radiological modality used to evaluate disease spread.

Some paediatric abdominal tumours, most notably Wilms' tumour and adrenal carcinoma, have a propensity to invade the inferior vena cava (IVC) and occasionally result in tumour thrombus extending into the right atrium. This is regarded as local extension of tumour and not metastatic disease.

13.5
Mediastinal Tumours

13.5.1
Germ Cell Tumours

Primary germ cell tumours account for up to 10% of all mediastinal masses in children and are second only to lymphoma as a cause of a thymic mass. They are thus most often located in the anterior mediastinum (DULMET et al. 1993). Up to a half of all patients have no symptoms at the time of diagnosis (SASAKA et al. 1998). Conversely, large tumours causing tracheal compression or superior vena caval obstruction are also well recognised. Germ cell tumours which include teratomas, teratocarcinomas, seminomas, dysgerminomas, embryonal cell carcinomas, endodermal sinus tumours and choriocarcinomas, typically present no earlier than the second decade of life. Overall, germ cell tumours are malignant in about 10% of cases. Malignant germ cell neoplasms are frequently associated with elevated serum levels of human chorionic gonadotropin or alpha-foetoprotein. Teratomas account for the vast majority of mediastinal germ cell lesions in children and they can have varied amounts of mature and immature somatic tissues. Teratomas are characteristically composed of well-differentiated ectodermal, mesodermal and endodermal derivatives. Mature teratomas are benign lesions. Immature teratomas are potentially malignant but in patients less than 15 years of age have biological and clinical behaviour similar to mature teratomas (DULMET et al. 1993).

CT attenuation values and MR signal intensity for all these tumours are highly variable depending on the amount of fat, calcium or soft tissue in the mass (Fig. 13.7). Most teratomas have well-defined margins, thick walls and some fatty tissue or calcification or both. In fact, fat and calcification in an anterior mediastinal mass almost invariably indicate a germ cell origin. Seminomas typically have more homogeneous, soft-tissue attenuation while the more malignant lesions frequently have large necrotic components but there is wide variation in the appearance of all these tumours.

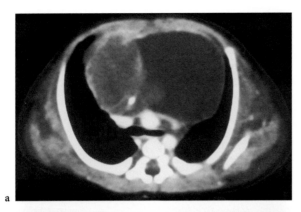

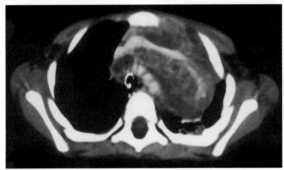

Fig. 13.7a, b. Germ cell tumours. **a** Contrast-enhanced CT, at the level of the carina, showing a typical anterior mediastinal teratoma with variable attenuation and one dense focus of calcification near the posteriorly displaced major vessels. **b** CT after intravenous contrast-enhancement in another child revealing a complex cystic and fatty immature teratoma causing compression of the left brachiocephalic vein

Teratomas may rupture into adjacent structures such as the pleural space, pericardium, lung parenchyma or tracheobronchial tree. Up to one third of mature benign mediastinal teratomas are reported to rupture, with malignant lesions having a significantly lesser tendency to leak their contents (SASAKA et al. 1998). Severe symptoms such as chest pain or haemoptysis are more commonly found in ruptured than in unruptured tumours (CHOI et al. 1998). Proteolytic or digestive enzymes and sebaceous materials within these teratomas are thought to play a role in their tendency to rupture and cause adjacent non-infectious inflammation. High amylase levels have been found in pleural effusions and in the tumour contents (SASAKA et al. 1998). Ruptured tumours have a tendency to display more heterogeneity in their internal components than unruptured teratomas. Ancillary findings in ruptured tumours depend on the space into which the rupture occurs. Rupture into the lung or through the tracheobronchial tree

may cause a chemical pneumonitis or fat-containing masses in the adjacent lung parenchyma. Haemoptysis with expectoration of hair or sebaceous material indicates a fistula between the tumour and the tracheobronchial tree and is said to be pathognomonic of a mature teratoma (SASAKA et al. 1998). Rupture into the pleura or pericardium results in pleural or pericardial effusions (CHOI et al. 1998). Adjacent consolidation or atelectasis is suspicious for rupture but can also be seen with compressive atelectasis from any large mass. Rupture is important to recognise or suspect as inflammatory changes and adhesions secondary to extravasation of tumour contents may result in more hazardous and extensive surgery than had been anticipated.

13.5.2
Thymoma

Epithelial tumours of the thymus are classified as thymoma or thymic carcinoma, according to the absence or presence of clear-cut cytological atypia to the neoplastic epithelial cell component (PESCARMONA et al. 1992). Thymomas are uncommon in children accounting for less than 5% of mediastinal tumours, and the vast majority are benign lesions. True thymic carcinomas are very rare. The radiological findings of thymomas vary from a small focal heterogeneous mass adjoining either thymic lobe to a large lobulated tumour which replaces the whole thymus and distorts the mediastinal structures (Fig. 13.8).

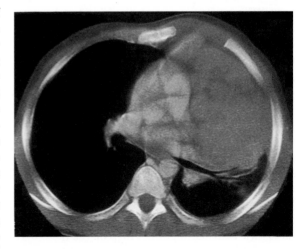

Fig. 13.8. Thymoma. Relatively homogeneous but non-enhancing left thymic mass proven to be a thymoma after resection and histological assessment

Variable low attenuating lesions with moderate contrast enhancement are characteristic. Calcification is uncommon. Thymoma in childhood usually occurs in isolation and is only rarely associated with myasthenia gravis. Malignant lesions tend to be more invasive with pleural encasement or pulmonary metastases. As with many mediastinal masses, an associated pericardial effusion is often an indicator of an aggressive tumour with intrapericardial invasion.

13.5.3
Neuroblastoma

The majority of posterior mediastinal masses in children are neurogenic tumours arising from the paravertebral sympathetic chain. Although neurofibromas are seen in paediatric patients, most occur in children with neurofibromatosis. The major childhood neurogenic tumours are neuroblastoma, gan-

glioneuroblastoma and ganglioneuroma. Neuroblastoma and ganglioneuroblastoma occur in the first decade of life whereas the more benign ganglioneuroma is seen in older children and adolescents. Thoracic neuroblastoma accounts for 15% of all cases of neuroblastoma. There is typically less advanced malignancy than in primary abdominal neuroblastoma with an associated better outcome. In one series of 96 children with thoracic neuroblastoma, the median age at presentation was at 0.9 years, only 20% had metastatic disease, and actuarial survival was 88% at 4 years (ADAMS et al. 1993). Interestingly, in that study a posterior mediastinal mass was diagnosed incidentally on chest radiographs performed for non-tumour related symptoms in half the cases.

In most instances the chest film suggests the correct diagnosis, particularly when posterior rib erosion is seen indicating a posterior mediastinal mass (Fig. 13.9). On CT most tumours are well-circumscribed, fusiform masses oriented vertically in a para-

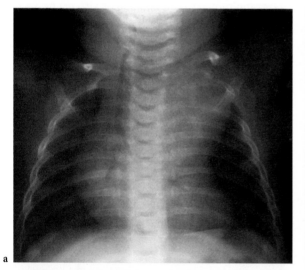

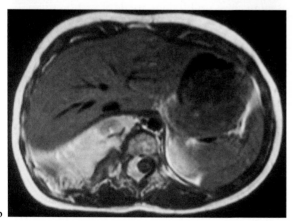

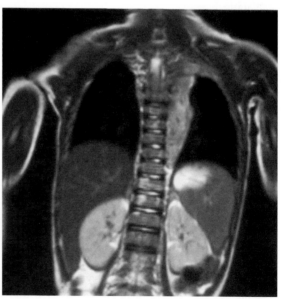

Fig. 13.9a–c. Neuroblastoma. **a** Chest radiograph in an infant showing an opacity in the left upper zone, posterior rib erosion and distortion typical of a posterior mediastinal mass. Tracheal shift to the right is also seen. **b** Axial T1 W MRI after gadolinium administration in another child revealing that a large right-sided chest tumour extends into the abdomen with displacement of the right diaphragmatic crus anteriorly. Note enhancing tumour within the spinal canal displacing the thecal sac to the left. **c** Coronal T2 W MRI demonstrating a left paraspinal mass extending from the apex to virtually the lung base. There is marked heterogeneity to the vertebral marrow due to widespread metastatic neuroblastoma

spinal location. Approximately 40% contain some calcification. Enlargement of intervertebral neural foramina and spread into the abdomen via the aortic or oesophageal hiatus or by direct invasion may also be evident (Fig. 13.9). Delineation of extent of disease is necessary for correct staging and is now most readily accomplished with MRI (SLOVIS et al. 1997). Bone marrow involvement is also easily recognised on MRI. When MRI is not possible, then contrast-enhanced CT must be performed to best assess tumour margins and intraspinal extension. As only 50% of children with intraspinal extension of tumour are symptomatic at the time of diagnosis, it is mandatory that intraspinal invasion is looked for in all patients (Fig. 13.9). Although less common, it is also important that lymph node or chest wall involvement is recognised in order to help select the optimal therapeutic approach. Abdominal sonography, Tc99m-MDP bone and metaiodobenzylguanidine (MIBG) scintigraphy should also be routinely performed in all neuroblastoma patients to identify or exclude metastatic disease.

Ganglioneuroma in older children is indistinguishable radiologically from neuroblastoma – all patients need histological confirmation and staging to rule out metastatic disease. When histological assessment is unclear, biopsy not feasible or the diagnosis uncertain, MIBG scanning should be considered. Positive uptake will be seen in over half of all cases, will confirm a neural crest tumour and simultaneously screens for metastases.

13.5.4
Lymphangioma

Most lymphangiomas (cystic hygromas) occur in the neck with up to 10% having an intrathoracic extension. Such larger lesions have varying amounts of lymphangiomatous and haemangiomatous components. These masses tend to be uniformly hyperintense on T2 W MRI and the haemangiomatous component in particular characteristically displays vivid enhancement after gadolinium administration. Coronal and sagittal MRI clearly depict the degree of great vessel and airway displacement and mediastinal infiltration. Occasionally intraspinal extension is also seen. CT will display a lymphangioma as a predominantly low attenuation mass but MRI is preferred for better overall assessment.

Lymphangiomatous malformations arising within the mediastinum and pulmonary parenchyma in children are being increasingly recognised (WUNDERBALDINGER et al. 2000; AVIV and McHUGH 2000). Simultaneous chylous pleural effusion and pulmonary interstitial thickening have now been described in a number of these paediatric patients. Ectatic lymphatic channels that weep chyle into the pleural space, or diffuse involvement of the visceral and parietal pleura, with or without a mediastinal mass, are the likely causative processes. Although lymphangiomas are benign lesions, those patients with generalised lymphangiomatosis and a chylothorax associated with osteolytic lesions have a poor prognosis. Intractable effusions and respiratory failure frequently supervene. We believe there is a spectrum of angiomatous disease processes that includes lymphangiomatosis and vanishing bone disease and have seen patients with proven lymphangiomatosis and non-contiguous bone resorption. Cross-sectional imaging has increased our awareness of the extent of soft tissue abnormality in the mediastinum and elsewhere in these patients.

Intrapulmonary lymphangiomas also occur. They are a rare form of localised lymphangectasia and are again part of the spectrum of lymphatic lung malformations. A pulmonary lymphangioma is typically seen in an older child or teenager. Imaging techniques generally show a large dense mass with varying cystic components which usually defies preoperative diagnosis (DRUT and MOSCA 1996).

13.6
Chest Wall Tumours

13.6.1
Benign

Benign chest wall lesions are dealt with in Chap. 15.

13.6.2
Malignant

13.6.2.1
Ewing's Sarcoma/Primitive Neuroectodermal Tumour

Chest wall Ewing's sarcoma and primitive neuroectodermal tumours (PNET), also known as Askin tumours, albeit separate histological entities, are recognised as biologically related lesions (SALLUSTIO et al. 1998). A classification that is gaining acceptance is to label all these tumours as 'malignant small round cell type'. From a radiological perspective they all generally manifest as peripheral chest wall masses, with or without associated rib destruction, and cannot be separated on imaging criteria alone.

Typically the chest radiograph will suggest the likely tumour based on the finding of a mass with intrathoracic growth, rib and chest wall involvement and concomitant pleural effusion (Fig. 13.10). Rib destruction essentially excludes a benign process and should be actively sought on plain radiography and CT (actinomycosis and rib osteomyelitis are uncom-

mon in childhood and generally present a different clinical picture). In a recent review of 29 PNETs from our institution, there were 11 chest PNETs in four of whom the whole hemithorax was occupied by tumour (Dick et al. 2001). The average diameter of the thoracic masses was 7 cm. A solid heterogeneous mass is characteristic with the larger lesions having more low attenuating or necrotic centres on CT (Fig. 13.10). Regional lymphadenopathy is usually absent although retrocrural nodal enlargement was seen in three of our patients. Calcification within the tumour is uncommon and when present is relatively unremarkable. Ultrasound of these peripheral chest masses has on occasion proved superior to CT and MRI in excluding tumour infiltration of the lung or diaphragm. PNETs tend to displace adjacent structures such as the bronchi or major vessels rather than encase them (Dick et al. 2001). The tumours are characteristically hyperintense on T2 W MRI and of intermediate signal on T1 W sequences. Contrast enhancement is variable. MRI is probably superior in assessing tumour extent and local invasion but to some degree CT and MRI are complimentary studies, bearing in mind that CT is helpful in assessing adjacent rib changes and in evaluating the lung parenchyma for metastases. There are conflicting reports regarding the prognostic significance of local rib and chest wall invasion (Dick et al. 2001; Sallustio et al. 1998). All these patients also merit routine Tc99m-MDP bone scans for staging purposes. Patients with distant skeletal metastases at diagnosis have a poor outcome.

13.6.2.2
Rhabdomyosarcoma and Other Sarcomas

Rhabdomyosarcoma is the most common soft tissue sarcoma in childhood, accounting for up to 10% of solid paediatric malignancies (McHugh and Boothroyd 1999). Primary intrathoracic rhabdomyosarcoma is, however, rare in the paediatric age group as other primary sites are much more common. Rhabdomyosarcoma can arise from virtually any compartment in the chest including the lung and chest wall. The thorax is regarded as an unfavourable primary site for rhabdomyosarcoma with a tendency towards more alveolar (and less embryonal) histology, advanced disease at presentation and tumours occurring in older children. All these factors are known to be associated with a worse outcome in rhabdomyosarcoma patients. These tumours most commonly present as large or rapidly enlarging solid masses, and a

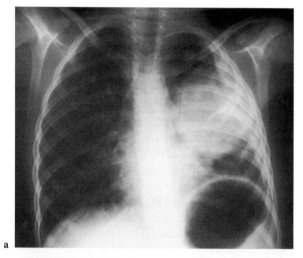
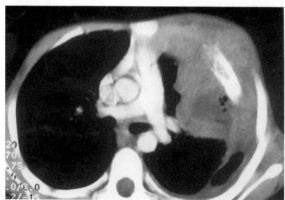

Fig. 13.10a, b. Ewing's sarcoma. **a** Chest X-ray displaying a rounded left mid-zone opacity with an elevated hemidiaphragm. Note lytic changes and expansion to the anterior third left rib in keeping with a malignant, aggressive lesion. **b** Axial enhanced CT in the same patient showing a thickened rib surrounded by a large chest wall mass. Gas bubbles are secondary to a percutaneous biopsy. A pleural effusion is noted and contralateral pulmonary metastases were evident on lung window settings

pleural effusion is not infrequent. Irregular contrast enhancement with variable areas of low attenuation are typical on CT examination (Fig. 13.11). Calcification within the mass is not a feature but destruction of adjacent ribs is occasionally seen.

Fibrosarcoma, unspecified sarcoma, and thoracic rhabdomyosarcomas are all indistinguishable radiologically, relying on histological examination for their differentiation. A leiomyosarcoma could also appear similar but increasingly now would typically be seen in a young AIDS patient. The whole group of sarcoma tumours accounts for one fifth of all intrapulmonary malignancies in children. The majority of sarcomas are, however, chest wall masses.

13.6.2.3
Mesothelioma

Although there is some controversy regarding the nomenclature and origin, mesothelioma in childhood does occur (FRAIRE et al. 1988). Primary tumours may originate from the pleura, pericardium or peritoneum with two thirds of cases arising in the pleural space. Diffuse tumours are more common than localised lesions. Benign and malignant mesothelioma cannot be differentiated on histological or radiological grounds, although diffuse or invasive masses are more likely to be malignant and, of course, lesions that metastasise are by definition malignant. Some tumours in childhood may have an indolent course, and disease-free survival is possible. FRAIRE et al. (1988) were of the opinion that childhood mesothelioma is a sporadic, distinct entity separate from adult mesothelioma. There has been some specula-

tion that either asbestos or isoniazid exposure or irradiation may predispose to these tumours in childhood, but the available evidence to date does not support a direct causal link.

13.7
Tumours of the Diaphragm

Primary tumours arising in the diaphragm are extremely rare in childhood. Tumours derived from muscle, blood vessels, fat or fibrous tissue are possible. Fibrosarcoma is the most common malignant diaphragmatic tumour reported in adults. Four primary rhabdomyosarcomas of the diaphragm have been described in children to date (GUPTA et al. 1999). A pronounced diaphragmatic 'hump' on a frontal chest radiograph is said to be the classic sign of a primary tumour arising from the diaphragm. Diaphragmatic masses, however, can mimic an elevated hemidiaphragm or eventration but ultrasound evaluation should easily demonstrate a mass lesion thus excluding those more common diagnoses. If there is no hepatic invasion the mass should be seen to move separately from the liver on sonography. Malignant tumours may present with a pleural effusion which may obscure an underlying mass lesion. In the case reported by GUPTA et al. the tumour was clearly located cranial to the liver on axial CT and sharply demarcated from it indicating an extrahepatic origin. Coronal or sagittal MRI would be the optimal method for demonstrating a neoplasm arising from the diaphragm. MRI is generally more useful, however, in demonstrating the site of origin of a large mass abutting the hemidiaphragm, the relationship of the diaphragm to the mass including diaphragmatic integrity and in delineating the extent of such a mass lesion.

13.8
Conclusions

The above-mentioned thoracic tumours are all relatively uncommon in childhood. Nevertheless, when there is failure to respond to the usual medical treatment, and particularly when there is mediastinal compression or displacement or rib changes, the possibility of neoplasia increases significantly. Some other even rarer chest tumours (Fig. 13.12) inevitably also occur from time to time and often merit

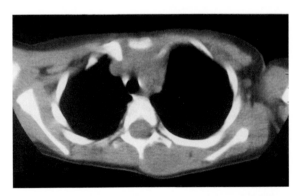

Fig. 13.11. Rhabdomyosarcoma. Unenhanced CT showing enlargement of the left erector spinae muscles due to a biopsy proven rhabdomyosarcoma. The extent and margins of this tumour would be best evaluated by CT after intravenous contrast enhancement, or more preferably by MRI

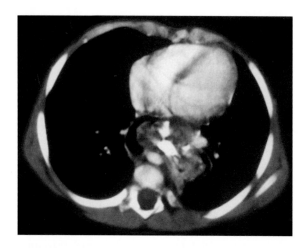

Fig. 13.12. Esophageal teratoma. Teratomas may rarely occur in the posterior mediastinum but seldom involve the esophagus to this degree. Contrast-enhanced CT here demonstrates a large, calcified mass anterior to the descending thoracic aorta within the lumen of a markedly distended esophagus

individual case reports but have not been detailed here. Vertebral neoplasms have not been discussed as these are generally categorised and dealt with in skeletal texts.

Cardiac tumours are also extremely rare in paediatrics and fall predominantly within the practice of the paediatric cardiologist. Cardiac rhabdomyomas are the commonest of these neoplasms, usually occurring in children with tuberous sclerosis (TS) or a family history of TS (LIANG et al. 2000). In symptomatic neonates cardiac rhabdomyomas are generally fatal. Patients with no major dysrhythmia or haemodynamic obstruction, however, have an excellent prognosis. Over half of all tumours completely or partially regress over time, and in children who can be managed conservatively other lesions tend to remain stable (LIANG et al. 2000).

Although improvements in CT and MRI will undoubtedly aid diagnosis in patients with thoracic tumours in the future, mention should also be made of positron emission tomography, or so-called PET, scanning. Many different types of tumour have now been found to exhibit high levels of fluorodeoxyglucose uptake and thus can be imaged with a PET scanner (SHULKIN 1997). PET scanning can frequently differentiate benign from malignant lesions and in some paediatric patients has identified unexpected pulmonary metastases (SHULKIN 1997). PET holds great promise in the evaluation of childhood malignancies not only for detection but also staging and assessing response to therapy. As the technique is

becoming more "paediatric-friendly" it seems likely that it will play an increasing role in the management of childhood thoracic tumours in the future.

References

Adams GA, Shochat SJ, Smith EI et al (1993) Thoracic neuroblastoma: a Pediatric Oncology Group study. J Pediatr Surg 28:372–377

Agrons GA, Rosado-de-Christenson ML, Kirejczyk WM et al (1998) Pulmonary inflammatory pseudotumor: radiologic features. Radiology 206:511–518

Aviv R, McHugh K (2000) Mechanisms of chylous effusions in lymphangiomatosis. AJR 175:1191

Brown G, Shaw DG (1995) Inflammatory pseudotumours in children: CT and ultrasound appearances with histopathological correlation. Clin Radiol 50:782–786

Chadwick EG, Connor EJ, Guerra Hanson C et al (1990) Tumours of smooth muscle origin in HIV-infected children. JAMA 263:3182–3184

Choi S-J, Lee JS, Song KS, Lim T-H (1998) Mediastinal teratoma: CT differentiation of ruptured and unruptured tumors. AJR 171:591–594

Coakley FV, Cohen MD, Johnson MS et al (1998) Maximum intensity projection images in the detection of simulated pulmonary nodules by spiral CT. Br J Radiol 71:135–140

Cohen MD (1996) Commentary: imaging and staging of Wilms' tumors: problems and controversies. Pediatr Radiol 26:307–311

Connolly BL, Chait PG, Duncan DS, Taylor G (1999) CT-guided percutaneous needle biopsy of small lung nodules in children. Pediatr Radiol 29:342–346

Cowie F, Corbett R, Pinkerton CR (1997) Lung involvement in neuroblastoma: incidence and characteristics. Med Ped Oncol 28:429–432

Crisp AJ, Babyn PS, Weitzman S, Thorner P (1996) Significance of lung nodules at CT in children with solid malignant tumours. Presented at International Pediatric Radiology, Boston

Curtis JM, Lacey D, Smyth R, Carty H (1998) Endobronchial tumours in childhood. Eur J Radiol 29:11–20

de Chadarevian J-P, Wolk JH, Inniss S et al (1997) A newly recognised cause of wheezing: AIDS-related bronchial leiomyomas. Pediatr Pulmonol 24:106–110

Dehner LP, Watterson J, Priest J (1995) Pleuropulmonary blastoma: a unique intrathoracic-pulmonary neoplasm of childhood. Perspect Pediatr Pathol 18:214–226

Dick EA, McHugh K, Kimber C, Michalski A (2001) Radiology of non-central nervous system primitive neuroectodermal tumours: diagnostic features and correlation with outcome. Clin Radiol (in press)

Dickstein PJ, Amaral SMM, Silva AMLF et al (1993) Bronchial mucous gland adenoma presenting as a bronchogenic cyst. Pediatr Pulmonol 16:370–374

Diederich S, Lenzen H, Windmann R et al (1999) Pulmonary nodules: experimental and clinical studies at low dose CT. Radiology 213:289–298

Drut R, Mosca HH (1996) Intrapulmonary cystic lymphangioma. Pediatr Pulmonol 22:204–206

Dulmet EM, Macchiarini P, Suc B, Verley JM (1993) Germ cell tumours of the mediastinum: a 30 year experience. Cancer 72:1894–1901

Fraire AE, Cooper S, Greenberg SD et al (1988) Mesothelioma of Childhood. Cancer 62:838–847

Gross E, Chen MK, Hollabaugh RS, Joyner RE (1996) Tracheal hamartoma: report of a child with a neck mass. J Pediatr Surg 31:1584–1585

Guest AR, Strouse PJ, Chung Hiew C, Arca M (2000) Progressive esophageal leiomyomatosis with respiratory compromise. Pediatr Radiol 30:247–250

Gupta AK, Mitra DK, Berry M (1999) Primary embyonal rhabdomyosarcoma of the diaphragm in a child: case report. Pediatr Radiol 29:823–825

Hancock BJ, Di Lorenzo M, Youssef S et al (1993) Childhood primary pulmonary neoplasms. J Pediatr Surg 28:1133–1136

Hartman GE, Shochat SJ (1983) Primary pulmonary neoplasms of childhood: a review. Ann Thorac Surg 36:108–119

Hedlund GL, Navoy JF, Galliani CA, Johnson WH Jr (1999) Aggressive manifestations of inflammatory pseudotumor in children. Pediatr Radiol 29:112–116

Jayne D, Bridgewater B, Lawson RAM (1997) Endobronchial inflammatory pseudotumour exacerbating asthma. Postgrad Med J 73:98–99

Karnak I, Akcoren Z, Senocak ME (2000) Endobronchial leiomyoma in children. Eur J Pediatr Surg 10:136–139

Kaste SC, Pratt CB, Cain AM et al (1999) Metastases detected at the time of diagnosis of primary pediatric extremity osteosarcoma: imaging features. Cancer 86:1602–1608

Kim CK, Chung CY, Koh YY (2000) Primary small cell bronchogenic carcinoma in a 14 year old boy. Pediatr Pulmonol 29:317–320

Kim WS, Lee KS, Kim IO et al (1997) Congenital cystic adenomatoid malformation of the lung: CT-pathologic correlation. AJR 168:47–53

Kramer SS, Wehunt WD, Stocker JT, Kashima H (1985) Pulmonary manifestations of juvenile laryngotracheal papillomatosis. AJR 144:687–694

Liang CD, Ko SF, Huang SC (2000) Echocardiographic evaluation of cardiac rhabdomyoma in infants and children. J Clin Ultrasound 28:381–386

Mas Estelles F, Andres V, Vallcanera A et al (1995) Plasma cell granuloma of the lung in childhood: atypical radiologic findings and association with hypertrophic osteoarthropathy. Pediatr Radiol 25:369–372

Maziak DE, Todd TR, Keshavjee SH et al (1996) Adenoid cystic carcinoma of the airway: thirty-two year experience. J Thorac Cardiovasc Surg 112:1522–1531

McHugh K, Boothroyd AE (1999) The role of radiology in childhood rhabdomyosarcoma. Clin Radiol 54:2–10

Meisel JA, Guthrie KA, Breslow NE et al (1999) Significance and management of computed tomography detected pulmonary nodules: a report from the National Wilms Tumor Study Group. Int J Radiation Oncol Biol Phys 44:579–585

Paulussen M, Ahrens S, Craft AW et al (1998) Ewing's tumour with primary lung metastases: survival analysis of 114 (European Intergroup) Cooperative Ewing's Sarcoma Studies patients. J Clin Oncol 16:3044–3052

Pescarmona E, Giardini R, Brisigotti M et al (1992) Thymoma in childhood: a clinicopathological study of five patients. Histopathology 21:65–68

Priest JR, McDermott MB, Bhatia S et al (1997) Pleuropulmonary Blastoma: a clinicopathologic study of 50 cases. Cancer 80:147–161

Romeo C, Impellizzeri P, Grosso M et al (1999) Pleuropulmonary blastoma: long-term survival and literature review. Med Pediatr Oncol 33:372–376

Sallustio G, Pirronti T, Lasorella A et al (1998) Diagnostic imaging of primitive neuroectodermal tumour of the chest wall (Askin tumour). Pediatr Radiol 28:697–702

Sasaka K, Kurihara Y, Nakajima Y et al (1998) Spontaneous rupture: a complication of benign mature teratomas of the mediastinum. AJR 170:323–328

Senac MO Jr, Wood BP, Isaacs H, Weller M (1991) Pulmonary blastoma: a rare childhood malignancy. Radiology 179:743–746

Shulkin BL (1997) PET applications in pediatrics. Q J Nucl Med 41:281–291

Slovis TL, Meza MP, Cushing B et al (1997) Thoracic neuroblastoma: what is the best imaging modality for evaluating extent of disease? Pediatr Radiol 27:273–275

Tagge EP, Mulvihill D, Chandler JC et al (1996) Childhood pleuropulmonary blastoma: caution against nonoperative management of congenital lung cysts. J Pediatr Surg 31:187–190

van den Bosch JMM, Wagenaar SS, Corrin B et al (1987) Mesenchymoma of the lung (so called hamartoma): a review of 154 parenchymal and endobronchial cases. Thorax 42:790–793

Verbeke JIM, Verbene AAPH, den Hollander JC, Robben SGF (1999) Inflammatory myofibroblastic tumour of the lung manifesting as progressive atelectasis. Pediatr Radiol 29:816–819

Wang LT, Wilkins EW Jr, Bode HH (1993) Bronchial carcinoid tumors in pediatric patients. Chest 103:1426–1428

Wright JR Jr (2000) Pleuropulmonary blastoma. Case report documenting transition from type I (cystic) to type III (solid). Cancer 88:2853–2858

Wunderbaldinger P, Paya P, Partik B et al (2000) CT and MR imaging of generalised cystic lymphangiomatosis in pediatric patients. AJR 174:827–832

14 Thoracic Manifestations of Systemic Diseases

Alan S. Brody

CONTENTS

14.1
Introduction

This chapter will concentrate on the evaluation of the thorax in children with systemic disorders. Following a discussion of examination techniques, specific systemic conditions that have known thoracic manifestations will be discussed. For each condition or group of conditions, the general features of the condition will be described, followed by a review of the imaging characteristics of thoracic manifestations. Imaging evaluation will emphasize advanced imaging techniques and recent developments. The reader is encouraged to review the overall description of the different conditions as well as the specific imaging information. Knowledge of the clinical and laboratory features of these diseases may allow the radiologist to be the first

Alan S. Brody, MD
Professor of Radiology and Pediatrics, Department of Radiology, Children's Hospital Medical Center, 3333 Burnet Avenue, Cincinnati, Ohio 45229-3039, USA

to suggest an underlying systemic disease in a child with a thoracic abnormality. Knowledge of the associated pulmonary abnormalities frequently narrows the differential of lung findings in these children.

In addition to specific associated thoracic abnormalities, many systemic diseases produce effects that can be reflected by thoracic findings on diagnostic imaging. Increased central venous pressure or decreased capillary oncotic pressure can result in pulmonary edema. Abnormal host defenses frequently result in both an increased incidence of pulmonary infection and a change in the spectrum of infection. Abnormalities of muscle strength or the nervous system can result in aspiration with direct chemical insult to the lungs as well as an increase in infection. The likelihood of such effects should be borne in mind, as in the proper clinical situation these abnormalities may be more common than pathologies associated with a specific systemic disease.

14.2
Examination Techniques

14.2.1
Plain Radiographs and Computed Radiography

Plain radiographs remain the most common imaging study of the chest. Pediatric chest radiography requires expertise on the part of the radiology technologist in order to obtain correct patient position, lung volume, lack of motion, and correct technique. Interstitial lung disease is frequently very subtle in children. In addition, viral infections are very common, and produce findings of interstitial lung disease that are frequently indistinguishable from noninfectious causes.

Computed radiography is replacing film radiography at many sites. The resolution of computed radiography is lower than that of film/screen radiography. No studies have specifically compared the two systems in the evaluation of pediatric interstitial lung disease. Radiologists must be aware that computed radiography and PACS incorporate factors including imaging plate characteristics, system resolution, and image compression that can all impact the ability to detect subtle lung disease (KIDO et al. 1996).

14.2.2
Computed Tomography

Computed tomography (CT) is the primary cross-sectional imaging modality for evaluating the thorax. All components of the thorax can be well evaluated with CT. There are specific areas that are better evaluated with magnetic resonance imaging (MRI), but MRI cannot currently fully evaluate the lung parenchyma and does not provide a complete means of evaluating the chest.

Numerous studies have demonstrated the superiority of CT over chest radiographs in detecting thoracic abnormalities (NATHANSON et al. 1991; KUHN 1993; LYNCH et al. 1999). Due to the increased sensitivity and specificity of CT compared to chest radiographs, CTs may be ordered either to better evaluate radiographic abnormalities or to definitively assess the presence and extent of a suspected complication of systemic disease. CT scanning can show parenchymal abnormalities when chest radiographs are normal. With increasing therapeutic options in many systemic diseases, the additional information provided by CT scanning is of increasing value to clinicians. This has resulted in a marked increase in the number of chest CTs ordered. Examination technique must be carefully planned to minimize radiation exposure while maximizing image quality.

Low dose techniques have been applied to both helical CT and high-resolution CT (HRCT) in children, using techniques as low as 32 mAs (ROGALLA et al. 1999; LUCAYA et al. 2000). At our institution we have decreased mAs for all CT scanning, using between 40 and 150 mAs in children from infancy to young adulthood. A lower dose is used when imaging the lung than when imaging the abdomen. In general, 120 kVp is used for all studies. The shortest scan time that uses complete gantry rotation should be used. The use of partial arc scanning, which decreases scan speed by obtaining less data for each slice should be evaluated for its effect on noise and artifacts. These effects will likely differ with different CT scanners. We use the same dose for helical and HRCT. Helical CT should be performed with a pitch of 1.3 or greater.

HRCT directly irradiates a much smaller amount of the chest than helical CT. This results in a further dose reduction when HRCT is used.

Motion blurring will markedly degrade CT images, particularly HRCT images. We have found, however, that HRCT may still provide more information than helical CT despite the presence of some motion blurring. It is very important to limit gross body movement, but images obtained during quiet respiration can often provide useful information. Many children can be studied without sedation, but the ability to adequately sedate patients is an important component of the pediatric imaging department. The use of a "stop ventilation " technique that images sedated young children during a respiratory pause induced by mask ventilation can produce a striking improvement in image quality (LONG et al. 1999).

HRCT is the method of choice for the evaluation of diffuse parenchymal disease. Evaluation of the mediastinum and chest wall should be performed with helical CT. If both evaluations are needed, helical CT can be performed first with limited HRCT images performed subsequently, using the helical CT to suggest appropriate levels. The use of intravenous contrast will not degrade HRCT images.

14.2.3
Magnetic Resonance Imaging

Recent reports have shown that nodules as small as 3 mm can be detected, but parenchymal characteristics useful in the evaluation of these patients such as interstitial fibrosis or ground glass increased density can not be seen with MRI (HATABU et al. 1999). While MRI does not provide a complete evaluation of the lung parenchyma, it has been used in specific clinical situations. MRI has been used clinically to demonstrate pulmonary hemorrhage (HSU et al. 1992). In a study of immunocompromised patients, MRI was found to be superior to CT in demonstrating early necrotizing pneumonia (LEUTNER et al. 2000).

MRI has a greater scope of application in evaluating the chest wall, where it is the most sensitive means of evaluation and is better able to demonstrate soft tissue inflammation and bone marrow changes in the ribs than CT. When spinal abnormalities are suspected, MRI is usually the modality of choice.

Mediastinal vascular anatomy is well demonstrated by both modalities. Mediastinal masses can be evaluated with either modality. MRI is preferred in posterior mediastinal masses because it more accurately evaluates spinal involvement. In the anterior and middle mediastinum, both modalities are useful with CT preferred to identify calcification, and MRI better able to discriminate mediastinal masses from normal mediastinal tissues. Cardiac and pericardial masses are best evaluated with MRI.

As well as imaging considerations, differences in imaging time and environment may be factors in choosing between CT and MRI. MRI requires longer imaging time and frequently requires sedation. At most institutions availability is limited compared to CT. Support equipment may be more difficult to maintain in the MRI environment.

A new MRI technique currently being investigated at several sites is the use of hyperpolarized helium. The patient inhales this gas which fills the ventilated lung and has a very short T1 that produces strong signal on appropriate pulse sequences. Dynamic imaging can be performed to evaluate wash in and wash out of gas as well as overall ventilation (DONNELLY et al. 1999). This is a potentially powerful technique to combine the resolution of MRI with the functional information usually provided by nuclear medicine lung scanning. The hyperpolarized helium must be generated using dedicated equipment, and has a short half-life. This may limit the general availability of this technique.

14.2.4
Nuclear Medicine

Nuclear medicine adds functional information to the morphological information provided by CT and MRI. Gallium imaging can be used to assess disease activity (KAPALA et al. 1983). Single photon emission CT (SPECT) is becoming increasingly available and markedly improves the localization of abnormalities seen with nuclear medicine. Imaging time for nuclear medicine studies is longer than for CT and more often requires sedation. Pediatric expertise is important, particularly when studies require cooperation, for example when performing ventilation scans.

14.3
Connective Tissue Diseases

The connective tissue diseases (CTDs) are a group of diseases characterized by immune system abnormalities and inflammation affecting different sys-

tems and tissues. Common CTDs in children include juvenile rheumatoid arthritis (JRA), dermatomyositis (DM) and systemic lupus erythematosus (SLE). Patients may present with features of multiple CTDs. This presentation has been called mixed connective tissue disease (MCTD) or overlap syndrome.

Lung involvement varies with the type of CTD. Clinically apparent pulmonary abnormalities are very rare in JRA, rare in DM, and more common in SLE (CERVERI et al. 1992). Overlap syndromes also more commonly show lung involvement (Fig. 14.1). In a study of pulmonary function in children with CTD, pulmonary function abnormalities were found in the majority of children with active disease, although none had abnormalities on chest radiographs (CERVERI et al. 1992).

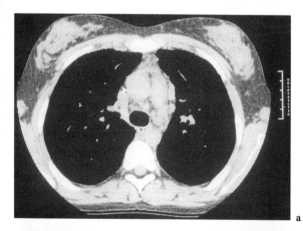

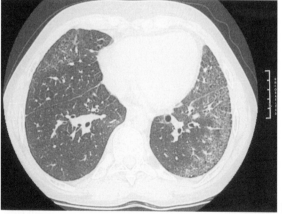

Fig. 14.1a,b. High-resolution computed tomography image through the lower lungs in a 13-year-old with mixed connective tissue disease. **a** Mediastinal windows show multiple small lymph nodes throughout the mediastinum. **b** Lung windows show peripheral small cystic spaces separated by well-seen fibrous walls. This honeycombing appearance suggests pulmonary fibrosis. These changes have been slowly progressing for several years. The patient has only minimal pulmonary symptoms

Clinically evident pulmonary disease is rare in JRA, occurring in 4% in one study (ATHREYA et al. 1980). However, when pulmonary function tests were performed in 16 children with JRA, 10 had abnormalities (WAGENER et al. 1981). Among imaging findings, pleural and pericardial effusions were the most common abnormalities, occurring in five of 191 children studied by ATHREYA et al. (1980) (Fig. 14.2). Lymphocytic interstitial pneumonitis (LIP) occurred in two children in this group. In two additional cases, LIP preceded other symptoms of JRA by as much as 2 years (LOVELL et al. 1984; UZIEL et al. 1998). These reports describe nonspecific interstitial infiltrates on chest radiographs. No report of CT findings is given. The reported appearance of LIP on HRCT shows predominantly ground glass opacity with associated consolidation, nodules, and cysts also seen (LYNCH et al. 1999).

Scleroderma is characterized by fibrotic infiltration of connective tissues. Involvement of the skin and the gastrointestinal tract, particularly the esophagus, is most common. The term systemic sclerosis is used to describe disseminated disease. Scleroderma presents most commonly in adult women, but 10% of patients present in the pediatric age. Both pulmonary function test abnormalities and parenchymal abnormalities are common in scleroderma. In a study of 11 patients aged 5–19 years old, eight had interstitial lung disease on HRCT. A broad range of abnormalities was described. The most common were ground

glass opacity in eight, subpleural nodules in seven, peripheral linear opacities in six, and honeycombing in five. Chest radiographs were positive in only two patients (SEELY et al. 1997).

SLE is a multisystem disease characterized by the production of numerous autoantibodies. The prevalence of SLE in childhood is 5–10 per 100,000 children. Approximately one fifth to one sixth of SLE patients present before the age of 16 years (ARKACHAISRI and LEHMAN 1999). Recent advances in genetics suggest that SLE results from a combination of genetic and environmental factors.

Lung disease is common in children with SLE, probably occurring in more than half of patients. The most common abnormality is restrictive lung disease detected on pulmonary function tests. Clinically apparent disease is less common, with estimates as low as 5%. The most common abnormality is pleural disease with resulting effusions. HRCT reliably identifies parenchymal lung disease more frequently than chest radiographs in adults with SLE (BANKIER et al. 1995). No current study has evaluated the lungs in children with SLE. Lupus pneumonitis is a rare condition that can be difficult to diagnose due to a nonspecific presentation of shortness of breath and a variable appearance of parenchymal opacity (Fig. 14.3). Massive pulmonary hemorrhage is more common and of greater clinical concern. This condition is not seen in other CTDs. Patients present with parenchymal abnormalities and a decrease in hematocrit. Hemoptysis may not occur. This frequently fatal complication can be treated with steroids and cytotoxic agents, so identification is clinically important (SCHWAB et al. 1993). Alveolar opacities and a reticulonodular appearance can be seen on radiographs. CT appearance also includes ground glass opacity. The appearance of pulmonary hemorrhage is not specific on plain radiographs or CT. Lupus pneumonitis and infection can produce the same appearance, and cannot reliably identify pulmonary hemorrhage. MRI has been reported as a means of specifically identifying hemorrhage by T2 shortening (HSU et al. 1992).

"Shrinking lung syndrome" is a term used to describe a progressive decrease in lung volume seen in some patients with SLE. This is usually identified on chest radiographs as a progressive elevation of the diaphragm despite attempted full inspiration. The etiology is unknown, but may relate to a combination of pleural restriction due to recurrent pleural inflammation, pulmonary restriction due to fibrosis, and muscle weakness of the diaphragm and chest wall. African American patients are most commonly affected.

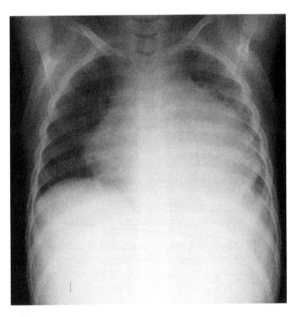

Fig. 14.2. Large pericardial effusion and small left pleural effusion in an 8-year-old boy with juvenile rheumatoid arthritis

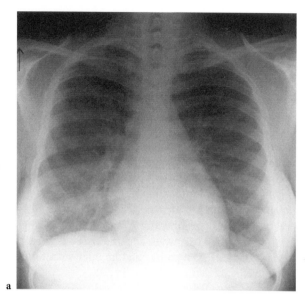

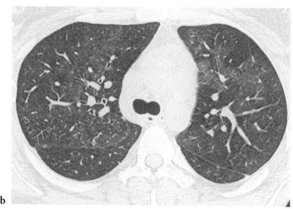

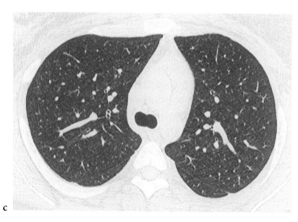

Fig. 14.3a–c. Lupus pneumonitis in a 17-year-old young woman with systemic lupus erythematosus who presented with short-ness of breath. **a** Chest radiograph showed questionable basilar increased markings without other abnormality. **b** Initial high-resolution computed tomography (HRCT) demonstrates bilat-eral areas of ground glass attenuation throughout both lungs. No other abnormality was seen. **c** HRCT following steroid treat-ment shows resolution of the parenchymal abnormalities

In addition to the pulmonary parenchymal abnor-malities described above, pulmonary hypertension has been reported in JRA, scleroderma, and SLE.

14.3.1
Immune Deficiencies

Defenses against infection include physical barriers, B cells, T cells, natural killer cells, phagocytes, and compliment proteins. Defects in all of these occur, and result in increased infections. The lungs are directly exposed to infectious agents and are frequently the site of infection in children with abnormal infection fighting ability. Involvement of the lungs is seen to varying degrees in all of the immunodeficiencies.

The radiologist has several roles when evaluating the lungs of children who may have an immunodefi-ciency. These include suggesting the possibility of an immunodeficiency, identifying imaging characteris-tics consistent with a certain immunodeficiency, and evaluating infections as part of the acute care of these patients. The radiologist may be the first to suggest the possibility of immunodeficiency, by noticing fre-quent infections such as recurrent pneumonia and by identifying unusual patterns of disease or slow res-olution of infections. In suspected immunodeficien-cies, imaging findings such as the presence of the thymus or lymphadenopathy may limit the differen-tial diagnosis. The most common request is to evalu-ate the lungs for infection, and to suggest a likely etiol-ogy. The pathogens most likely to cause disease differ in different immunodeficiency syndromes, again nar-rowing the differential diagnosis.

Increased understanding of the molecular basis of the immune system as well as immunogenetics is allowing a far more detailed understanding of the immunodeficiency syndromes (JONES and GASPAR 2000). With this increased understanding has come increased complexity in evaluating and classifying these children. The radiologist will now likely be increasingly faced with new or extremely uncommon syndromes.

When interpreting imaging studies on these patients, it is frequently of benefit to ask the clini-cians to relate the patients disease to one or more of the well-described immunodeficiency syndromes included at the end of this section. This will allow the radiologist to both limit the differential diagnosis, and to point out inconsistencies between the imag-ing appearance in a specific child and the expected appearance of the syndrome.

The primary role of thoracic imaging in children with immunodeficiencies is the evaluation of pulmonary infections. Plain radiographs remain the most frequently obtained imaging study. CT scanning is both more sensitive (Padley et al. 1995) and specific (Mathieson et al. 1989) than chest radiographs. Active mycobacterium infection will frequently show a "tree in bud" appearance of infectious material filling and dilating distal bronchioles. Invasive aspergillosis may show a "halo" appearance of ground glass opacity surrounding parenchymal nodules (Seely et al. 1997). Pneumocystis has a broad range of appearances. In a review of adult patients, a patchy distribution of ground glass opacity was most common, followed by cystic spaces and bullae (Kuhlman et al. 1990). Other features included adenopathy and pleural effusions . In an evaluation of 40 interpretations of 13 different biopsy proven diffuse lung diseases, Lynch et al. were able to make a confident diagnosis in 25 cases with CT scanning, compared to five cases on chest radiographs (Lynch et al. 1999). When a specific etiology is needed, CT can be used to guide bronchoscopy and fine needle biopsy in order to increase the yield of these more invasive procedures (Spencer et al. 1996).

14.3.2
Immunodeficiency Syndromes

14.3.2.1
B Cell Disorders

B cells are named for their association with the bursa of Fabricius in chickens. In humans, B cells are associated with the bone marrow. The fetal liver may act as a bursal equivalent in humans. B cell disorders result from a decreased ability to form immunoglobulins and are the most frequent primary immunodeficiencies. IgA deficiency occurs as frequently as 1 in 333 blood donors. Agammaglobulinemia occurs in approximately 1 in 50,000.

14.3.2.1.1
Selective IgA Deficiency

IgA is the immunoglobulin secreted onto epithelial surfaces. It is present in smaller amounts in serum as well. IgA deficiency can be seen in people with no increase in infections. Increased infections are frequently present and are usually limited to the respiratory, gastrointestinal, and genitourinary systems.

14.3.2.1.2
X-Linked (Bruton) Agammaglobulinemia

Infants with X-linked agammaglobulinemia present clinically after maternally transmitted IgG antibodies decrease in the second half of the first year of life. Without IgG therapy, recurrent bacterial infections occur. Organisms include streptococci, pneumococci, *H. influenza*, and mycoplasma. Hepatitis and enterovirus infections are increased, while other viral infections are usually handled normally. *Pneumocystis carinii* and fungal infections are rare. The adenoids, tonsils, and lymph nodes are usually small. The lateral airway radiograph can be very helpful in suggesting this diagnosis when adenoid tissue is absent. Beware the patient who has had an adenoidectomy, of course.

14.3.2.1.3
Common Variable Immunodeficiency

Common variable immunodeficiency is usually less severe than agammaglobulinemia, but otherwise similar in clinical manifestations. The tonsils, adenoids, and lymph nodes are normal in size. Splenomegaly is seen in about 25% of cases. Lymphadenopathy is common.

14.3.2.2
T Cell Disorders

T lymphocytes are named for their association with the thymus. T cells function in the initial response to antigen and in limiting the potentially harmful immune response. T cells are responsible for delayed hypersensitivity reactions and for graft rejection as well as infection fighting. Children with T cell disorders have more severe problems with infection than infants with B cell disorders.

Children with T cell disorders are susceptible to infections with acid fast bacilli, fungi, viruses, and *Pneumocystis carinii* (Fig. 14.4).

14.3.2.2.1
Thymic Hypoplasia (DiGeorge's Syndrome)

The combination of thymic absence, hypocalcemia, and immune deficiency form DiGeorge's syndrome. The thymus and parathyroid glands are usually hypoplastic rather than absent. Presentation in the neonatal period is more often due to hypocalcemia induced seizures than to immunodeficiency. The later

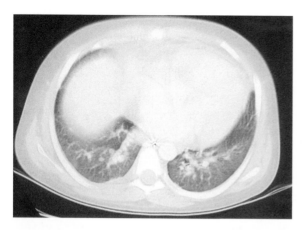

Fig. 14.4. A 9-year-old with T-cell deficiency. Computed tomography demonstrates multiple bilateral basilar nodules due to aspergillus infection

clinical course is similar to children with severe combined immunodeficiency (SCID).

14.3.2.2.2
X-Linked Immunodeficiency with Hyper IgM

These children are identified by an elevated IgM and decreased IgG and IgA in serum. While this would suggest a B cell defect, the B cells in these children can form normal immunoglobulins when they are tested with normal T cells. Immunohistochemical staining shows normal numbers of circulating B cells. Presentation is similar to agammaglobulinemia.

14.3.2.3
B and T Cell Combined Disease

14.3.2.3.1
Severe Combined Immunodeficiency

This is the most severe of the immunodeficiencies with absent T and B cell function. Without bone marrow transplantation, survival beyond the second year of life is rare. A number of different genetic defects underlie SCID including autosomal recessive and X-linked forms. SCID is rare, occurring in less than 1:100,000 live births.

The role of radiology of the thorax in these children is in the evaluation of the recurrent infections that are the primary cause of mortality (Fig. 14.5). While these patients have a small thymus, imaging is not usually helpful in suggesting this diagnosis prior to the onset of infections.

14.3.2.3.2
Combined Immunodeficiency (Nezelof's Syndrome)

In these patients, antibody formation is decreased but not absent. Neutropenia is common. Immunoglobulins are usually increased. Chronic pulmonary infections, chronic diarrhea, and failure to thrive are common. This syndrome can be confused with pediatric AIDS.

14.3.2.3.3
Wiskott-Aldrich Syndrome

This syndrome consists of recurrent infections, eczema, and thrombocytopenia. Infections due to organisms with polysaccharide capsules including pneumococcus are common. Herpes virus infections and skin superinfections occur. *Pneumocystis carinii* and pneumococcus are common causes of pulmonary infection in these children.

14.3.3
Chronic Granulomatous Disease

Children with chronic granulomatous disease (CGD) have a phagocyte defect that interferes with microorganism killing. The phagocytes are otherwise normal, but after engulfing a microorganism, the superoxide burst necessary for killing does not occur. CGD occurs in both X-linked and autosomal forms.

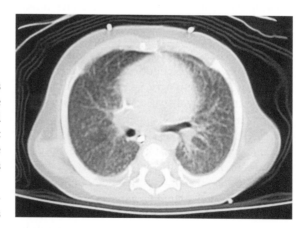

Fig. 14.5. An 8-month-old boy with severe combined immunodeficiency syndrome and cytomegalovirus pneumonia. High-resolution computed tomography shows diffuse ground glass attenuation with fine nodules throughout the lungs

Symptoms usually develop in the first 2 years of life. Presentation and ongoing complications are related to granuloma and abscess formation (Fig. 14.6). Suppurative lymphadenopathy is common, as are chronic skin infections. These manifestations are likely due to ongoing inflammatory response to viable microorganisms. Histopathologic studies have shown that the granulomas in these patients may contain relatively few organisms with the largest component caused by an exuberent inflammatory response (Mos-KALUK et al. 1994).

Staphylococcus aureus is the most commonly cultured organism, with enteric bacilli frequently isolated. Streptococcal disease is relatively rare in these patients (JOHNSTON and McMURRY 1967). Fungi and atypical mycobacteria are other causes of infection.

Thoracic manifestations are most commonly pneumonias and abscesses. The lungs are the most common site of infection (MOSKALUK et al. 1994). Infections involving both the lungs and the chest wall may suggest the diagnosis (Fig. 14.6). The chronicity of lung lesions in this disease may lead to development of a systemic blood supply to areas of pulmonary infection, also referred to as pseudosequestration (MATSUZONO et al. 1995).

14.3.4
Sickle Cell Disease

The sickle hemoglobinopathies all include the presence of hemoglobin S within red blood cells. A substitution of valine for glutamic acid in the hemoglobin beta chain changes the structure of hemoglobin allowing the hemoglobin to crystalize under conditions of low oxygen state, dehydration, and acidosis. When the hemoglobin crystalizes, the red blood cell becomes less flexible and assumes the familiar sickle shape. These sickle cells have a decreased life span with a resulting hemolytic anemia. These nondeformable cells often obstruct small capillaries where slow flow increases the changes that encourage further sickling in a cascade effect.

Homozygous hemoglobin (Hgb) S produces the most severe disease. Different mutations are associated with different amounts of hemoglobin F. Higher levels of Hgb F are associated with decreased disease severity. Compound heterozygous conditions present a spectrum of disease severity depending on the non-S hemoglobin. The most common are hemoglobin S with hemoglobin C (Hgb S/C) and hemoglobin S with b hemoglobin thalassemia (Hgb S/B). Hemo-

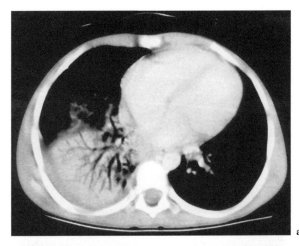

a

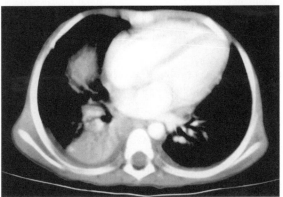

b

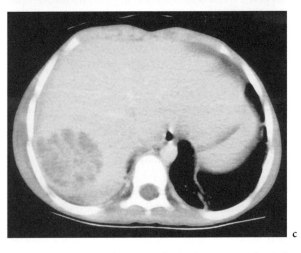

c

Fig. 14.6a–c. Computed tomography (CT) images performed on a boy with chronic granulomatous disease. At age 3 years, a CT scan (**a**) showed right middle lobe pneumonia with effusion and calcification. At age 5 years, CT again shows a right middle lobe pneumonia (**b**), with an hepatic abscess (**c**). Drainage procedure demonstrated a *Staphylococcus aureus* infection extending through the diaphragm

globin S with homozygous b thalassemia is similar to HgbSS, while S plus heterozygous b thalassemia and Hgb SC disease will often have preserved splenic function and less risk of occlusive crisis and infection. Heterozygous hemoglobin S and hemoglobin A is the asymptomatic carrier state.

Infants show no abnormalities, with symptoms developing as fetal hemoglobin is replaced by defective adult type hemoglobin. Early presentation is commonly with hand-foot syndrome, a painful swelling of the hands and feet. Soft tissue swelling and periosteal new bone formation are seen radiographically. Anemia and painful crises in other locations then develop. Decreased splenic function causes an increased susceptibility to infection. The most common organisms affecting the lung are pneumococcus and nontypable hemophilus species.

The two most common chest complications of sickle cell disease are pneumonia and the acute chest syndrome. Functional asplenia can occur as young as 6 months of age. Children are then particularly susceptible to infections caused by bacteria with polysaccharide capsules. Pneumococcal infections are the most common cause of death in young children with sickle cell disease.

The most common thoracic findings in children with sickle cell disease are mild cardiomegaly and increased lung markings. Biconcave vertebral bodies develop due to endplate microinfarcts resulting in softening of the bone that is then impressed by the nucleus pulposus of the intervertebral disk.

Lung function can be abnormal from an early age. Evidence of obstructive pulmonary disease has been shown on pulmonary function tests in infants and young children (KOUMBOURLIS et al. 1997). The presence of myocardial perfusion abnormalities in children has also been reported (ACAR et al. 2000).

The acute chest syndrome (ACS) is a major cause of morbidity and mortality in sickle cell disease This is a largely descriptive term applied to the clinical situation where the patient with sickle cell disease develops a new infiltrate on chest radiograph accompanied by chest pain, fever, and respiratory symptoms. ACS accounts for 30% of deaths in sickle cell patients under 10 years old (MARTIN and BUONOMO 1997). In a prospective study of 538 patients admitted for ACS, overall mortality was 3% (VICHINSKY et al. 2000). A specific cause can be identified in ACS in 40%–70% of cases. Etiologies include infection, fat embolism, and pulmonary infarction (VICHINSKY et al. 2000). Rib infarctions have also been identified in ACS (GELFAND et al. 1993) (Fig. 14.7).

The infiltrates of ACS must occupy at least one complete bronchopulmonary segment without evidence of volume loss. The appearance of the individual infiltrates is not helpful in suggesting an etiology. Longitudinal evaluation may be of benefit. A lack of resolution of parenchymal infiltrates was associated with the presence of an infectious etiology and longer clinical course (MARTIN and BUONOMO 1997). The presence of infiltrates in four or more lobes on the admission chest radiograph was associated with an incidence of complications nine times that of involvement in one lobe (VICHINSKY et al. 2000). Increasing infiltrates over the first days of hospitalization are also associated with an increase in complications and prolonged hospitalization.

CT has also been studied in ACS. Using 3-mm thick sections, BHALLA et al. found evidence of decreased peripheral pulmonary vessels in children with ACS (BHALLA et al. 1993). This decrease was not seen in children without sickle cell disease whose CT scans were used as controls. These findings suggest that there is a component of microvascular occlusion in these children.

14.3.5
Langerhan's Cell Histiocytosis

Langerhan's cell histiocytosis (LCH) is characterized by tissue infiltration by cells of bone marrow origin with characteristic large histiocytes. These cells are monocytes that can be identified by the presence of Birbeck granules in the cytoplasm or immunohistochemically by CD-1 positivity.

Previous classification into eosinophilic granuloma, Letterer-Siwe disease, and Hand-Schüller-Christian disease are no longer used. The current classification divides these patients into those with single system involvement, and those with multisystem involvement. The presence of multisystem involvement requires more intensive therapy than single system involvement.

In a review of 42 children with LCH, eight had pulmonary abnormalities on chest radiographs. In this study, all those with pulmonary abnormalities had multisystem disease (SMETS et al. 1997). Four had lung lesions at the time of diagnosis and six of the eight were symptomatic. One presented with bilateral pneumothoraces.

All children showed interstitial changes, predominantly reticulonodular densities. Follow up CT scans were performed in four of the eight, and revealed

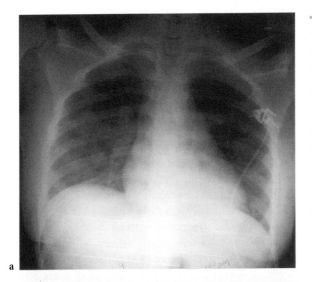

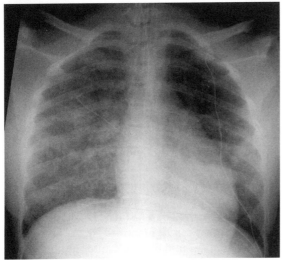

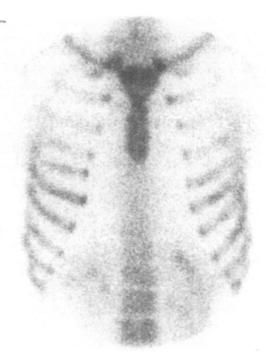

Fig. 14.7a–c. Acute chest syndrome in a 17-year-old young woman with sickle cell/b thalassemia. The patient was admitted with a painful crisis. Initial chest radiograph showed clear lungs. On the second day of admission the patient complained of chest pain. The patient became increasingly hypoxic and was intubated the next day. She was hospitalized for 3 weeks. a Chest radiograph on the second day of admission demonstrates confluent opacity in the left lower lobe and less well-defined opacity at the right lung base. b Chest radiograph performed on the fourth day of admission demonstrates diffuse, ill-defined, and nodular opacities throughout both lungs. The patient was intubated. c Technetium-99m methylene diphosphanate bone scan shows increased uptake in multiple ribs indicating rib infarcts

nodules, a mediastinal mass, and lung cysts. Two patients developed macronodules up to 4 cm in size associated with increasing disease in other systems. Isolated pulmonary involvement has been reported (CHATKIN et al. 1993). Other unusual findings include mediastinal lymphadenopathy (SHAKER et al. 1995).

The most specific CT findings of LCH are pulmonary cysts (Fig. 14.8). Most reports describe small cysts with thin or imperceptible walls. During active stages of disease, cysts and nodules coexist and cavitating nodules may be seen. Lung involvement by laryngeal papillomatosis and cavitating lung metastases are other causes of this appearance. A highly suggestive feature of LCH cysts in adults is the irregular shapes formed by the cysts, likely due to coalescence of smaller cysts.

14.3.6
Cystic Fibrosis

The lungs of an infant born with cystic fibrosis (CF) are histologically completely normal. Within a few months, the presence of airway inflammation and infection can be identified (KHAN et al. 1995). Bronchiectasis and mucous plugging follow and become the distinctive features of CF lung disease. Born with normal lungs, 95% of people with CF will die of respiratory complications with a mean life expectancy of 31 years. The presence of normal lungs at birth presents the opportunity to eliminate these respiratory complications if an early cure can be found. Even without a cure as yet, the history of CF is one of dramatic advances. This progress is reflected in the fact that the factor best predicting life expectancy in CF is the patient's year of birth.

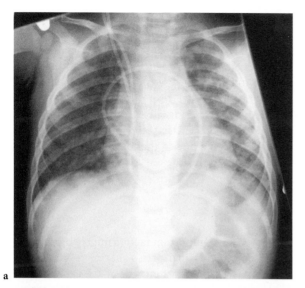

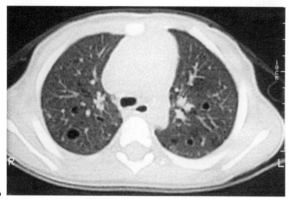

Fig. 14.8a,b. A 1-year-old child who presented with fever and tachypnea. **a** Initial chest radiograph demonstrated bilateral nodular parenchymal opacities. These opacities resolved over several weeks. Biopsy of a bone lesion revealed Langerhan's cell histiocytosis. **b** High-resolution computed tomography performed 3 months later demonstrates multiple bilateral small cysts with thin walls

Children with CF are a more heterogeneous group than originally described. Pulmonary and pancreatic disease are the primary abnormalities in CF, but 15% of patients have adequate pancreatic function. The severity of lung disease in CF is also more variable than often appreciated. The range of disease in patients with homozygous delta508 mutations ranges from the development of bronchiectasis in the first few years of life to a 20-year-old patient with normal pulmonary function tests and chest radiograph. Complete bilateral absence of the vas deferens (CBAVD) is the mildest form of the CF spectrum. At the present time genotype predicts phenotype in pancreatic sufficiency, but not the severity or pattern of respiratory disease.

14.3.6.1
Genetics

CF is an autosomal recessive disease that affects approximately 1 in 4000 live births in the United States. CF occurs most commonly in Caucasians where the incidence is 1 in 2500 live births, with progressively lower frequency in black, Hispanic, and Asian populations. The gene for CF is located on the long arm of chromosome 7. The CF gene encodes the CF transmembrane conductance regulator (CFTR). CFTR is a single chain protein that forms a membrane bound regulated chloride channel activated by cyclic adenosine monophosphate (cAMP). CFTR functions primarily at the apical cell membrane where it regulates fluid balance across the cell membrane with effects on both chloride and sodium. The most common mutation is a three base pair deletion that causes a deletion of phenylalanine at position 508 of the protein product. This delta508 mutation is present in 90% of those with CF (FOUNDATION 2000). Homozygous delta508 is responsible for 70% of cases of CF (FOUNDATION 2000). Nearly 1000 additional mutations of the CF gene have been identified.

14.3.6.2
Diagnosing CF

Of the children with CF, 70% present within the first year, 80% by 4 years, and 90% by the age of 12 years. The mean age at diagnosis of all patients with CF listed in the Cystic Fibrosis Patient Registry in 1999 was 3 years with a median age of 6 months (FOUNDATION 2000). In the first year, gastrointestinal findings are more common than respiratory disease. In North America, nearly all Caucasian infants with meconium ileus have CF. In a series of 1175 infants with CF, 13% presented with meconium ileus. In 1999 19% of infants diagnosed with CF had meconium ileus (FOUNDATION 2000). Gastrointestinal findings after the neonatal period and within the first year include malabsorbtion and failure to thrive. CF should be suspected in children with these symptoms without regard to the presence of pulmonary disease.

After the first year, respiratory complaints increase, becoming the most common reason to suspect CF. By the age of 6 years, pulmonary function tests show an effect on lung function with mean forced expiratory volume in 1 s approximately 70% of expected, and forced vital capacity approximately 80% of expected (FITZSIMMONS 1993).

One of the earliest characteristics of the child with CF was the salty taste of the child's skin. Abnormal sweat chloride was reported in 1953 (DI SANT'AGNESE et al. 1953). Sweat chloride determination remains the most common diagnostic test for CF. This test requires careful technique and should only be performed at centers expert in sweat chloride determination. Greater than 60 mEq/ml is generally regarded as positive, 40–60 mEq/ml indeterminate, and less than 40 mEq/ml negative. Other methods of making the diagnosis include genotyping and neonatal screening.

In 1999, 7% of children diagnosed with CF were identified by neonatal screening (FOUNDATION 2000). Neonatal screening is performed by measuring the level of immunoreactive trypsinogen in a dried blood spot. Positive screening tests must be confirmed by further tests including meconium lactase, sweat chloride, or genotyping. A controlled trial of neonatal screening in Wisconsin has shown improved growth and nutritional status in children with CF identified by neonatal screening (FARRELL et al. 2001). A study in Australia demonstrated improvement in both nutrition and pulmonary function (WATERS et al. 1999).

A report by MASSIE et al. (2000) found that in a screened population CF is still detected on clinical grounds. In this group, gastrointestinal symptoms remain more common at presentation than pulmonary symptoms. Of nine children diagnosed with CF after negative neonatal screening, eight presented with failure to thrive or steatorrhea, and one with respiratory symptoms.

14.3.6.3
Pulmonary Pathophysiology of CF

Abnormal CFTR causes a change in the composition of the fluid lining the airways which results in numerous changes in the normal function of the airway epithelium. Mucous is abnormal with resulting plugging of airways and decreased mucocilliary clearance. Abnormal mucous in CF likely results both from abnormal mucous produced by the mucous glands, and the presence of cellular degradation products from white blood cells. Deoxyribonucleic acid is a major component of the degradation products, and is a major contributor to the increased viscosity and tendency of the mucous to form long strands. Both infection and inflammation result in increased proteolytic enzymes that damage the epithelium and the supporting structure of the airways.

Repeated infection and increased inflammatory response cause airway damage which makes the airways more susceptible to infection. Infection then increases in both frequency and severity, inciting greater inflammatory response. A snowball effect results in progressive respiratory compromise. The hallmarks of CF lung disease are bronchiectasis secondary to obstruction and airway damage and mucous plugging due to the tenacious mucous produced in CF.

14.3.6.4
Lung Care in CF

One of the most important factors improving longevity in CF patients in North America is the use of skilled care through a network of CF centers. Two important concepts of care are routine monitoring and early intervention. Pulmonary exacerbations are treated with aggressive pulmonary physiotherapy and parenteral antibiotics.

Regular pulmonary care in CF has also traditionally been directed at the clearance of lower airway secretions and the treatment of infection. In the last decade, numerous new techniques have become available. In addition to manual external percussion, mechanical airway clearance techniques include airway oscillators and high frequency chest compression with an inflatable vest. The tenacity of secretions can be treated by the administration of recombinant human deoxyribonuclease which breaks up DNA strands, decreasing the stickiness of CF mucous (Fig. 14.9). Inhaled bronchodilators and hypertonic salines can be administered.

In addition to oral antibiotics, inhaled antibiotics have been shown to improve pulmonary function in initial short term trials (RAMSEY et al. 1999). Airway inflammation can also be directly treated. In a 4-year study, KONSTAN and colleagues have shown that inhaled ibuprofen decreased the decline of pulmonary function in CF. This effect was most marked in children (KONSTAN et al. 1995).

For many patients, the progression of lung disease results in respiratory insufficiency that persists despite medical treatment. Lung transplantation is the treatment for end stage CF pulmonary disease. Both cadaveric transplantation and living donor lobe transplantation are used. In the 1999 CF registry, 114 bilateral lung transplant recipients and 27 lobe transplant recipients are listed.

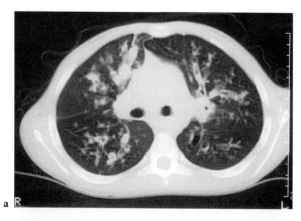

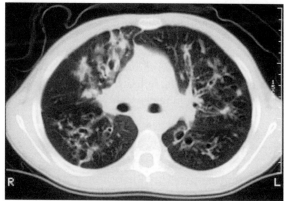

Fig. 14.9a,b. High-resolution computed tomography images in an 11-year-old boy with cystic fibrosis showing improvement in mucous plugging following treatment with human recombinant DNase. a Images obtained prior to beginning daily inhalation therapy with DNase show bronchiectasis, bronchial wall thickening, and multiple areas of mucoid impaction seen as large tubular structures. b Images obtained after several months of daily DNase therapy. Mucous has cleared from many of the ectatic bronchi

14.3.6.5
Imaging in Cystic Fibrosis

The role of imaging in the care of children with CF is changing. Historically, care has been based on clinical evaluation, with plain radiographs used to confirm clinical impressions, and as an indicator of overall disease severity. Plain radiographs remain the most common imaging study performed in patients with CF. CF center directors report that CT is frequently obtained, although little has been written on the use of CT in the care of patients with CF. Nuclear medicine evaluation has been reported primarily as a research tool. A preliminary study of an experimental MRI technique providing both airway and parenchymal evaluation has been published.

14.3.6.5.1
Plain Radiographs

Children with CF are born with normal lungs, but rapidly develop a cycle of infection and inflammation that causes airways disease and eventually parenchymal damage. Radiographs in the first year are usually normal. Abnormal chest radiographs will show changes typical of airways disease. The appearance is the same as seen with viral or atypical infections. Features more typical of CF including bronchiectasis and mucous plugging are not seen in the first several years.

Scoring systems for the evaluation of lung disease on chest radiographs include the Chrispin-Norman (CHRISPIN and NORMAN 1974; BRASFIELD et al. 1979, 1980) and NIH (SOCKRIDER et al. 1994) scores. Comparison between the Brasfield and NIH scores found that the behavior of the two systems is similar (SAWYER et al. 1994). While these scores correlate with disease severity in older patients, they are insensitive when used in young children (WEATHERLY et al. 1993). A new chest radiograph scoring system was specifically developed for use in young children with CF (WEATHERLY et al. 1993). Despite continued development of this system since 1993, early chest radiographs do not correlate well with clinical changes in young children with mild disease (KOSCIK et al. 2000).

No pediatric study has been performed to evaluate the ability of plain radiographs to reflect changes due to treatment. In an adult study, GREENE and colleagues (GREENE et al. 1994) found that chest radiographs obtained during an acute exacerbation could not be differentiated from radiographs obtained when the patients were clinically well.

14.3.6.5.2
Computed Tomography

Currently, HRCT is the most accurate means of evaluating the morphologic changes of CF lung disease. HRCT can detect and quantify the changes seen in children with CF including bronchiectasis, peribronchial thickening, mucous plugging, parenchymal air trapping, and lung destruction.

In 1986, JACOBSEN et al. compared chest radiographs and CT in 12 adult patients with CF. The authors found that CT was more sensitive for the detection of bronchiectasis, mucous plugging, and hilar adenopathy (JACOBSEN et al. 1986). In 1990, BHALLA et al. described a scoring system for HRCT in CF (BHALLA et al. 1991). This scoring system evaluates the severity of bronchiectasis and peribronchial thickening, and the extent of bronchiectasis, mucous plugging, sacculations or abscesses, bullae, emphysema, and collapse or consolidation. The authors found again that CT was more accurate than chest radiographs in detecting abnormalities. The score correlated with the pulmonary function test ration of forced expiratory volume in 1 min to forced vital capacity (FEV1/FVC). In the same year, NATHANSON published a scoring system for CF using electron beam CT in a pediatric population. This scoring system correlated well with pulmonary function tests and clinical scores (NATHANSON et al. 1991). A scoring system devised by MAFESSANTI and colleagues (MAFFESSANTI et al. 1996) has been adopted and used by several authors.

More recent efforts have evaluated the ability of HRCT to evaluate progression of disease and response to treatment. An adult study showed that the findings differed when HRCTs obtained during exacerbations were compared to those obtained when patients were at their baseline health. HRCT scores were higher during exacerbations. Air fluid levels in ectatic bronchi during exacerbation resolved on follow-up scans. Centrilobular nodules and mucous plugging improved in about one third of the cases (SHAH et al. 1997).

In a pediatric study, the HRCT appearance was compared between admission and discharge for treatment of an acute pulmonary exacerbation (BRODY et al. 1999). In this study, the HRCT appearance improved in 13 of 15 admissions. Peribronchial thickening, mucous plugging, and the overall appearance were all significantly improved on the discharge HRCT.

A study that included patients aged between 2 and 32 years evaluated the change in HRCT appearance over time. The authors found that HRCT scores increased significantly when the interval between studies was more than 18 months, with no significant change over shorter intervals (HELBICH et al. 1999).

The above information provides support for the continued development of HRCT as part of the clinical care of children with CF. At the time of writing, however, no studies had evaluated the impact of using HRCT as part of the care of these children. One report has pointed out that useful patient care information can be obtained with a combination of pulmonary function tests and chest radiographs, as well as with HRCT (SANTAMARIA et al. 1998).

14.3.6.5.3
Nuclear Medicine

The functional information provided by nuclear medicine imaging has been used to evaluate pulmonary ventilation/perfusion relationships, aerosol deposition, and mucous clearance in patients with CF (LAUBE et al. 1992; SIRR et al. 1986). The findings of nuclear medicine pulmonary blood flow have been shown to correlate with HRCT images (DONNELLY et al. 1997). The relative sensitivities of the two modalities have not been determined.

These studies have been primarily used in a research context, with lung scanning used clinically in some cases of pretransplant lung evaluation to determine relative lung function and to identify areas of nonfunctioning lung.

14.3.6.5.4
Magnetic Resonance Imaging

Several studies of MRI in CF have been published. One early study demonstrated the ability of MRI to detect hilar adenopathy and bronchiectasis with mucous plugging. Bronchiectasis with bronchial wall thickening could also be detected (FIEL et al. 1987). A study in 1994 compared conventional axial CT to MRI and found that the resolution of MRI did not allow adequate evaluation of the gross features of CF lung disease (CARR et al. 1995). The lack of adequate signal from the lung parenchyma does not allow conventional MRI to evaluate parenchymal abnormalities.

A new MR technique is the use of hyperpolarized helium-3. This gas has a very strong MR signal. When inhaled, all ventilated portions of the lung show this high signal. Unperfused areas are seen as focal defects. The appearance is grossly similar to nuclear medicine ventilation scans, but with much higher resolution (Fig. 14.10). No ionizing radiation is used. Hyperpolarized helium-3 has a short half-life. The availability of the gas will likely limit the use of this technique.

A preliminary report using helium-3 and conventional proton MR in four patients with CF (DONNELLY et al. 1999) found extensive ventilation defects that were frequently much more striking than associated morphologic defects. The small number did not allow statistical analysis but MR scores were higher in patients with higher Brasfield chest radiograph scores. MR scores were also higher in patients with

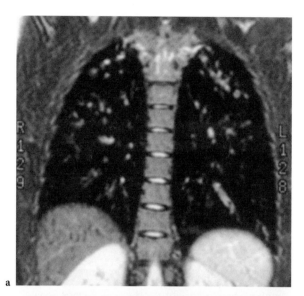

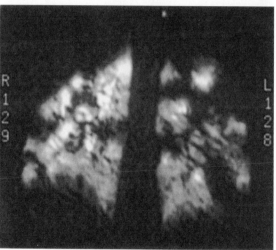

Fig. 14.10a,b. Coronal 10-mm thick magnetic resonance (MR) images of the posterior lungs in a patient with cystic fibrosis. **a** Fast spin echo T2-weighted MR images demonstrate nodular and linear areas of increased signal greatest at the lung apices corresponding to mucous filled ectatic bronchi. **b** Helium-3 MR images demonstrate multiple filling defects in the high signal due to the inhaled helium-3 indicating areas of absent or decreased ventilation. These defects are much greater than the airway abnormalities seen on the conventional MR image. (Images courtesy of LANE F. DONNELLY, MD)

lower FEV1. This is a new area of investigation that may well provide a new and valuable outcome surrogate for CF.

14.3.7
Phacomatoses

14.3.7.1
Tuberous Sclerosis

Tuberous sclerosis (TS) is one of the neurocutaneous syndromes that include neurofibromatosis and Sturge-Weber syndrome. TS is a genetic disease with autosomal dominant transmission and variable penetration. The incidence is approximately 1:30,000.

The classic clinical triad includes mental retardation, seizures, and adenoma sebaceum. The characteristic rash has been described as a butterfly rash over the cheeks with a narrower affected area on the nose. TS, however, affects multiple organ systems. In addition to the central nervous system abnormalities, abnormal cellular proliferation results in angiomyolipomas of the kidneys, rhabdomyomas of the heart, and lymphangioleiomyomatosis (LAM) of the lungs.

LAM affects women of reproductive age, with most patients presenting in the third decade; however, children as young as 11 years old have been diagnosed with LAM. Clinical presentation is with dyspnea or spontaneous pneumothorax. LAM is not seen on chest radiographs until extensive fibrosis has developed late in the course of the disease. The early appearance of LAM is characterized by the presence of multiple small cysts with thin or imperceptible walls. These cysts are evenly distributed through the lungs. Unlike the cysts of LCH, cysts in LAM are round and do not usually coalesce. Useful in differentiating these cysts from other causes of destructive lung disease is the presence of normal lung parenchyma between the cysts.

The reported incidence of LAM in TS is less than 1%. We have recently completed a prospective HRCT screening study of young women with TS. In our group, the incidence of lung cysts was 30%. This higher incidence likely reflects a high incidence of mild findings that will not present clinically or be apparent on chest radiographs (Fig. 14.11).

The incidence of cardiac rhabdomyomas in TS is 20%–30%. Half of all cardiac rhabdomyomas are found in patients with TS. This is the most common cardiac tumor of childhood (BECKER 2000). Cardiac

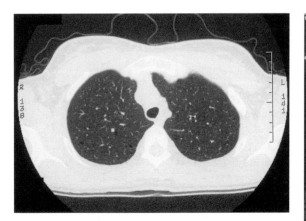

Fig. 14.11. High-resolution computed tomography image through the upper lungs in an asymptomatic young adult woman with tuberous sclerosis. Multiple cysts of less than 1 cm with imperceptible walls are seen in the right lung. These likely represent early changes of lymphangioleiomyomatosis

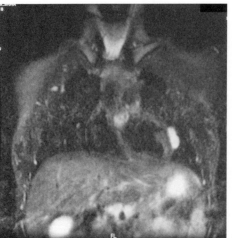

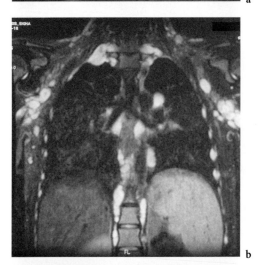

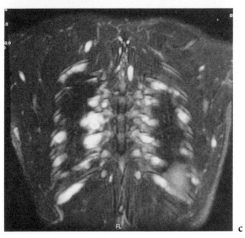

rhabdomyomas usually present in the first year. Obstruction of blood flow, reduced overall contractility, and interference with electrical conduction can all cause symptoms. Clinical presentations include prenatal demise and sudden death. The most common presentations are cardiac, including congestive heart failure and arrhythmias. Asymptomatic tumors have been found on screening echocardiography. Regression of these tumors has also been reported (SALLEE et al. 1999). Cardiac rhabdomyomas are frequently multiple, and are usually located in the ventricles.

Rhabdomyomas are most often detected on echocardiography. MRI is usually performed to further evaluate these masses. The MRI appearance is variable with most lesions showing increased signal compared to the myocardium on short TR/short TE images (LUND et al. 1989). Rhabdomyomas may be isointense on multiple pulse sequences, as well as before and after contrast administration (SEMELKA et al. 1992). For this reason, small, intramural lesions may not be detected on MRI. Cardiac lipomas and fibromas are less common than rhabdomyomas, but can be seen in children with TS. The characteristic signal patterns of fat and fibrosis may suggest the presence of one of these lesions when assessing cardiac masses in TS.

14.3.7.2
Neurofibromatosis

Neurofibromatosis is the most common of the phacomatoses with a prevalence of 1 in 2–4000. Neurofi-

Fig. 14.12a–c. A 17-year-old girl with neurofibromatosis type 1. Coronal magnetic resonance images (fast spin echo T2 with fat saturation) through the anterior (**a**), middle (**b**), and posterior (**c**) chest show multiple high signal neurofibromas throughout the mediastinum, chest wall, and arising from the pericardium

bromatosis is transmitted as an autosomal dominant, but one half of cases arise from a new mutation. Two distinct forms of neurofibromatosis are designated NF-1 and NF-2. NF-1 accounts for 90% of cases of neurofibromatosis and can present in many different ways including café-au-lait spots, axillary or inguinal freckling, Lisch nodules of the iris, neurofibromas, bone lesions, and optic gliomas. NF-2 is associated with bilateral acoustic neuromas.

Thoracic manifestations in children include neurofibromas, rib erosions, scoliosis, and spinal erosions (Fig. 14.12). Spinal erosions can occur secondary to dural ectasia, neurofibromas, or lateral meningoceles. Lateral meningoceles and neurofibromas can be differentiated on CT scanning by administering intravenous contrast, with neurofibromas showing enhancement (ROSSI et al. 1999). On MRI, a characteristic target appearance can be seen on T2-weighted sequences with a low signal center and very high signal peripherally. Contrast-enhanced T1-weighted sequences can also be used to distinguish meningoceles from neurofibromas.

Pulmonary manifestations in adults include pulmonary fibrosis and bulla formation (WEBB and GOODMAN 1977; BURKHALTER et al. 1986). Neither of these findings has been reported in children. The presence of interstitial abnormalities in children has been mentioned anecdotally by several observers. It is possible that the adult disease begins in the first two decades, but does not become symptomatic or evident on chest radiographs until later.

References

Acar P, Sebahoun S, de Pontual L et al (2000) Myocardial perfusion in children with sickle cell anaemia. Pediatr Radiol 30(5):352–354

Arkachaisri T, Lehman TJ (1999) Systemic lupus erythematosus and related disorders of childhood. Curr Opin Rheumatol 11(5):384–392

Athreya BH, Doughty RA, Bookspan M et al (1980) Pulmonary manifestations of juvenile rheumatoid arthritis. A report of eight cases and review. Clin Chest Med 1(3):361–374

Bankier AA, Kiener HP, Wiesmayr MN et al (1995) Discrete lung involvement in systemic lupus erythematosus: CT assessment. Radiology 196(3):835–840

Becker AE (2000) Primary heart tumors in the pediatric age group: a review of salient pathologic features relevant for clinicians. Pediatr Cardiol 21(4):317–323

Bhalla M, Turcios N, Aponte V et al (1991) Cystic fibrosis: scoring system with thin-section CT. Radiology 179(3):783–788

Bhalla M, Abboud MR, McLoud TC et al (1993) Acute chest syndrome in sickle cell disease: CT evidence of microvascular occlusion. Radiology 187(1):45–49

Brasfield D, Hicks G, Soong S et al (1979) The chest roentgenogram in cystic fibrosis: a new scoring system. Pediatrics 63(1):24–29

Brasfield D, Hicks G, Soong S et al (1980) Evaluation of scoring system of the chest radiograph in cystic fibrosis: a collaborative study. AJR Am J Roentgenol 134(6):1195–1198

Brody AS, Molina PL, Klein JS et al (1999) High-resolution computed tomography of the chest in children with cystic fibrosis: support for use as an outcome surrogate. Pediatr Radiol 29(10):731–735

Burkhalter JL, Morano JU, McCay MB et al (1986) Diffuse interstitial lung disease in neurofibromatosis. South Med J 79(8):944–946

Carr DH, Oades P, Trotman-Dickenson B et al (1995) Magnetic resonance scanning in cystic fibrosis: comparison with computed tomography. Clin Radiol 50(2):84–89

Cerveri I, Bruschi C, Ravelli A et al (1992) Pulmonary function in childhood connective tissue diseases. Eur Respir J 5(6):733–738

Chatkin JM, Bastos JC, Stein RT et al (1993) Sole pulmonary involvement by Langerhans' cell histiocytosis in a child. Eur Respir J 6(8):1226–1228

Chrispin AR, Norman AP (1974) The systematic evaluation of the chest radiograph in cystic fibrosis. Pediatr Radiol 2:101–106

di Sant'Agnese PA, Darling RC, Perera GA et al (1953) Sweat electrolyte disturbance associated with childhood pancreatic disease. Am J Med 15:777–784

Donnelly LF, Gelfand MJ, Brody AS et al (1997) Comparison between morphologic changes seen on high-resolution CT and regional pulmonary perfusion seen on SPECT in patients with cystic fibrosis. Pediatr Radiol 27(12):920–925

Donnelly LF, MacFall JR, McAdams HP et al (1999) Cystic fibrosis: combined hyperpolarized 3He-enhanced and conventional proton MR imaging in the lung–preliminary observations. Radiology 212(3):885–889

Farrell PM, Kosorok MR, Rock MJ et al (2001) Early diagnosis of cystic fibrosis through neonatal screening prevents sever malnutrition and improves long-term growth. Pediatrics 107:1–13

Fiel SB, Friedman AC, Caroline DF et al (1987) Magnetic resonance imaging in young adults with cystic fibrosis. Chest 91(2):181–184

FitzSimmons SC (1993) The changing epidemiology of cystic fibrosis (see comments). J Pediatr 122(1):1–9

Foundation CF (2000) Annual data report. Cystic Fibrosis Foundation patient registry. Cystic Fibrosis Foundation, Bethesda, pp 1–22

Gelfand MJ, Daya SA, Rucknagel DL et al (1993) Simultaneous occurrence of rib infarction and pulmonary infiltrates in sickle cell disease patients with acute chest syndrome. J Nucl Med 34(4):614–618

Greene KE, Takasugi JE, Godwin JD et al (1994) Radiographic changes in acute exacerbations of cystic fibrosis in adults: a pilot study. AJR Am J Roentgenol 163(3):557–562

Hatabu H, Gaa J, Tadamura E et al (1999) MR imaging of pulmonary parenchyma with a half-Fourier single-shot turbo spin-echo (HASTE) sequence. Eur J Radiol 29(2):152–159

Helbich TH, Heinz-Peer G, Fleischmann D et al (1999) Evolution of CT findings in patients with cystic fibrosis. AJR Am J Roentgenol 173(1):81–88

Hsu BY, Edwards DK, Trambert MA et al (1992) Pulmonary

hemorrhage complicating systemic lupus erythematosus: role of MR imaging in diagnosis. AJR Am J Roentgenol 158(3):519–520

Jacobsen LE, Houston CS, Habbick BF et al (1986) Cystic fibrosis: a comparison of computed tomography and plain chest radiographs. Can Assoc Radiol J 37(1):17–21

Johnston RB, Jr., McMurry JS (1967) Chronic familial granulomatosis. Report of five cases and review of the literature. Am J Dis Child 114(4):370–378

Jones AM, Gaspar HB (2000) Immunogenetics: changing the face of immunodeficiency. J Clin Pathol 53(1):60–65

Kapala GB, Chusid MJ, Sty JR et al (1983) Ga-67 chest imaging. Chronic granulomatous disease. Clin Nucl Med 8(12):632

Khan TZ, Wagener JS, Bost T et al (1995) Early pulmonary inflammation in infants with cystic fibrosis (see comments). Am J Respir Crit Care Med 151(4):1075–1082

Kido S, Ikezoe J, Kondoh H et al (1996) Detection of subtle interstitial abnormalities of the lungs on digitized chest radiographs: acceptable data compression ratios. AJR Am J Roentgenol 167(1):111–115

Konstan MW, Byard PJ, Hoppel CL et al (1995) Effect of high-dose ibuprofen in patients with cystic fibrosis (see comments). N Engl J Med 332 13:848–854

Koscik RE, Kosorok MR, Farrell PM et al (2000) Wisconsin cystic fibrosis chest radiograph scoring system: validation and standardization for application to longitudinal studies. Pediatr Pulmonol 29(6):457–467

Koumbourlis AC, Hurlet-Jensen A, Bye MR et al (1997) Lung function in infants with sickle cell disease. Pediatr Pulmonol 24(4):277–281

Kuhlman JE, Kavuru M, Fishman EK et al (1990) Pneumocystis carinii pneumonia: spectrum of parenchymal CT findings. Radiology 175(3):711–714

Kuhn JP (1993) High-resolution computed tomography of pediatric pulmonary parenchymal disorders. Radiol Clin North Am 31(3):533–551

Laube BL, Chang DY, Blask AN et al (1992) Radioaerosol assessment of lung improvement in cystic fibrosis patients treated for acute pulmonary exacerbations. Chest 101(5):1302–1308

Leutner CC, Gieseke J, Lutterbey G et al (2000) MR imaging of pneumonia in immunocompromised patients: comparison with helical CT. AJR Am J Roentgenol 175 2:391–397

Long FR, Castile RG, Brody AS et al (1999) Lungs in infants and young children: improved thin-section CT with a noninvasive controlled-ventilation technique – initial experience. Radiology 212(2):588–593

Lovell D, Lindsley C, Langston C et al (1984) Lymphoid interstitial pneumonia in juvenile rheumatoid arthritis. J Pediatr 105(6):947–950

Lucaya J, Piqueras J, Garcia-Peña P et al (2000) Low-dose high-resolution CT of the chest in children and young adults: dose, cooperation, artifact incidence, and image quality. AJR Am J Roentgenol 175(4):985–992

Lund JT, Ehman RL, Julsrud PR et al (1989) Cardiac masses: assessment by MR imaging. AJR Am J Roentgenol 152(3):469–473

Lynch DA, Hay T, Newell JD et al (1999) Pediatric diffuse lung disease: diagnosis and classification using high- resolution CT. AJR Am J Roentgenol 173(3):713–718

Maffessanti M, Candusso M, Brizzi F et al (1996) Cystic fibrosis

in children: HRCT findings and distribution of disease. J Thorac Imaging 11(1):27–38

Martin L, Buonomo C (1997) Acute chest syndrome of sickle cell disease: radiographic and clinical analysis of 70 cases. Pediatr Radiol 27(8):637–641

Massie J, Wilson J, Freezer N et al (2000) Clinical diagnosis of cystic fibrosis in a screened community: 1989–1998 (abstract). Pediatr Pulmonol 20:436

Mathieson JR, Mayo JR, Staples CA et al (1989) Chronic diffuse infiltrative lung disease: comparison of diagnostic accuracy of CT and chest radiography. Radiology 171(1):111–116

Matsuzono Y, Togashi T, Narita N et al (1995) Pulmonary aspergillosis and pseudosequestration of the lung in chronic granulomatous disease. Pediatr Radiol 25(3):201–203

Moskaluk CA, Pogrebniak HW, Pass HI et al (1994) Surgical pathology of the lung in chronic granulomatous disease. Am J Clin Pathol 102(5):684–691

Nathanson I, Conboy K, Murphy S et al (1991) Ultrafast computerized tomography of the chest in cystic fibrosis: a new scoring system. Pediatr Pulmonol 11(1):81–86

Padley S, Gleeson F, Flower CD et al (1995) Review article: current indications for high resolution computed tomography scanning of the lungs. Br J Radiol 68(806):105–109

Ramsey BW, Pepe MS, Quan JM et al (1999) Intermittent administration of inhaled tobramycin in patients with cystic fibrosis. Cystic Fibrosis Inhaled Tobramycin Study Group. N Engl J Med 340(1):23–30

Rogalla P, Stover B, Scheer I et al (1999) Low-dose spiral CT: applicability to paediatric chest imaging. Pediatr Radiol 29(8):565–569

Rossi SE, Erasmus JJ, McAdams HP et al (1999) Thoracic manifestations of neurofibromatosis-I. AJR Am J Roentgenol 173(6):1631–1638

Sallee D, Spector ML, van Heeckeren DW et al (1999) Primary pediatric cardiac tumors: a 17 year experience. Cardiol Young 9(2):155–162

Santamaria F, Grillo G, Guidi G et al (1998) Cystic fibrosis: when should high-resolution computed tomography of the chest Be obtained? Pediatrics 101(5):908–913

Sawyer SM, Carlin JB, DeCampo M et al (1994) Critical evaluation of three chest radiograph scores in cystic fibrosis (see comments). Thorax 49(9):863–866

Schwab EP, Schumacher HR Jr, Freundlich B et al (1993) Pulmonary alveolar hemorrhage in systemic lupus erythematosus. Semin Arthritis Rheum 23(1):8–15

Seely JM, Effmann EL, Muller NL et al (1997) High-resolution CT of pediatric lung disease: imaging findings. AJR Am J Roentgenol 168(5):1269–1275

Semelka RC, Shoenut JP, Wilson ME et al (1992) Cardiac masses: signal intensity features on spin-echo, gradient-echo, gadolinium-enhanced spin-echo, and TurboFLASH images. J Magn Reson Imaging 2(4):415–420

Shah RM, Sexauer W, Ostrum BJ et al (1997) High-resolution CT in the acute exacerbation of cystic fibrosis: evaluation of acute findings, reversibility of those findings, and clinical correlation. AJR Am J Roentgenol 169(2):375–380

Shaker KG, Umali CB, Fraire AE et al (1995) Langerhans' cell histiocytosis of the lung in association with mediastinal lymphadenopathy. Pathol Int 45(10):762–766

Sirr SA, Elliott GR, Regelmann WE et al (1986) Aerosol penetration ratio: a new index of ventilation. J Nucl Med 27(8):1343–1346

Smets A, Mortele K, de Praeter G et al (1997) Pulmonary and mediastinal lesions in children with Langerhans cell histiocytosis. Pediatr Radiol 27(11):873–876

Sockrider MM, Swank PR, Seilheimer DK et al (1994) Measuring clinical status in cystic fibrosis: internal validity and reliability of a modified NIH score. Pediatr Pulmonol 17(2):86–96

Spencer DA, Alton HM, Raafat F et al (1996) Combined percutaneous lung biopsy and high-resolution computed tomography in the diagnosis and management of lung disease in children (see comments). Pediatr Pulmonol 22(2):111–116

Uziel Y, Hen B, Cordoba M et al (1998) Lymphocytic interstitial pneumonitis preceding polyarticular juvenile rheumatoid arthritis. Clin Exp Rheumatol 16(5):617–619

Vichinsky EP, Neumayr LD, Earles AN et al (2000) Causes and outcomes of the acute chest syndrome in sickle cell disease. National Acute Chest Syndrome Study Group (see comments). N Engl J Med 342(25):1855–1865

Wagener JS, Taussig LM, DeBenedetti C et al (1981) Pulmonary function in juvenile rheumatoid arthritis. J Pediatr 99(1):108–110

Waters DL, Wilcken B, Irwing L et al (1999) Clinical outcomes of newborn screening for cystic fibrosis. Arch Dis Child Fetal Neonatal Ed 80(1):F1–F7

Weatherly MR, Palmer CG, Peters ME et al (1993) Wisconsin cystic fibrosis chest radiograph scoring system. Pediatrics 91(2):488–495

Webb WR, Goodman PC (1977) Fibrosing alveolitis in patients with neurofibromatosis. Radiology 122(2):289–293

15 Radiology of the Chest Wall

Georg F. Eich, Christian J. Kellenberger, Ulrich V. Willi

CONTENTS

15.1
Introduction

The chest wall of a child can give rise to a variety of lesions or pseudolesions that can be classified into normal variant, malformation, trauma, infection, and tumor. These lesions pertain to the skin and subcutaneous tissue (superficial layer), muscles and bones of the shoulder girdle and the pectoralis region (intermediate layer), and/or the deep layer, which includes the dorsal spine, the ribs and intercostal spaces, the sternum, several fascial layers, and the parietal pleura. Pathology of the breast and the diaphragm are excluded from this review.

This chapter is structured according to the nosological entities mentioned above. We will discuss alterations in the shape of the chest that may be associated with functional or esthetic problems or that may mimic a tumor. The appropriate imaging technique for assessment of a *deformity* or *variant* is emphasized. Infections of the chest wall can originate from penetrating wounds or hematogenous spread within bone,

Georg F. Eich
Division of Pediatric Radiology, Kantonsspital, 5001 Aarau, Switzerland
Christian J. Kellenberger
Division of Pediatric Radiology, The University Children's Hospital, Steinwiestrasse 75, 8032 Zürich, Switzerland
Ulrich V. Willi
Division of Pediatric Radiology, The University Children's Hospital, Steinwiestrasse 75, 8032 Zürich, Switzerland

joint, or soft tissue. The importance of imaging in defining the exact topography of the focus and its extent is stressed. Chest wall tumors are essentially mesenchymal tumors. Both benign and malignant neoplasms occur. The Ewing sarcoma family of tumors and rhabdomyosarcoma are the most prevalent malignant tumors of the chest wall. The chest may be exposed to *trauma* (accidental or non-accidental). The imaging findings of both types of injuries will be discussed, with particular emphasis on sternoclavicular fractures, which are difficult to diagnose both clinically and with conventional radiology.

15.2
Normal Variant, Congenital Abnormality and Deformity

15.2.1
Anatomic Variants

The normal shape of the chest is fairly symmetrical and narrower in its upper portion than in the lower three fourths. Normal infants have a relatively wide anteroposterior diameter of the chest compared to older children. The *thoracic index* (widest anteroposterior diameter/widest transverse diameter) is about 0.85 in infants compared to 0.72 in older children (Nathanson 1994). The thoracic index is decreased in pectus excavatum and in a child with an idiopathic flat chest. In the latter condition, the chest is flat and wide, normal thoracic kyphosis is reduced, the heart is located slightly to the left, but the sternum is normal in position. The thoracic index is increased in pectus carinatum.

Infants have a prominent double curvature of the clavicle that can simulate a fracture on chest radiographs taken with the child in a rotated position. The sternal end of the clavicle may show marked cupping during the second decade, which should not be misinterpreted as osteoarthritis (Fig. 15.1).

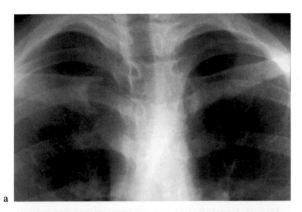

a

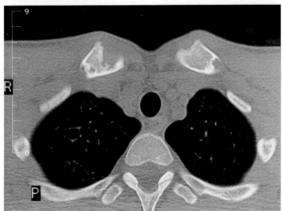

b

Fig. 15.1a, b. Normal variant of clavicles in a 15-year-old boy with fever of unknown origin. **a** Chest X-ray; close-up view of upper median aspect shows irregular sclerosis of right medial clavicular concavity, initially mistaken for osteomyelitis. **b** Axial CT scan through upper chest area at level of medial clavicular ends shows correlating irregular clavicular contours, especially on the right. No local soft tissue swelling. Subsequently, scintigraphy demonstrated osteomyelitis in the right distal femoral metaphysis

Isolated rib anomalies are common incidental findings, usually of no clinical importance, with an estimated frequency of about 2% (COURY and DEL-APORTE 1954). Such anomalies include partial aplasia or agenesis of ribs, bridging between two adjacent ribs by synostosis or pseudoarticulation, bifid ribs, and supernumerary ribs. Unilateral or bilateral cervical ribs may arise from the seventh cervical vertebra and can sometimes cause a thoracic outlet syndrome by compression of the brachial plexus or the subclavian artery. Intrathoracic rib is a rare anomaly that can be seen on chest radiographs (see Chap. 3, Fig. 3.19) (KAMARUDDIN et al. 1995). Eleven pairs of ribs occur in isolation or as a manifestation of various syndromes like trisomy 18, Down's syndrome, and

cleidocranial dysplasia (TAYBI and LACHMAN 1996).

Anatomic variations of the anterior chest wall are very common (DONNELLY et al. 1999). Up to one third of all children show asymmetry in the shape or size of the rib cartilage or in the position of the sternum. Usually a palpable anterior chest wall bump is the cause for concern. The underlying anatomical cause may be a tilted sternum, or various anomalies of the rib cartilage, such as a prominent anterior convexity, localized thickening, bifid cartilage, or a parachondral nodule. Even a mild degree of pectus excavatum or carinatum can produce a circumscribed protrusion that quite frequently prompts referrals for imaging studies. Of 27 children who underwent computed tomography (CT) or magnetic resonance imaging (MRI) for an asymptomatic, palpable chest wall bump, all had either benign lesions or normal variants of bone or cartilage formation in the anterior chest wall (DONNELLY et al. 1997). Ultrasound (US) is an alternative method that can easily show the underlying anatomic variant and rule out a malignant chest wall mass for anxious parents and referring physicians (Fig. 15.2).

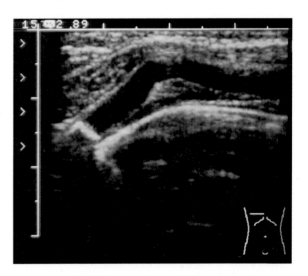

Fig. 15.2. Rib deformity in a 9-year-old boy with chest wall lump. Transverse US scan through right upper thoracic area shows redundancy of cartilaginous anterior rib portion (hockey stick shape)

15.2.2
Malformation and Deformity

Malformation of the chest wall may be a manifestation of a syndrome or skeletal dysplasia (TAYBI and LACHMAN 1996). Of particular interest is asphyxiating thoracic dystrophy (Jeune Syndrome), which may be diagnosed at any age. Affected patients usually have varying degrees of chest narrowing and rib shortening.

A small thorax with thin ribs and small lungs can be a feature of neuromuscular disorders, particularly myasthenia gravis, myotonia, spinal muscular atrophy and other myopathies. Thin ribs can be a feature of progeria and the trisomies 8, 13, and 18. Preterm infants show gracile ribs with posterior thinning. Thick ribs can be a manifestation of thalassemia (Cooley's anemia), mucopolysaccharidosis and other disorders. Inferior rib notching is due to abnormalities of the intercostal neurovascular bundle, such as arterial or venous collaterals (e.g. coarctation of the aorta, superior vena cava syndrome), and to neurogenic tumors (e.g. neurofibromatosis).

Rib aplasia or hypoplasia, when isolated, is of little clinical significance. Multiple hypoplastic ribs with or without additional spinal segmentation defects cause asymmetric deformity of the chest. Hypoplasia or aplasia of the lung can also cause an asymmetric thoracic cage.

Kyphoscoliosis can be idiopathic or congenital (due to vertebral segmentation defects), or it may be a complication of a neuromuscular disorder. The chest shows crowding of ribs on the concave side of the curvature and assessment of the heart and lung may become difficult. It is not uncommon to find a smaller lung volume and atelectasis on the convex side. Spiral CT with three-dimensional (3D) reconstruction is helpful for delineating vertebral anomalies and chest wall morphology (BUSH and KALEN 1999). MRI may be indicated if there is suspected spinal cord pathology.

Poland syndrome is characterized by unilateral partial or complete absence of the pectoralis muscles, hypoplasia of subcutaneous or breast tissues, hypoplasia or absence of ribs, and anomalies of the ipsilateral upper limb. On plain films the affected hemithorax appears hyperlucent. In the preoperative assessment of Poland syndrome, CT or MRI may help in defining the extent of the musculoskeletal and soft tissue anomalies and in showing the available muscles for reconstructive surgery (WRIGHT et al. 1992) (Fig. 15.3).

Cleidocranial dysplasia, an autosomal dominant inherited syndrome, is characterized by hypoplasia or absence of one or both clavicles resulting in hypermobile, drooping shoulders. Other features of the chest wall include small scapulae, deficient sternal ossification, posterior wedging of thoracic vertebrae, scoliosis, kyphosis and short ribs with prominent

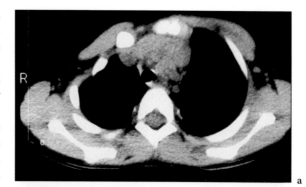

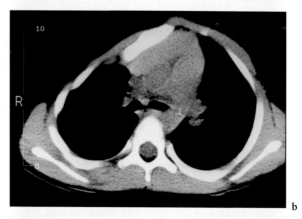

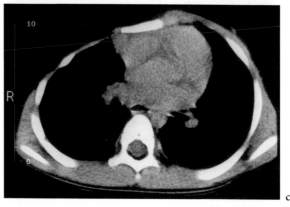

Fig. 15.3a–c. Poland syndrome in a 4-year-old boy. Unenhanced axial CT scans at three different levels (**a–c**) show hypoplasia of major and minor right pectoralis muscles and right hemithorax with asymmetry of rib cage and sternum

downward slope. Leading features of cleidocranial dysplasia are brachycephaly, wide sutures, persistence of the anterior fontanelle, abnormal dentition, absent or delayed ossification of pubic bones, and wide pubic symphysis (TAYBI and LACHMAN 1996).

Congenital pseudarthrosis of the clavicle is an isolated anomaly of the clavicle. This rare anomaly presents in infancy with a painless palpable mass. The clavicle shows a smoothly marginated defect in the middle third, virtually always on the right side. There is no history of a prior trauma. Pseudarthrosis may be caused by the failure of two primary ossification centers to fuse (CADILHAC et al. 2000).

In Sprengel's deformity the scapula fails to descend from its cervical origin and becomes fixed to the cervical spine by a fibrous band or an omovertebral bone. The scapula is high in position medially and rotated. Anomalies of ribs or vertebrae are frequently present (Klippel-Feil syndrome). Spiral CT with 3D reconstructions can be helpful in delineating the deformity and in planning corrective surgery (Fig. 15.4) (CHO et al. 2000).

Pectus excavatum, also known as "funnel chest," is the most common chest wall deformity. It is usually an isolated lesion that occurs sporadically or it may be inherited with an autosomal dominant trait. It can be associated with Turner syndrome, osteogenesis imperfecta, muscular dystrophy, or with connective tissue disorders like Marfan and Ehlers-Danlos syndromes. The lower portion of the sternum shows an inward curvature with a relative protrusion of the attached costal cartilages on each side. The sternum is usually rotated to the right. The characteristic radiographic findings are easily recognized (Fig. 15.5). On the anteroposterior view of the chest radiograph, the anterior rib ends have a steep downward course, while the posterior ribs are more horizontally oriented. The heart is shifted to the left and rotated. The right parasternal soft tissues produce a paracardial density and partially obscure the right heart border by a silhouetting effect. This should not be mistaken for middle lobe disease. On the lateral view the chest is narrow and the degree of sternal depression is easily seen. CT is useful to determine and quantify the severity of the deformity and to assess the results of surgery (Fig. 15.5) (PRETORIUS et al. 1998). For this purpose we use the pectus index, the ratio of the transverse diameter to the narrowest anteroposterior diameter that can be calculated from a single axial scan or a limited CT study (HALLER et al. 1987; CHUANG and WAN 1995). In rare cases respiratory or cardiac symptoms may be present, but most patients with pectus excavatum are asymptomatic and surgical correction is performed for cosmetic reasons. Restrictive lung volumes may not change following surgery, but cardiorespiratory function can improve secondary to higher cardiac output (HALLER and LOUGHLIN 2000).

Pectus carinatum or "pigeon breast" is a congenital or acquired deformity that develops with growth and

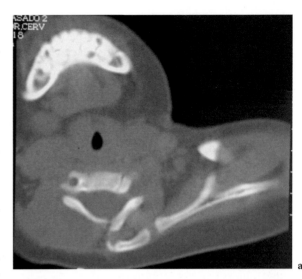

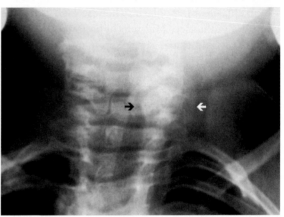

Fig. 15.4a, b. Sprengel's deformity in Klippel-Feil syndrome in a 2-year-old girl. **a** Anteroposterior radiograph shows the elevated left scapula and a rounded density superimposed on the cervical spine (*arrows*) corresponding to the omovertebral bone. Both are better demonstrated on the CT scan (**b**). The patient had associated cervical spinal abnormalities

is frequently associated with congenital heart disease (*voussure cardiaque*) (Fig. 15.6). Other causes include long-standing obstructive lung disease, Marfan syndrome, Ehlers-Danlos syndrome, Noonan syndrome, Morquio syndrome, or prune belly syndrome, among others. The deformity seems to be caused by a growth disturbance of both the sternum and costal cartilages with premature sternal fusion. The short sternum and costal cartilages protrude anteriorly with flattening of the chest laterally (Fig. 15.7). Most patients with a congenital pectus carinatum are asymptomatic. Surgery can correct the deformity.

Herniation of thoracic contents occurs when there is a defect in bony or soft tissue structures of the

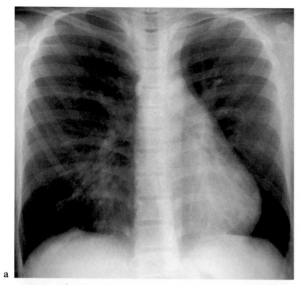

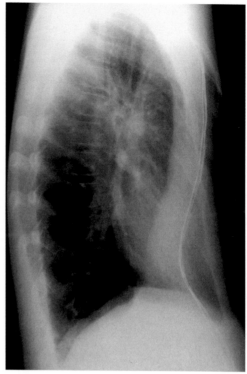

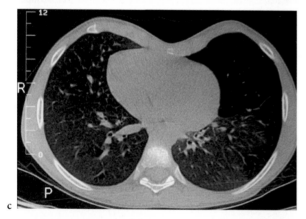

Fig. 15.5a–c. Pectus excavatum. **a, b** Postero-anterior (**a**) and lateral (**b**) chest X-rays in a 14-year-old boy show steep course of elongated anterior ribs, cylindrical shape of chest and displacement of heart to the left due to reduced mid-sagittal diameter of chest. **c** Axial CT scan of lower chest region in a 9-year-old boy shows less severe anterior chest concavity and no displacement of the heart. A hyperlucent left pulmonary upper lobe due to a congenital lobar emphysema is also seen

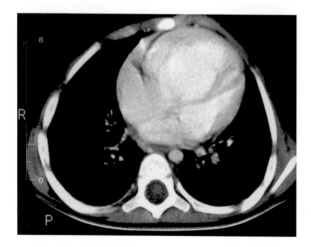

Fig. 15.6. Cor pulmonale ("*voussure cardiac*") in a 2.5-year-old boy. Axial contrast-enhanced CT scan through lower thoracic region shows (chronic) cardiac enlargement leading to increased sagittal diameter with additional left-sided protuberance of the chest. The child had primary pulmonary hypertension

chest wall. Cleft sternum is a rare congenital lesion caused by partial or complete failure of sternal fusion at an early stage of embryonic development. Depending on the location and degree of the defect, herniation of thymus or the heart may occur (ectopia cordis). Craniofacial hemangiomas and omphalocele are common associated anomalies (FOKIN 2000). Lung hernia is a protrusion of pulmonary tissue through a defect of the chest wall. It may be cervical or intercostal in location. Most intercostal hernias are acquired secondary to prior chest tube placement, surgery, trauma, chest wall neoplasm, or infection, but they can also be congenital (Fig. 15.8). Cervical or apical hernia is associated with chronic obstructive lung disease in adults. In infants and children it arises spontaneously as a result of a congenital defect in the costovertebral fascia. The main symptom is an intermittent bulging in the supraclavicular or intercostal area that appears with crying, coughing, or straining.

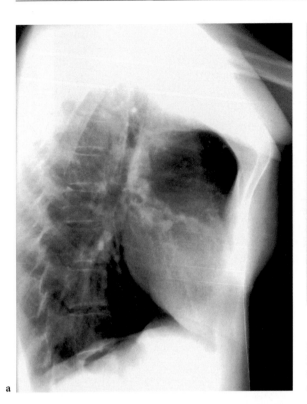

a

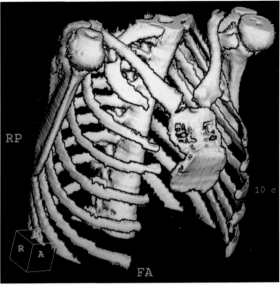

b

Fig. 15.7a, b. Pectus carinatum in a 17-year-old girl. a Lateral X-ray view of thorax shows protrusion of upper and mid portions of the sternum. b Three-dimensional CT reconstruction demonstrates correlating severe sternum deformity

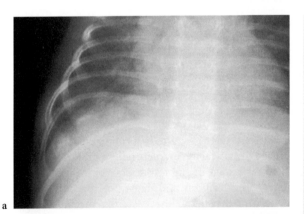

a

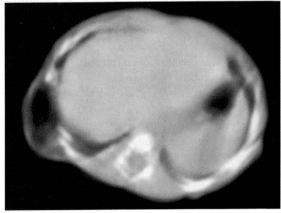

c

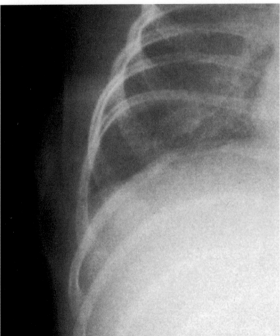

b

Fig. 15.8a–c. Lung herniation in a 4-week-old girl. a Chest X-ray at rest shows increased space between right ribs 9 and 10 and no lung prolapse. b On repeated chest X-ray while crying, lung herniates between the two ribs. c Axial CT while crying shows the herniated lung

Chest radiographs or CT performed during inspiration may fail to show the lung herniation. Fluoroscopy during crying, coughing or Valsalva maneuver is valuable for diagnosing lung hernias (THOMPSON 1976).

15.3
Infection

Primary infection of the chest wall is relatively rare in children, but it is potentially fatal since secondary sepsis or spread to the pleural spaces, the mediastinum (Fig. 15.9), or pericardium can occur. Chest wall infection originates from hematogenous spread of organisms with sepsis or bacteremia, or from direct extension from a wound after injury or surgery (sternotomy) to the chest. *Staphylococcus aureus* is the most prevalent organism in chest wall infections of patients from Europe or North America (SHARIF et al. 1990). *Mycobacterium tuberculosis* (Fig. 15.10) may be more prevalent in other areas of the world. Other micro-organisms (*Actinomyces*, *Blastomyces*, *Nocardia*, and *Aspergillus* species) and cat-scratch disease can occasionally cause chest wall infections (GOLLODAY et al. 1985; LEW and WALDVOGEL 1997). Chest wall infections are especially common in immunocompromised patients.

Clinical symptoms include fever, pain, and focal signs of inflammation such as edema, erythema, hyperthermia, and occasionally fistulous tracts. Infection can involve the soft tissues and/or bone and cause abscess formation, cellulitis and/or granulation tissue formation. Depending on the structure preferentially affected it is called pyomyositis when muscles are involved, (necrotizing) fasciitis when only subcutaneous fat and fascia are affected, osteomyelitis when there is bone involvement, and pyogenic arthritis where there is joint involvement.

Clinical recognition of a chest wall infection can be difficult, particularly when it is located in the intermediate or deep layers of the chest wall. The underlying process is often underestimated by physical examination alone. A suspected (or unsuspected) infection of the chest wall is usually first imaged with chest radiographs, which may show a mass lesion within the chest wall or the extrapleural space. Additional signs that may also be present include rib destruction and/or sclerosis, pulmonary infiltrate, pleural effusion, and calcifications, air, or gas within the soft tissues (Figs. 15.9–11). US, CT, and MRI help

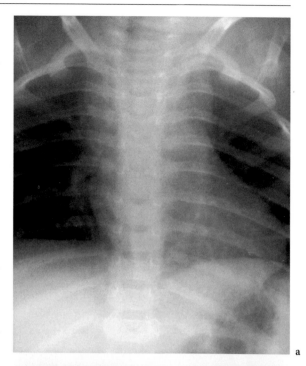

a

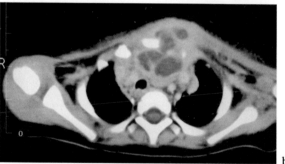

b

Fig. 15.9a, b. Sternoclavicular osteoarthritis in an 11-month-old girl. **a** Medial segment of chest X-ray shows widening of upper mediastinum; medial aspect of left clavicle not well seen. **b** Contrast-enhanced axial CT scan through upper chest area demonstrates large inflammatory mass containing large septated abscess involving left sternoclavicular region with severe osteolytic changes; mass reaches deeply into posterior mediastinum displacing trachea to the right

to confirm the presence, location, and extent of the single or multiple infectious foci (Figs. 15.9–15.12). Positron emission tomography (PET) is a very sensitive tool for detecting clinically silent foci of infection in immunocompromised patients. US, CT, and MRI show fluid collections and rib destruction, and can guide percutaneous aspiration or drainage. US is usually sufficient for diagnosing small, superficial and well-delineated lesions, while CT or MRI are the techniques of choice for imaging large, complex, and

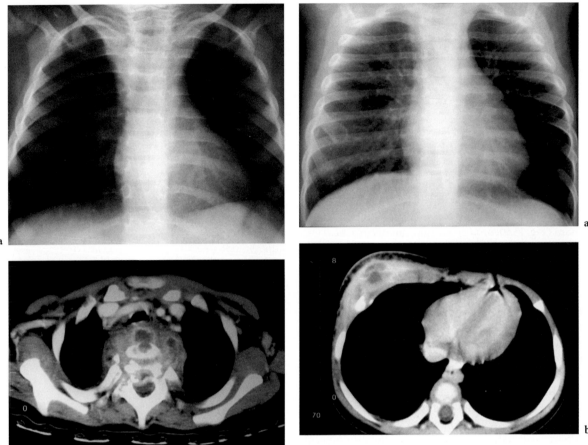

Fig. 15.10a, b. TBC abscess with vertebral osteomyelitis in a 2.5-year-old girl. **a** Chest X-ray shows unusual prominent shape of upper mediastinal region. **b** Contrast-enhanced axial CT scan through upper chest area shows complex paraspinal inflammatory mass with multiple abscesses involving vertebra, spinal arch and spinal canal

Fig. 15.12a, b. Osteomyelitis of anterior rib in an 8-month-old boy. **a** Chest X-ray shows well defined osteolytic lesion in the anterior bony aspect of sixth right rib. **b** Contrast-enhanced axial CT demonstrates mainly local inflammatory swelling of right anterolateral chest wall with central abscess and related osteolytic rib changes

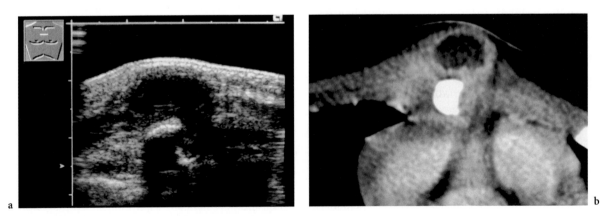

Fig. 15.11a, b. Osteomyelitis of sternum in a 2.5-year-old girl. **a** Transverse ultrasound scan through lower presternal area demonstrates subcutaneous abscess and narrowed lower sternal body. **b** Contrast-enhanced axial CT at the same level shows abscess correlate, complete osteolysis of left part of lower sternal body, and surrounding inflammatory soft tissue changes

deep-seated lesions for which surgery is considered. Epidural extension may only be visible with CT or MRI (see Fig. 15.10).

An abscess appears as a sonolucent area on US with increased through-transmission and absence of blood flow centrally. Contrast-enhanced CT shows an iso- or hypodense, nonenhancing center and an enhancing rim (Figs. 15.9–15.12) (FARO et al. 1993), similar to that seen on T1-weighted MRI sequences. T2-weighted and short tau inversion recovery (STIR) sequences show a high signal intensity collection. A moderate increase in signal intensity on T2-weighted sequences may be present in mycotic infection (SHARIF et al. 1990). MRI is very sensitive for detecting osteomyelitis and is often more accurate than bone scans for differentiating between soft tissue inflammation and acute osteomyelitis. Chronic osteomyelitis is recognized on radiographs and CT as an area of destruction and reparative sclerosis within and around the affected part of bone. Inflammation of the surrounding soft tissues (cellulitis) appears as thickening in all modalities. In addition to this, US shows increased soft tissue echogenicity and perfusion, while CT and MRI show contrast enhancement. Soft tissue inflammation is best delineated by MRI with fat-suppressed T2-weighted or STIR sequences, or T1-weighted sequences following administration of contrast material, which provide better differentiation from the unaffected subcutaneous fat. In our experience septic arthritis of the sternoclavicular joint is usually associated with osteomyelitis of the adjacent clavicle or sternum. CT and MRI show the joint effusion and osteolytic changes of the affected bone more readily than US and they can confirm or exclude posterior extension of the process into the mediastinum (see Fig. 15.9).

Tuberculous spondylitis is relatively rare in developed countries, but it is the commonest vertebral infection in other parts of the world. The spinal infection mostly stems from primary pulmonary tuberculosis. One or several segments of the spine may be involved, particularly in the thoracic and lumbar region. Usually the infection is limited to the body of the vertebra, which may become destroyed along with the contiguous intervertebral disc and an adjacent or distant vertebra. Paraspinal abscesses, usually bilateral, are the rule. Calcification within a paraspinal abscess can occur in long-standing cases (SILVERMAN and KUHN 1992). Vertebral collapse can lead to kyphosis and/or scoliosis and even to cord compression. The radiographic changes of tuberculous spondylitis are nonspecific, but the indolent presentation

may be suggestive of tuberculosis. CT and MRI can show the epidural extension of the process and delineate the topography of an abscess (see Fig. 15.10).

Friedrich's disease is a disorder of unknown origin thought to be an aseptic necrosis with clinical and radiologic features that can mimic infection at the sternoclavicular joint (LEVY et al. 1981). The lesion is usually unilateral but may be bilateral. Tender swelling at the sternoclavicular region is the typical presenting symptom. The erythrocyte sedimentation rate may be elevated. Radiographs show destruction and repair at the medial end of a clavicle (Fig. 15.13). Histology discloses necrosis of the clavicular epiphyseal region without evidence of infection. Aspiration cultures are negative. The symptoms usually subside spontaneously without treatment over several months. Radiological features improve very slowly. Our experience has shown that it may take up to 18 months for the clavicles to become radiologically normal.

There are some similarities between Friedrich's disease and SAPHO syndrome, a disorder characterized by a variable combination of synovitis, acne, pustulosis, hyperostosis, and osteitis. The different aseptic skin abnormalities are associated with chronic recurrent multifocal osteomyelitis, a rare, mostly symmetrical, non-purulent inflammation of bone. Although it can involve other bones, the inflammation has a predilection for the anterior chest wall where it can cause tenderness, and swelling. Radiographic abnormalities include sclerosis and periostitis with expansion of the affected bone (LETTS et al. 1999).

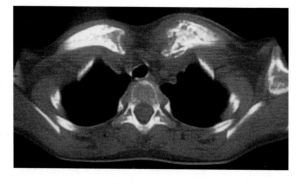

Fig. 15.13. Friedrich's disease in a 9-year-old girl. Axial CT scan through upper chest inlet area shows symmetrical changes of clavicles at their medial aspects from chronic inflammatory process

15.4
Tumors

The chest wall can give rise to a wide variety of benign and malignant tumors that are primarily mesenchymal in origin, in keeping with the predominant tissue components of the chest wall. Tumors of the chest wall are relatively infrequent during infancy and childhood, but a high proportion is malignant (KUMAR et al. 1977; SHAMBERGER and GRIER 1994; SHAMBERGER et al. 1989). The tumors often present as a palpable mass, or, less frequently, with pain, cough, or respiratory distress from a large pleural effusion or an extensive intrathoracic component. Secondary involvement of the chest wall from an intrathoracic mass is rare in childhood (Table 15.1).

Table 15.1. Nosology of chest wall tumors (SHAMBERGER and GRIER 1994)

Benign lesions	Malignant lesions
Chondroma	Chondrosarcoma
Osteochondroma	Osteochondrosarcoma
Osteoma	Osteosarcoma
Fibroma	Fibrosarcoma
Lipoma	Mesenchymal sarcoma
Eosinophilic granuloma	Ewing's sarcoma (Askin's tumor)
Hemangioma	Rhabdomyosarcoma
Mesenchymal hamartoma	Leiomyosarcoma
Aneurysmal bone cyst	Lymphoma
Fibrous dysplasia	

The lesion may be located within the bones and/or within the soft tissues of the chest wall. A sharply marginated osteolytic lesion usually signifies a slow-growing (benign) process; however, differentiation from a malignant lesion is not always possible, and biopsy may be required (KOZLOWSKI et al. 1989). Multifocal Langerhans' cell histiocytosis (eosinophilic granuloma) with typical osteolytic lesions of the skull vault or vertebra plana allow a confident clinical diagnosis (Fig. 15.14).

Hemangiomas and lymphangiomas are the most common soft tissue tumors in children, particularly in neonates, infants, and young children. Lymphangiomas are called cystic hygromas when dilated lymphatic vessels lead to the formation of cysts. Lymphangiomas are usually present at birth and are found in the neck and chest wall region. Extension into the mediastinum and axilla can occur. The growth of lymphangiomas is often self-limited. Hemangiomas, however, may increase in size and subsequently involute spontaneously. When located beneath the skin, hemangio-

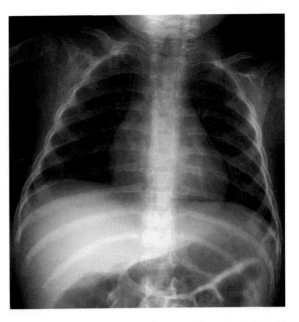

Fig. 15.14. Langerhans' cell histiocytosis in a 14-month-old girl. Chest X-ray shows numerous osseous changes involving almost all ribs, mainly anterior portions, but also scapulae, clavicles, humeri, as well as multiple skeletal parts not shown on this film

mas may exhibit the typical strawberry red color. Both lymphangiomas and blood vessel tumors can be multifocal, and lesions composed of lymphatic vessels and blood capillaries are found on occasion. Hemangiomas and lymphangiomas can become large and disfiguring or compress blood vessels, the trachea and/or other vital structures (STOUT and LATTES 1967). They therefore may require imaging for staging purposes before surgery or radiologic intervention. Solitary lymphangiomas of bone are rare; radiographically they are usually osteolytic single or multiloculated lesions. Hemangiomas may have a similar radiographic appearance or present as a radiolucent slightly expansile lesion possessing a radiating lattice-like or web-like trabecular pattern (Figs. 15.15, 15.16).

An association between lymphangiomas and hemangiomas with massive osteolysis has been noted in children and young adults particularly in the thoracic and pelvic region. This "vanishing bone disease" or "Gorham-Stout syndrome" is a rare condition in which spontaneous, progressive resorption of bone occurs. The involved bones show osteoporosis and partial or complete destruction without evidence of reaction. Joints may be crossed and pleural effusion with thoracic involvement may be present (Fig. 15.17). MRI can show the underlying vascular tumor (ASSOUN et al. 1994).

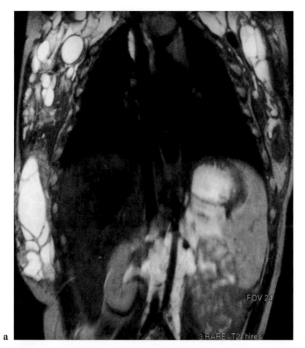

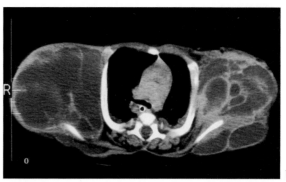

Fig. 15.15a, b. Multifocal lymphangioma in a 3-month-old boy. a Coronal T2-weighted (rapid acquisition relation enhancement) fat-saturated MRI view of posterior thorax and abdomen demonstrates extensive bilateral involvement of the chest wall and right abdominal wall by complex lymphangioma, as well as involvement of the retroperitoneum with encasement of lower abdominal portions of the inferior vena cava and aorta and extending into the left renal fossa posteriorly. b Axial CT view through the chest at carina level shows grotesque expansion of the chest wall by septated lymphangioma involving soft tissues of the back

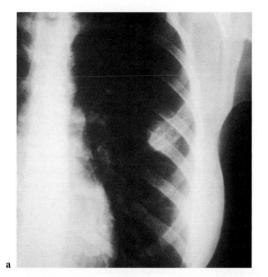

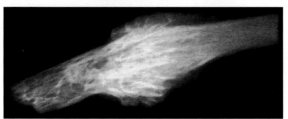

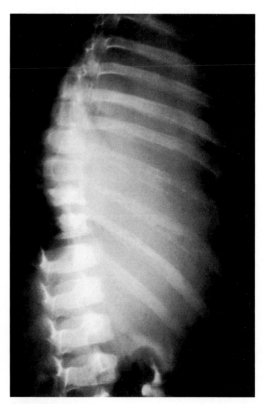

Fig. 15.16a, b. Rib hemangioma in a 10-year-old girl. X-ray of left hemithorax (a) and X-ray of the resected rib specimen (b) show enlarged and sclerotic anterior portion of eighth rib with a radiating lattice-like pattern

Fig. 15.17. Gorham disease in a 2.5-year-old girl. Left posterior oblique chest X-ray demonstrating multiple osteolytic and expansive rib lesions. Several affected dorsal vertebral bodies show a loss of height

Osteochondroma is a common benign tumor of the growing skeleton and probably the most common benign bone tumor of the chest wall. It is composed of cortical and medullary bone with a cartilaginous cap and is continuous with the underlying parent bone. It usually projects from the metaphysis of a tubular bone, but a rib, vertebra, clavicle, scapula, and the sternum may also be involved. The rib is most frequently affected near the costochondral junction (Fig. 15.18). Osteochondromas of the ribs may produce pleural effusion or hemothorax. Plain radiographs, CT, and MRI are able to depict the exostosis and its origin from the parent bone.

Mesenchymal hamartoma, also known as mesenchymoma, is a rare benign lesion of infants and young children, usually identified at birth. It is characterized by focal overgrowth of soft tissues and skeletal elements of the chest wall. The lesion may be bilateral or multicentric. On radiographs it appears as a partially calcified mass of the chest wall with involvement of one or more ribs. The rib deformity consists of partial or complete destruction, erosion, and enlargement. There may be focal calcification of cartilage. The tumors are well delineated, often lobulated, and measure up to 8 cm in diameter. The mass may decrease in size without treatment and the prognosis of the patients is excellent (SHAMBERGER and GRIER 1994; AYALA et al. 1993) (Fig. 15.19).

Lipoblastoma is a benign soft tissue tumor composed of fatty tissue, fibrovascular septa, and myxoid stroma. It is encountered in infants and young children, while lipoma is usually found in older individuals (STOUT and

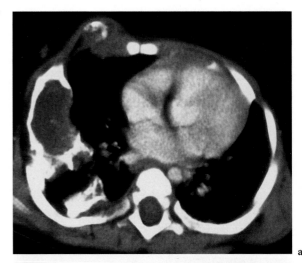

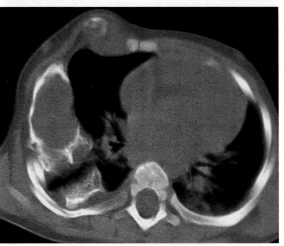

Fig. 15.19a, b. Benign mesenchymoma in an 11-month-old boy. Contrast-enhanced axial CT view of chest at mid-level shows severe complex right rib alterations due to multifocal bulky expansion from the mesenchymal tumor and associated pleural changes. **a** Soft tissue view; **b** bone view

LATTES 1967). The imaging features of a lipoblastoma consist of a fatty tumor containing areas of stroma that may enhance with intravenous contrast (Fig. 15.20).

Fibrous tumors and tumor-like lesions, a large and diverse group of distinct entities that differ greatly in their clinical behavior, are relatively frequent, particularly in infants and young children, mostly boys. Most fibrous tumors are benign or intermediate in their biologic behavior. The chest wall may be affected by extraabdominal fibromatosis (desmoid or aggressive fibromatosis), which can involve the muscle and overlying fascia of the shoulder girdle of adolescents and young adults. The tumor has the potential to grow to a large size, to recur, and to infiltrate neighboring tis-

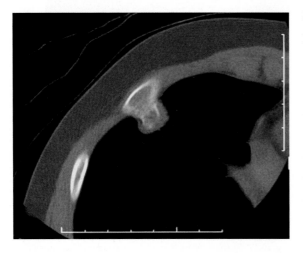

Fig. 15.18. Osteochondroma in a school-aged child. Close up section of axial chest CT scan shows ossified chondroma coming off the rib toward the chest inside

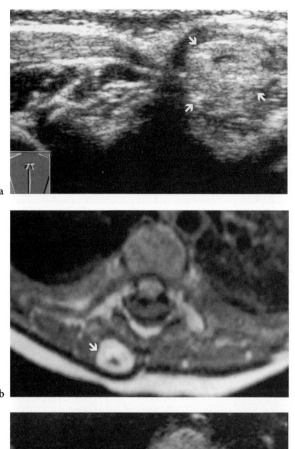

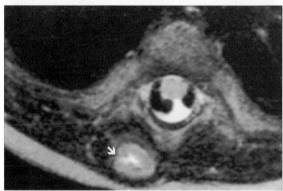

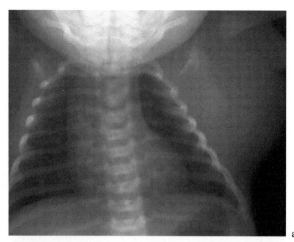

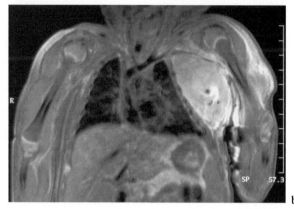

Fig. 15.21a, b. Congenital fibrosarcoma in a 3-day-old boy. a Chest X-ray shows large left extrathoracic soft tissue mass with severe displacement of ipsilateral scapula and deforming left hemithorax. b Coronal T1-weighted contrast-enhanced MRI view of the thorax with suboptimal fat saturation demonstrates diffusely enhancing left-sided extrathoracic soft tissue mass impinging left lateral chest wall

Fig. 15.20a–c. Lipoblastoma in a 5-month-old girl. a Transverse ultrasound (US) view of upper back region (prone position) shows right paramedian round and mostly hyperechoic structure (*arrows*) with small hypoechoic inner portion. b, c Axial T1- and T2-weighted MRI scans show well defined fatty tumor (*arrows*) with small central liquid content, correlating with US

sues. The imaging features are usually nonspecific, but low signal intensity on T1- and T2-weighted sequences may suggest a fibrous tumor. Other fibrous lesions that can affect the chest wall include fibrous hamartoma of infancy, infantile myofibromatosis, juvenile hyaline fibromatosis, and infantile or adult type fibrosarcoma (EICH et al. 1998) (Fig. 15.21).

Neurogenic tumors, such as schwannomas and neurofibromas (particularly in patients with neurofibromatosis) or neuroblastoma and its variants (ganglioneuroblastoma and ganglioneuroma) may involve the intercostal nerves or the sympathetic ganglia. They may lead to erosion, thinning, destruction, and separation of adjacent ribs (Figs. 15.22, 15.23). Patients with neurofibromatosis type I may suffer from extensive involvement of the chest wall by plexiform neurofibromas or malignant neurofibrosarcoma. In addition to these features, such patients may show widening of the ribs (twisted ribbon appearance) and short segment kyphoscoliosis due to dysplastic vertebrae, with widening of the spinal canal

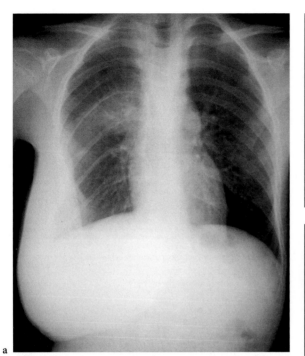

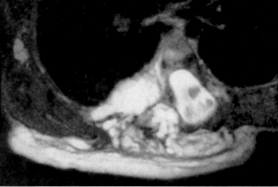

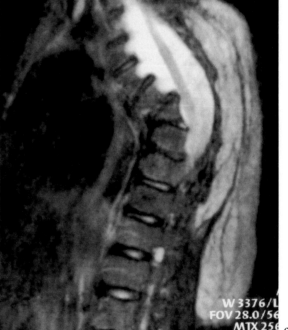

Fig. 15.22a–c. Plexiform neurofibroma (NF1) in an 11- year-old boy. **a** Chest X-ray demonstrates complex abnormality of right hemithorax with large extrathoracic soft tissue mass invading the pleural space, multiple dysplastic rib changes of varying degree, circumscribed density adjacent to the mediastinum and S-shaped scoliosis. **b** Axial T2-weighted (rapid acquisition relation enhancement) fat-saturated MRI view through the chest at mid-level shows multifocal and complex extra- and intrathoracic portions of neurofibroma with high fat content. Involvement of severely distended spinal canal. **c** Same technique as in (**b**); upper mid-sagittal view of the spine shows vertically extended neurofibroma within the soft tissues of upper back region as well as intraspinally; expansion of upper spinal canal due to severe dysharmonic thoracic hyperkyphosis from local vertebral wedge deformity, also caused by the underlying disease

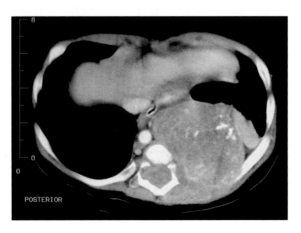

Fig. 15.23. Thoraco-abdominal neuroblastoma in a 5-month-old boy. Contrast-enhanced axial CT scan through lower chest area shows huge solid posterior mediastinal mass containing calcifications and extending extrathoracically through posterior chest wall as well as intraspinally. Notice expansive deformity of spinal canal due to long-standing neoplastic process. The child had neurological impairment that persisted after therapy

and intervertebral foramina, and dorsal scalloping of the vertebral bodies (SILVERMAN and KUHN 1992).

The most prevalent malignant tumors of the chest wall are the Ewing's sarcoma family of tumors, including Ewing's sarcoma, Askin's tumor and peripheral primitive neuroectodermal tumors (PNET) (Fig. 15.24) and the rhabdomyosarcomas. Of all malignant chest wall tumors in children approximately 50%–65% belong to the Ewing's sarcoma group, while up to 33% are either alveolar or embryonal rhabdomyosarcomas (SHAMBERGER and GRIER 1994; SHAMBERGER et al. 1989; DANG et al. 1999). These tumors are dealt with elsewhere in this book. Other malignant tumors are much less common, and metastases to the chest wall are exceedingly rare in children (Fig. 15.25).

The differential diagnosis of a "true tumor" includes pseudoneoplasms of other etiologies. Amongst these mention should be made of (recurrent) hematomas in

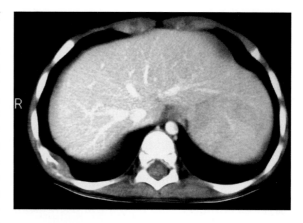

Fig. 15.25. Metastatic renal clear cell sarcoma in a 2.5-year-old boy. Contrast-enhanced axial CT scan through lower chest area shows destructive metastatic lesion in the postero-lateral aspect of the ninth right rib extending intra- and extrathoracically. This child had simultaneous vertebral, orbital and cranial vault metastases

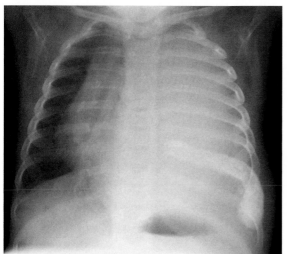

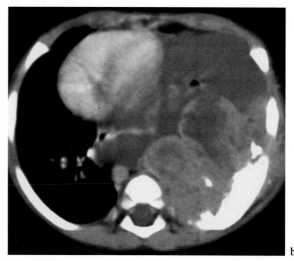

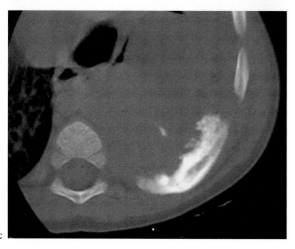

Fig. 15.24a–c. Primitive neuroectodermal tumor (PNET) in a 14-month-old boy. **a** Anteroposterior chest X-ray shows mass effect within left hemithorax with displacement of heart and mediastinal structures to the right. Diffusely hyperdense and enlarged eighth left rib. **b** Axial contrast-enhanced CT scan at mid-level of thorax demonstrates irregularly hypertrophic posterior aspect of eighth left rib associated with a huge intrathoracically growing heterogeneous soft tissue mass; anteriorly displaced left main stem bronchus with preserved lumen. **c** Close-up bone view shows osseous changes in more detail

a hemophiliac patient, which may present as a mass lesion (Fig. 15.26). Musculoskeletal hemorrhage of hemophiliac patients most commonly occurs within joints, but hemorrhage within bone and soft tissues can take place and cause local destructive bone changes. Subperiosteal hematomas can induce new bone formation or atrophy, or even complete destruction of the underlying bone. Such hemophiliac pseudotumors are relatively uncommon. They may extend from hemarthrosis under pressure, or develop from intraosseous, subperiosteal or soft tissue bleeding; or they may appear aggressive, as a large soft tissue mass with or without bone destruction (SILVERMAN and KUHN 1992).

Imaging is performed to detect a chest wall mass and to determine its location, size, and character. When a mass that originates in the chest wall expands into the chest cavity, it forms an obtuse angle with the adjacent chest wall. This feature might be recognized on radiographs, CT, or MRI. Masses that produce rib changes are extrapleural in location. Conventional radiographs are the first tools for imaging a chest wall mass in most places. Radiographs allow an approximate appreciation of the location of the lesion, its extension, rib destruction, and associated intrathoracic component, pleural effusion, or pulmonary metastases. Further imaging may be required in

large or aggressive-looking lesions for staging purposes. Both CT and MRI are able to delineate the mass, demonstrate osseous changes, and define the margin and internal structure of the lesion, lymphatic spread, and pleural effusion. Currently CT is better suited than MRI to show metastases to the lungs. Obviously when faced with a possibly malignant chest wall mass, an interdisciplinary approach should be used, and the choice of the imaging modality may vary with the availability of, and expertise in using, the local imaging tools.

15.5
Trauma

15.5.1
Accidental Trauma

With the exception of rib fractures and burns, traumatic lesions of the chest wall are usually part of a more complex injury to the chest. It may be caused by direct blunt contusion or compression, axial trauma to the spine, penetrating chest trauma, rapid deceleration or other mechanisms. Often, chest injuries are part of some polytrauma. Severe trauma to the

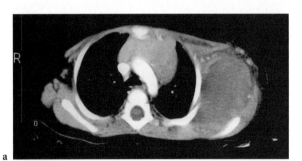

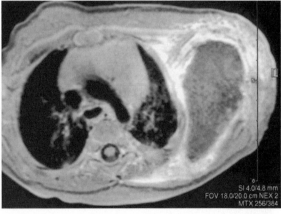

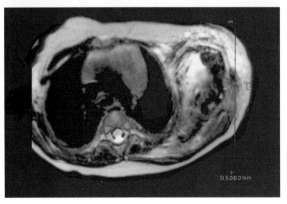

Fig. 15.26a–c. Acute bleeding in B-hemophilia in a 4-month-old boy. a Contrast-enhanced axial CT scan through chest at aortic arch level shows huge well defined "cystic lesion" in the left extrathoracic soft tissues displacing the scapula away from the chest wall and extending into the dorsal musculature. Mass contains contrast material. b, c Correlating axial T2-weighted (rapid acquisition relation enhancement) and T1-weighted fat-saturated contrast-enhanced MRI views demonstrate fluid and, respectively, blood content of the mass lesion with a peripheral rim of contrast due to inflammatory response

chest and/or other parts of the body involving the chest, as in polytrauma, commonly results in damage of multiple thoracic structures, including intrathoracic organs. Referral for imaging usually follows clinical assessment and stabilization of vital conditions. Plain films of the chest (and abdomen) may reveal life-threatening injuries, although CT is the method of choice to evaluate the chest in most situations of posttraumatic emergency.

This section focuses on the few traumatic injuries to the child's chest wall that are characteristic of some specific insult or are difficult to assess and diagnose. Rib fractures are easily overlooked on an initial chest film. The site of a rib fracture may point to an adjacent (i.e. locally-related) injury of the neighboring organs, which should be carefully examined. Trauma to the spine due to falls, motor vehicle accidents, or various sport activities is not uncommon. The injury usually consists of one or multiple vertebral compression fractures with paraspinal hemorrhage and edema (Fig. 15.27). The

paraspinal soft tissue mass from local hemorrhage may suggest the presence of associated aortic rupture. However, traumatic rupture of the thoracic or abdominal aorta is extremely rare in the pediatric age group and is usually excluded or demonstrated using contrast-enhanced CT and transesophageal echocardiography (LOWE et al. 1998; SPOUGE et al. 1991; TRACHIOTIS et al. 1996). Involvement of the spinal canal with neurological symptoms is uncommon and is less frequent in children and teenagers than in adults.

In children and adolescents and even in young adults, so-called sternoclavicular dislocation is, in fact, Salter type 1 or 2 medial clavicular epiphysiolysis (COPE et al. 1991; LEWONOWSKI and BASSETT 1992). It is uncommon and usually missed at the initial clinical examination. A fall on the shoulder, occurring during a bicycle accident or in contact sports, is the typical cause. If a sternoclavicular injury is suspected, contrast-enhanced CT is the diagnostic method of choice (COPE et al. 1991; YANG et al. 1996) (Figs. 15.28, 15.29).

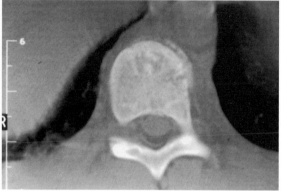

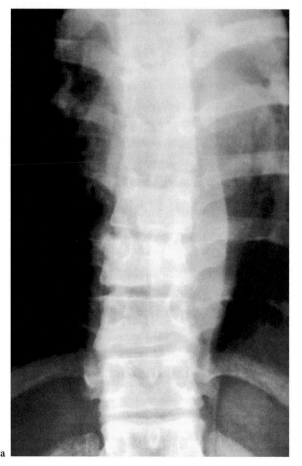

Fig. 15.27a, b. Roller blade accident: vertebral fracture in a 10-year-old boy. a Partial anteroposterior X-ray view of thoracic spine shows left paraspinal soft tissue mass at level of compressed vertebrae 9 and 10 and extending above this level. b Axial CT scan (bone window) at T-9 level shows vertebral compression fracture and left paraspinal hemorrhage/edema

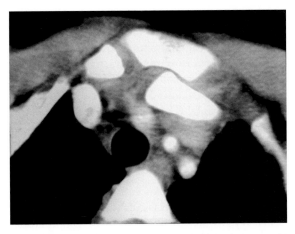

Fig. 15.28. Sternoclavicular dislocation (I) in a 15-year-old girl. Axial contrast-enhanced CT scan through sternoclavicular area demonstrates dislocation of left medial clavicular end behind manubrium of sternum and medially, thus space-occupying and explaining difficulty at swallowing

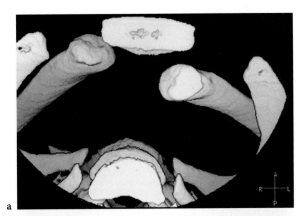

a

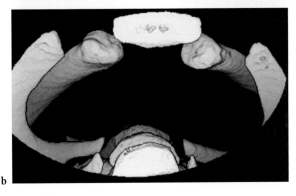

b

Fig. 15.29a, b. Sternoclavicular dislocation (II) in an 8-year-old boy. **a** Three-dimensional CT reconstruction demonstrates posterior dislocation of left clavicle. **b** Same technique as in (**a**) after closed reduction shows normal sternoclavicular relationship

Intravenous contrast is necessary to demonstrate compromise of the supracardiac vasculature, a complication of retrosternal clavicular dislocation that is less relevant in children than in adults. Dysphagia, however, is common. If CT is not available, plain films obtained with the Heinig projection, may provide significant diagnostic information, including posterior or anterior location of the dislocated clavicle (HEINIG 1968; LEE and GWINN 1974). This projection is, however, difficult to obtain and films often need to be repeated.

15.5.2
Non-accidental Trauma

Child abuse should be considered in any infant and young child with rib fractures, unless there is a plausible explanation, such as a motor vehicle accident, a metabolic, dysplastic, or syndromal bone disease or prematurity (BULLOCH et al. 2000; CADZOW and ARMSTRONG 2000). Rib fractures are due to typical mechanical factors involved in violence to the child's chest and may occur anywhere along the entire rib arc (KLEINMAN 1992; NG and HALL 1998). They are more common in its posterior part, especially close to the costovertebral joint. In child abuse, the rib fractures are commonly multiple and tend to be bilateral and somewhat symmetrical (Fig. 15.30). Ample specific information regarding the mechanism, pathophysiology, anatomic, and histologic findings in skeletal and soft tissue involvement of the entire body in child abuse has been collected and described by KLEINMAN (1996, 1998). If child abuse is suspected, a formal evaluation of the entire skeleton has to be performed and the information transmitted to the clinician(s) responsible for the child's care. Occasionally, rib lesions similar to the fractures in child abuse may be encountered in infants under physiotherapy while in intensive care. Rib fractures from cardiopulmonary resuscitation are unlikely in infants (SPEVAK et al. 1994).

Acknowledgements. We would like to acknowledge the contribution of imaging material by Drs. Paul Babyn and David Manson, The Hospital for Sick Children, Toronto, Dr. Kieran McHugh, The Hospital for Sick Children, London, and Dr. Javier Lucaya, HMI Vall d'Hebron, Barcelona.

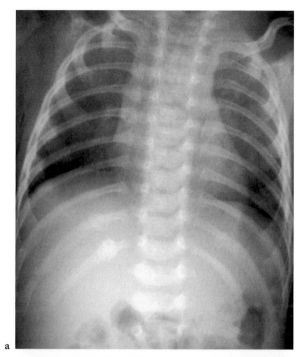

a

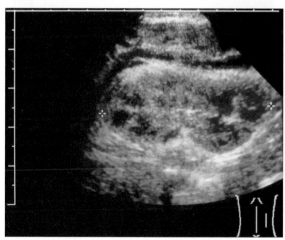

b

Fig. 15.30a, b. Rib fractures from non-accidental trauma in a 4-week-old boy. **a** Anteroposterior chest X-ray shows healing paraspinal fractures of the tenth and eleventh right and the tenth left ribs. **b** Previous posterior longitudinal ultrasound at 10 days had shown fluid behind right kidney and somewhat hyperechoic perirenal rim; but this had not been properly interpreted

References

Assoun J, Richardi G, Railhac JJ, Le Guennec P, Caulier M, Dromer C, Sixou L, Fournie B, Mansat M, Durroux D (1994) CT and MRI of massive osteolysis of Gorham. J Comput Assist Tomogr 18:981–984

Ayala AG, Ro JY, Bolio-Solis A, Hernandez-Batres F, Eftekhari F, Edeiken J (1993) Mesenchymal hamartoma of the chest wall in infants and children: a clinicopathological study of five patients. Skeletal Radiol 22:569–576

Bulloch B, Schubert CJ, Brophy PD, Johnson N, Reed MH, Shapiro RA (2000) Cause and clinical characteristics of rib fractures in infants. Pediatrics 105:E48

Bush CH, Kalen V (1999) Three-dimensional computed tomography in the assessment of congenital scoliosis. Skeletal Radiol 28:632–637

Cadilhac C, Fenoll B, Peretti A et al (2000) Congenital pseudarthrosis of the clavicle: 25 childhood cases. Rev Chir Orthop Reparatrice Appar Mot 86:575–580

Cadzow SP, Armstrong KL (2000) Rib fractures in infants: red alert! The clinical features, investigations and child protection outcomes. J Paediatr Child Health 36:322–326

Cho TJ, Choi IH, Chung CY et al (2000) The Sprengel deformity. Morphometric analysis using 3D-CT and its clinical relevance. J Bone Joint Surg Br 82:711–718

Chuang JH, Wan YL (1995) Evaluation of pectus excavatum with repeated CT scans. Pediatr Radiol 25:654–656

Cope R, Riddervold HO, Shore JL, Sistrom CL (1991) Dislocations of the sternoclavicular joint: anatomic basis, etiologies, and radiologic diagnosis. J Orthop Traum 5:379–384

Coury CH, Delaporte J (1954) Les anomalies congénitales des cotes. Formes anatomo-radiologiques et incidences pratiques (a propos de 288 cas). Sem Hop Paris 30:2656–2681

Dang NC, Siegel SE, Phillips JD (1999) Malignant chest wall tumors in children and young adults. J Pediatr Surg 34:1773–1778

Donnelly LF, Frush DP, Foss JN et al (1999) Anterior chest wall: frequency of anatomic variations in children. Radiology 212:837–840

Donnelly LF, Taylor CN, Emery KH et al (1997) Asymptomatic, palpable, anterior chest wall lesions in children: is cross-sectional imaging necessary? Radiology 202:829–831

Eich GF, Hoeffel JC, Tschäppeler H, Gassner I, Willi UV (1998) Fibrous tumours in children: imaging features of a heterogeneous group of disorders. Pediatr Radiol 28:500–509

Faro SH, Mahboubi S, Ortega W (1993) CT diagnosis of rib anomalies, tumors, and infection in children. Clin Imaging 17:1–7

Fokin AA (2000) Cleft sternum and sternal foramen. Chest Surg Clin North Am 10:261–276

Golladay ES, Hale JA, Mollitt DL, Seibert JJ (1985) Chest wall masses in children. South Med J 78:292–295

Haller JA, Kramer SS, Lietman SA (1987) Use of CT scans in selection of patients for pectus excavatum superior: a preliminary report. J Pediatr Surg 22:904–906

Haller JA, Loughlin GM (2000) Cardiorespiratory function is significantly improved following surgery for severe pectus excavatum. Proposed treatment guidelines. J Cardiovasc Surg (Torino) 41:125–130

Heinig CF (1968) Retrosternal dislocation of the clavicle: early recognition, x-ray diagnosis and management. J Bone Joint Surg (Am) 50:830

Kamaruddin K, Wright NB, Pilling DW (1995) Intrathoracic rib. Pediatr Radiol 25:60–61

Kleinman PK (1992) Fractures of the rib head in abused infants. Radiology 185:119–123

Kleinman PK (1996) Rib fractures in 31 abused infants: postmortem radiologic-histopathologic study. Radiology 200:807–810

Kleinman PK (1998) Diagnostic imaging of child abuse, 2nd edn. Mosby, St Louis

Kozlowski K, Campbell J, Morris L, Sprague P, Taccone A, Beluffi G, Marcinski A, Porta F, Stevens M (1989) Primary rib tumours in children (report of 27 cases with short literature review). Aust Radiol 33:210–222

Kumar AP, Green AL, Smith JW, Pratt CB (1977) Combined therapy for malignant tumors of the chest wall in children. J Pediatr Surg 12:991–999

Lee FA, Gwinn JL (1974) Retrosternal dislocation of the clavicle. Radiology 110:631–634

Letts M, Davidson D, Birdi N, Joseph M (1999) The SAPHO syndrome in children: a rare cause of hyperostosis and osteitis. J Pediatr Orthop 19:297–300

Levy M, Goldberg I, Fischel RE, Frisch E, Maor P (1981) Friedrich's disease. Aseptic necrosis of the sternal end of the clavicle. J Bone Joint Surg (Br) 63:539–541

Lew DP, Waldvogel FA (1997) Osteomyelitis. N Engl J Med 336:999–1007

Lewonowski K, Bassett GS (1992) Complete posterior sternoclavicular epiphyseal separation. A case report and review of the literature. Clin Orthop 281:84–88

Lowe LH, Bulas DI, Eichelberger MD, Martin GR (1998) Traumatic aortic injuries in children: radiologic evaluation. Am J Roentgenol 170:39–42

Nathanson I (1994) Chest wall abnormalities. In: Loughlin GM, Eigen H (eds) Respiratory disease in children: diagnosis and management. Williams and Wilkins, Baltimore, pp 533–541

Ng CS, Hall CM (1998) Costochondral junction fractures and intra-abdominal trauma in non-accidental injury (child abuse). Pediatr Radiol 28:671–676

Pretorius ES, Haller JA, Fishman EK (1998) Spiral CT with 3D reconstruction in children requiring reoperation for failure of chest wall growth after pectus excavatum surgery. Preliminary observations. Clin Imaging 22:108–116

Shamberger RC, Grier HE (1994) Chest wall tumors in infants and children. Semin Pediatr Surg 3:267–276

Shamberger RC, Grier HE, Weinstein HJ, Perez-Atayde AR, Tarbell NJ (1989) Chest wall tumors in infancy and childhood. Cancer 63:774–785

Sharif HS, Clark DC, Aabed MY, Aideyan OA, Haddad MC, Mattsson TA (1990) MR imaging of thoracic and abdominal wall infections: comparison with other imaging procedures. AJR Am J Roentgenol 154:989–95

Silverman FN, Kuhn J (1992) Caffey's pediatric X-Ray diagnosis, 9th edn. Mosby-Year Book, St Louis

Spevak MR, Kleinman PK, Belanger PL, Primack C, Richmond JM (1994) Cardiopulmonary resuscitation and rib fractures in infants. A postmortem radiologic-pathologic study. JAMA 272:617–618

Spouge AR, Burrows PE, Armstrong D, Daneman A (1991) Traumatic aortic rupture in the pediatric population. Role of plain film, CT and angiogaphy in the diagnosis. Pediatr Radiol 21:324–328

Stout AP, Lattes R (1967) Atlas of tumor pathology, second series, fascicle I: tumors of the soft tissues. Armed Forces Institute of Pathology, Washington DC

Taybi H, Lachman RS (1996) Radiology of syndromes, metabolic disorders, and skeletal dysplasias, 4th edn. Mosby, St Louis

Thompson JS (1976) Cervical herniation of the lung. Report of a case and review of the literature. Pediatr Radiol 4:190–192

Trachiotis GD, Sell JE, Pearson GD, Martin GR, Midgley FM (1996) Traumatic thoracic aortic rupture in the pediatric patient. Ann Thorac Surg 62:724–731

Wright AR, Milner RH, Bainbridge LC et al (1992) MR and CT in the assessment of Poland syndrome. J Comput Assist Tomogr 16:442–444

Yang J, al-Etani H, Letts M (1996) Diagnosis and treatment of posterior sternoclavicular joint dislocations in children. Am J Orthop 25:565–569

16 Current Imaging Status – Cardiac MRI

Taylor Chung

CONTENTS

16.1 Introduction

With the steady advances in the development of magnetic resonance imaging (MRI) technology, MRI has rapidly become the *non-invasive* imaging modality of choice for patients with congenital heart disease in whom echocardiography fails to fully depict the necessary clinically relevant anatomy (MARX and GEVA 1998). This is especially so for older patients and post-operative patients (ROEST et al. 1999) in whom the acoustic windows are poor. Since MRI can also provide physiologic information such as right (FOGEL 2000; HELBING et al. 1995, 1996; LORENZ 2000; PATTYNAMA et al. 1995) and left (CHUNG et al. 1988; FOGEL et al. 1996; FOGEL 2000; KATZ et al. 1988; LORENZ 2000; SAKUMA et al. 1993) ventricular function, and flow quantification (BRENNER et al. 1992; CAPUTO et al. 1991; HELBING et al. 1996; HUNDLEY et al. 1995; PELC et al. 1992; PELC 1995; POWELL and GEVA 2000; REBERGEN et al. 1993a,b, 1995; SIEVERDING et al. 1992; STEFFENS et al. 1994), one can quickly comprehend how powerful a diagnostic modality

MRI has become for the evaluation of selected patients with congenital heart disease. This chapter mainly focuses on techniques that are routinely available in most clinical MRI systems. Combining these techniques with a good understanding of the clinical questions to be answered, one can perform comprehensive and practical MRI examinations which include both morphologic and functional evaluation within reasonable scan times in most clinical environments.

16.2 Techniques

The following discussion reflects the author's recent clinical experience using Philips 1.5 T Gyroscan ACS-NT (version 6.2) and Philips 1.5 T Intera (version 7.1) (Philips Medical Systems, Best, Netherlands) at Texas Children's Hospital in Houston, Texas, USA.

16.2.1 Electrocardiographic Triggering

It has been said that if adequate electrocardiographic (ECG) waveform cannot be achieved with the patient inside the scanner, it is best not to initiate any form of examination. Although this statement is perhaps a bit exaggerated, especially when one can complete a contrast-enhanced MR angiogram without ECG-triggering, obtaining adequate ECG waveform in the MRI scanner can be a very frustrating experience for both the patient and the imager.

Due to the magnetohydrodynamic effect (DIMICK et al. 1987; KELTNER et al. 1990), the recorded ECG waveform from anteriorly placed electrodes can be contaminated by artifacts such that the T-wave may have high amplitude (so-called peaked T-wave) and lead to false triggering, especially in systems with rudimentary R-wave detection algorithm. One can

TAYLOR CHUNG, MD
Associate Professor of Radiology, Baylor College of Medicine, Edward B Singleton Department of Diagnostic Imaging, Texas Children's Hospital, 6621 Fannin St. MC 2–2521, Houston, TX 77030, USA

use posterior electrode positioning to significantly decrease these magnetohydrodynamic artifacts (DIMICK et al. 1987). However, the ECG waveform amplitude can be quite low, thus yielding poor signal-to-noise ratio (SNR). One solution is to place the electrodes anteriorly, but relatively low on the left chest (assuming levocardia). In a four-electrode system, use the left nipple as the landmark and place the left-arm electrode 1–2 cm above the nipple; place the right-arm electrode at a left parasternal position at the same craniocaudal level as the left-arm electrode; place the right-leg electrode approximately 2 cm below the left nipple; place the left-leg electrode over the left anterior axillary line at the same craniocaudal level as the right-leg electrode. In a three-electrode system, place the negative electrode at the right-arm electrode position, the positive electrode at the right-leg electrode position, and the ground lead at the left-leg electrode position. Equally important is the preparation of the skin surface and the actual placement of the individual electrodes. The skin needs to be clear of hair and rigorously cleaned either by rubbing with a dry gauze or by applying Nuprep (D.O. Weaver and Company, Aurora, Colorado, USA). Electrodes that have wet gel on their undersurface usually allow for good contact. The impedance to the ECG electric signal is then kept to a minimum.

Recently, fiber-optic ECG monitoring equipment has become available and is the technology of choice. It ensures the least contamination of the ECG signal by gradient noise. In addition, the theoretical chance of radio-frequency induced burns is almost non-existent. This is a very important point in pediatric MRI since patients who are sedated or under general anesthesia may not respond to pain. One vendor also provides a electronic filter with the fiber-optic system which can dampen the peaked T-wave effect and has been proven clinically to be effective in a small study of 12 patients with congenital heart disease and volunteers (BLOOMGARDEN et al. 1999). Unfortunately, despite these advances in technology, clinical experience has shown that such a system is not perfect and in some cases repositioning of electrodes is necessary. This is especially true in patients with complex congenital heart disease that have unusual spatial orientation of the ECG vectors.

Recently, a novel approach based on vector cardiography (VCG) (FRANK 1956) as opposed to standard frontal plane ECG signals (lead I, II, III) to achieve high quality/efficiency in ECG triggering has been introduced (CHIA et al. 2000a; FISCHER et al. 1999) and it is currently under clinical evaluation in selected centers. Vector cardiography has been classically used to analyze the electrical activity of the heart in four dimensions (x, y, z, time). This novel approach takes advantage of the fact that the vector loop in space of the electrical axis of the heart and that of the blood flow artifact originating from the magnetohydrodynamic effect have different orientations (CHIA et al. 2000b; DIMICK et al. 1987). The VCG-based R-wave triggering algorithms can then easily separate the native QRS vector loop from the flow artifact loop. In theory, this algorithm is independent of the direction of the electrical axis of the heart. Our initial clinical results with pediatric patients have been excellent, including results among a handful of patients with complex congenital heart diseases. The great advantage of this VCG-based triggering system is a standard, single method of electrode positioning for all patients (Fig. 16.1). In the small numbers of cases performed to date with this VCG system, we experienced excellent efficiency in R-wave triggering without having to re-position electrodes in a single case. *If this initial experience holds true, VCG-based triggering is likely to become the technique of choice in cardiac MRI.* There are also reports of early experiences using this technique in overcoming arrhythmia (CHIA et al. 2000b).

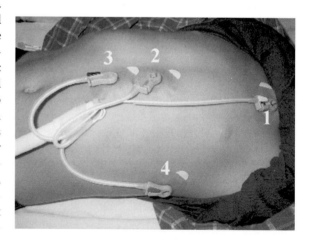

Fig. 16.1. Positioning of electrodes for the vector cardiogram (VCG) triggering system. On the chest of this sedated 5-year-old boy, electrodes *1–3* are placed along a left parasternal line with *1* at the level of the manubrium, *2* at level of the xiphoid, and *3* immediately below *2*. Electrode *4* is placed at the mid-axillary line at the same horizontal level as *2*. The electrode pairs (*1, 2*) and (*2, 4*) provide the vertical and horizontal components for the VCG, respectively, with electrode *3* being the reference lead

16.2.2
Choice of Coils

We favor the use of phased-array coils where or when possible. The major criteria in the choice of coil is the desired field-of-view (FOV) given the size of the patient and the ease of use. For example, previously, we would have used a quadrature head coil or head-neck coil for all infants who can fit into these coils. Recently, we have switched to using a two-element phased array shoulder coil (Fig. 16.2) in a small infant to get the desired FOV of 140–180 mm. For larger patients, we would use either a cardiac phased-array coil or body phased-array coil. Only for very large patients will we use the quadrature body coil.

16.2.3
Pulse Sequences for Morphology

Both black-blood and white-blood techniques have been used in the morphologic evaluation of patients with congenital heart disease (CHUNG 2000). Conventional spin-echo T1-weighted sequence with ECG-triggering and respiratory compensation (BAILES et al. 1985) has traditionally been the classical and robust sequence for black-blood imaging since the early days of cardiac MRI (FLETCHER et al. 1984; HERFKENS et al. 1983). More recently, the double- or triple-inversion recovery turbo spin-echo sequence has been shown to produce excellent quality black-blood images with high spatial resolution with scan

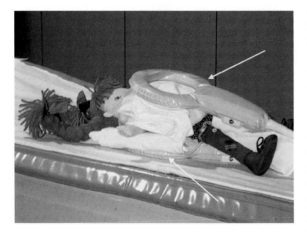

Fig. 16.2. Adapting a commercially available adult shoulder two-element phased-array coil for chest imaging in infants. The two coil elements (*arrows*) are positioned anteriorly and posteriorly. They need to be separated by a minimum distance usually equal to the diameter of the coil element

times of under 20 s. However, breath-holding is necessary which limits its utility in the pediatric population. One can run this sequence with multiple numbers of signal average (NSA) in a free-breathing mode with each image requiring approximately 1 min to acquire using four NSAs.

More recently, with the inherent flexibility in some scanner systems, an ECG-triggered, T1-weighted spin-echo sequence with a five-shot echo-planar-imaging (EPI) readout can be implemented on standard, commercially available scanner systems. With the EPI readout, scan time is significantly reduced, such that multiple signal averages can be used. The resultant images are of diagnostic quality with slightly more chemical shift artifacts than the conventional spin echo images (Fig. 16.3). However, the scan time for a similar range of anatomic coverage is shorter than the conventional spin echo sequence. For example, with a heart rate of 100 beats per minute, the spin echo EPI sequence with a matrix size of 256×192 and six NSAs takes 1 min 49 s to obtain 12 slices. The conventional spin echo with the same matrix size and the typical two NSAs takes 3 min 13 s to yield 12 slices.

For white-blood imaging, contrast-enhanced three dimensional (3-D) magnetic resonance angiography (CE-MRA) initially introduced in the early 1990s (PRINCE et al. 1993) is the most efficient sequence for the evaluation of extra-cardiac vascular anatomy in the chest (CHUNG et al. 1998). The current implementation of this sequence is in the form of 3-D acquisition of T1-weighted fast gradient echo or turbo field echo (TFE) using a flip angle of 40–45°, and the shortest repetition time (TR) and echo time (TE) available on the scanner. This sequence is typically run with multiple dynamics (or multiple phases). In our experience, the more complicated the extra-cardiac vascular anatomy is, the more useful this sequence seems to be. Although CE-MRA will yield the best images if the patient can suspend respiration, non-breathhold CE-MRA can also yield very good results (Fig. 16.4). As patients with complex congenital heart disease would have had palliative surgery with various venous shunts, in many instances, the later dynamic runs with mixed arterial and venous contrast are actually more informative than the early arterial phase in a CE-MRA sequence with multiple dynamics. Therefore, it follows that in a young patient who is sedated or who cannot hold breath, CE-MRA is a very simple sequence to use, especially when it is not critical to obtain pure arterial phase. If the MR scanner system does not have a robust method to check for the arrival of the contrast to the vessel of inter-

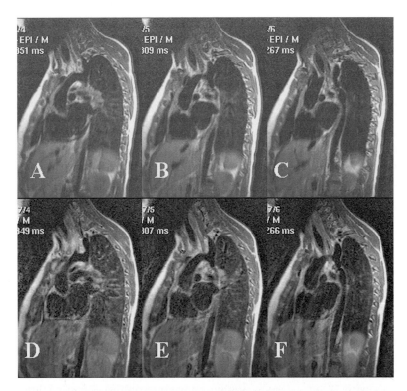

Fig. 16.3A–F. Oblique-sagittal images of a 9-year-old girl with unrepaired discrete coarctation. **A–C** ECG-triggered T1 echo-planar imaging (EPI) sequence, and (**D–F**) ECG-triggered T1 conventional spin echo sequence with respiratory compensation with an identical matrix size of 192+256, 280-mm FOV with 75% reduced FOV, 3-mm thick slices for ten slices with 10% skip, and identical TR/TE/flip angle of 571/21/90. The scan time for T1-EPI was 1 min 39 s, yielding ten slices using a five-shot EPI readout with six NSAs. The scan time for conventional spin echo with respiratory compensation was 2 min 55 s also yielding ten slices with two NSAs. The quality of the images is fairly similar with slightly more chemical shift artifact present in (**A–C**) and slightly more respiratory motion artifact in (**D–F**). The scan time is significantly shortened with T1-EPI

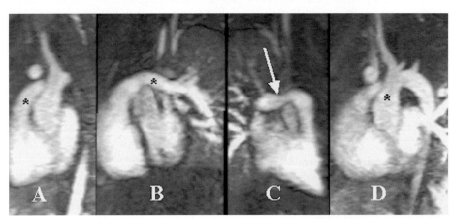

Fig. 16.4A–D. Multiple sub-volume maximum-intensity projections (MIPs) from a single three-dimensional contrast-enhanced magnetic resonance angiography (MRA) dataset obtained in a quietly breathing 7-year-old boy who underwent an arterial switch operation (Jatene procedure) for transposition of the great arteries. **A** Oblique-sagittal subvolume MIP showing patent neo-main pulmonary artery/right ventricular outflow (*asterisk*); **B** oblique-sagittal MIP along the patent left pulmonary artery (*asterisk*); **C** oblique-sagittal subvolume MIP along the right pulmonary artery showing mild stenosis (*arrow*); **D** oblique-sagittal subvolume MIP along the patent neo-ascending aorta (*asterisk*). Contrast-enhanced MRA with post-processing can be a very efficient technique to delineate the thoracic vascular anatomy

est, one can either estimate the arrival or simply start the acquisition with the injection of the contrast and run multiple dynamics. Test boluses of contrast can be used to more accurately determine the arrival time of the contrast. However, in young patients, the volume of contrast available is quite small and the test bolus volume is often a substantial percentage of the total volume of contrast.

Some recent scanner systems have a very sensitive method of tracking the contrast bolus (MEANEY et al. 1999). One can actually observe, in real time (two images per second), the contrast bolus arrive at the vascular region of interest and then manually initiate the acquisition of the CE-MRA sequence (Fig. 16.5). Valuable scan time can be saved by using real time tracking of the contrast bolus compared to using a test bolus. Another recent advance in rapid imaging is the use of a form of parallel imaging by taking advantage of the individual coil elements in phased-array coils. *Sensivity encoding* (SENSE) (PRUESSMANN et al. 1999) and *simultaneous acquisition of spatial harmonics* (SMASH) (SODICKSON and MANNING 1997) techniques have been introduced and preliminary clinical results in adults are very promising (SODICK-SON et al. 1999, 2000; WEIGER et al. 2000b). Our initial experience in pediatric patients with combining SENSE and CE-MRA has also been encouraging (Figs. 16.6 and 16.7). Depending on the imaging parameters and anatomic coverage, it is possible to reduce the acquisition time of a single dynamic of a CE-MRA to 4–10 s with the addition of the SENSE technique using a scan reduction factor of two with a standard four-element body phased-array coil. This technique may prove to be most advantageous in patients who are sedated and cannot hold breath (Fig. 16.6) or in patients who can only suspend respiration for a short

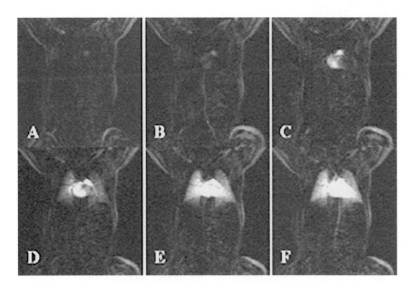

Fig. 16.5A–F. Bolus-tracking in a 5-kg, sedated infant. **A–F** are selected images from the bolus-tracking sequence which yields two images per second in real time with dynamic subtraction showing the 2 cc of gadolinium contrast bolus that was hand-injected into an intravenous line in the left foot coursing along the inferior vena cava in (**B**), to the right side of the heart and reaching the main pulmonary artery in (**C**), out to the lung parenchyma in (**D**) and (**E**), and finally returning to the left side of the heart and beginning to opacify the aorta in (**F**)

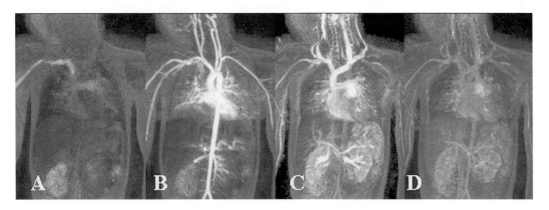

Fig. 16.6A–D. The SENSE technique with contrast-enhanced three-dimensional magnetic resonance angiography (3D-MRA) in a sedated, freely breathing 5-year-old boy. The MRA was set up with five dynamics and the acquisition was started with the initiation of an intravenous injection of 0.2 mmol/kg of gadolinium contrast agent. **A–D** Full-volume maximum intensity projection (MIP) images of the first through fourth dynamics of the dataset. Scan time of each dynamic or the acquisition time of each 3D set of data is 8 s. The parameters were: TR/TE/flip angle = 5.0/1.3/40, 20 partitions of 2.8 mm in thickness interpolated to 40 slices of 1.4 mm in thickness, field-of-view (FOV) of 400 mm with 80% reduced FOV, and a final in-plane matrix size of 256×211. The SENSE technique thus allows for faster MRA with higher in-plane resolution. Note the pure arterial contrast in the neck in (**B**) and the predominant venous phase contrast in (**C**)

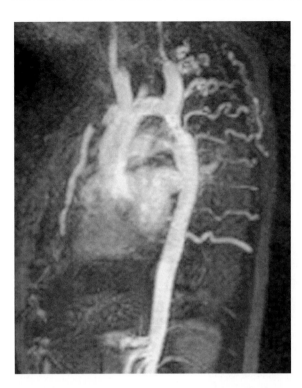

Fig. 16.7. Subvolume maximum intensity projection (MIP) image of contrast-enhanced three-dimensional magnetic resonance angiography (3D-MRA) with SENSE in the same patient as in Fig. 16.3. As the volume of acquisition was in an oblique sagittal slab only covering the thoracic aorta, each dynamic was just under 4 s long with an in-plane matrix of 256×213, field-of-view (FOV) of 350 mm with 70% reduced FOV. The discrete coarctation and collaterals are well seen even when the patient is breathing throughout the acquisition

period of time. For older patients who can breath-hold, multiple phases of the CE-MRA can be obtained within a single breathhold, thus improving the temporal resolution. Alternatively, one can use SENSE to increase the spatial resolution instead of decreasing the scan time (WEIGER et al. 2000b).

ECG-triggered cine fast gradient echo or cine TFE with segmented k-space filling is another robust white blood sequence for morphologic evaluation. This sequence can be used with multiple NSA on patients who cannot suspend respiration (HERNANDEZ et al. 1993) (Fig. 16.8), or can be used with one NSA on patients who can hold their breath (Fig. 16.9A). This cine sequence can yield multiple images within a cardiac cycle and thus have dynamic information not available from the static black blood sequences. In our experience, this cine sequence has replaced the traditional spin echo T1-weighted static black-blood sequence for morphologic evaluation.

This is usually implemented with the shortest TR, the shortest TE, and a small flip angle of 30°. Depending on the slice thickness and the matrix size, between two and four NSAs can yield adequate SNR. Scan time will also depend on the desired number of phases per cardiac cycle.

16.2.4
Pulse Sequences for Function

To evaluate ventricular function, the ECG-triggered cine TFE sequence mentioned previously can be used to obtain a series of images in the short-axis plane of the morphologic left ventricle from the apex to the base of both ventricles. A standardized method of obtaining the short-axis plane has been well-described and it is reproducible between studies and scanner operators (LORENZ et al. 1999). Many semi-automated post-processing software tools are available for the generation of ventricular function parameters such as ejection fraction, stroke volume, ventricular mass, etc. There are also normative data of right and left ventricular function for pediatric patients, although the number of patients is small (LORENZ 2000). As the use of MRI expands to the pediatric population, it will be important to accumulate a greater volume of normative data on ventricular function in a fashion similar to the development of normative data in echocardiography. For complex congenital heart conditions such as a single ventricle oriented in an unusual fashion, or in the evaluation of the morphologic right ventricle with its complex shape, multi-section cine sequences can yield accurate volume measurements (HELBING et al. 1995).

While the above-mentioned cine sequence is widely available and quite robust, one of the recent exciting advances in cardiac MRI techniques is the re-introduction of the balanced gradient-recalled echo technique (LEE and CHO 1988) and is more popularly known as the true FISP (free induction steady-state precession) sequence or balanced FFE (fast field-echo) or FIESTA (fast imaging employing steady state acquisition). This sequence has the advantage of being effectively flow independent and can produce images with excellent myocardial-blood pool distinction (Fig. 16.9B) and would be the sequence of choice for ventricular function evaluation. This pulse sequence is designed such that all the gradient lobes are completely balanced at read out and that it is essentially independent of TR. In fact, the shorter the TR can be, the less T2-weighted de-phasing artifacts

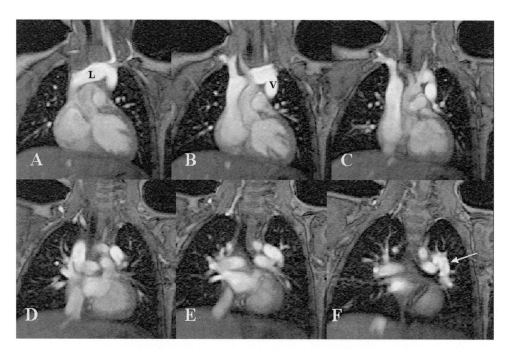

Fig. 16.8A–F. Segmented k-space cine turbo field echo (TFE) sequence with multiple NSAs in a sedated 18-month-old boy with partial anomalous pulmonary venous connection of left pulmonary vein (*arrow*) to left innominate vein (*L*) via a vertical vein (*V*). A–F (anterior to posterior) Selected coronal images of a cine sequence of the same phase in the cardiac cycle at different anatomic locations. The parameters were: TR/TE/flip angle = 8.4/3.0/30, field-of-view 180 mm, ten phases per cardiac cycle, 256×128 matrix, four lines per segment, two NSAs, scan time of 70 s per location

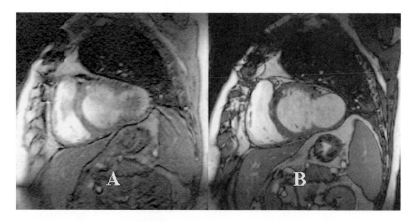

Fig. 16.9A,B. Comparison of (A) breath-hold segmented cine turbo field echo with (B) cine balanced fast field echo in an adult patient with left ventricular aneurysm. Note the significantly improved definition of the interface between the blood pool and the myocardium. (All images courtesy of Raja Muthupillai, PhD, of Philips Medical Systems, and Scott E. Flamm, MD, of St. Luke's Episcopal Hospital/Texas Heart Institute, Houston, Texas)

in the sequence. Since the latest scanning systems are capable of producing TR of well under 4 ms, this theory of balanced fast gradient echo sequence has become a clinical reality. This sequence is available with the latest scanner systems. The best results are obviously achieved with breath-hold imaging. However, this sequence can be implemented with multi- ple NSAs for free-breathing. Although the experience with this new sequence in the pediatric population is currently quite limited, it may be a potentially very powerful sequence if the image quality is adequate using multiple NSAs without breath-holding. In the limited experience among an adult population in selected centers, balanced FFE produces the optimal images of through-plane flow with the least amount of artifacts, while it is not as desirable with in-plane flow where flow artifacts can propagate in the phase-encode direction.

Another recent advance which should be mentioned is real time MRI. The latest scanner systems are fast enough to make real time MRI possible. For example, with an ultrafast segmented EPI sequence with real time reconstruction and display, adequate quality real time images have been achieved with 20 frames per second temporal resolution without view-sharing or interpolation (WEBER et al. 1999) (Fig. 16.10). Using the SENSE technique mentioned previously together with a special six-element receiver coil array WEIGER et al. reported multiple slice real-time imaging at a rate of 38 double-frames per second (WEIGER et al. 2000a). One of the applications is the evaluation of ventricular function without the need for ECG-triggering and respiratory suspension (WEBER et al. 1999; YANG et al. 1998). Most experience has been in the adult population, although Dr. Shi-joon Yoo (personal communication, November 2000) at the Hospital for Sick Children in Toronto, Canada, has recently started using real time MRI as one of the techniques in the morphologic evaluation of patients with congenital heart disease.

Non-invasive quantitative blood flow analysis is yet another extremely powerful tool that MRI has to offer. The most widely used pulse sequence is a retrospective ECG-triggered cine phase contrast (also known as velocity-encoded cine MRI) (BRENNER et al. 1992; CAPUTO et al. 1991; HELBING et al. 1996; HUNDLEY et al. 1995; POWELL et al. 2000; REBERGEN et al. 1993a,b, 1995; SIEVERDING et al. 1992; STEFFENS et al. 1994). This sequence make use of bipolar gradients such that flowing spins will accumulate a certain amount of net phase shift, whereas stationary spins will have a net phase shift of zero. This net phase shift is proportional to the velocity of the flowing spins (NAYLER et al. 1986; PELC et al. 1992; PELC 1995). Thus, one can prescribe an imaging plane perpendicular to the long axis of the vessel of interest and non-invasively interrogate for the velocity of blood flow in that vessel (Fig. 16.11). The accuracy of this technique has be validated both in vitro and in vivo (BOGREN et al. 1989; EVANS et al. 1993; FIRMIN et al. 1987; FRAYNE et al. 1995; KONDO et al. 1991; POWELL and GEVA 2000) and all have shown strong correlations with standard measurement methods. However, this is not to say that this sequence is perfect. Flow acceleration or other higher orders of velocity will induce phase incoherence and loss of signal. Accuracy will thus decrease in areas of flow turbulence. There are also other factors such as partial volume averaging at the edge of a vessel contributing to measurement errors. To minimize these errors, one can select a segment of the vessel that is straight, spend time setting up the imaging plane to be truly perpendicular to the long axis of the vessel, and use short echo times.

This is a very useful technique, especially when applied in older patients or post-operative patients with extracardiac shunts and conduits where there are poor acoustic windows for echocardiographic evaluation. Not only is MRI independent of having an acoustic window, the flow quantification can be performed in any plane in space and not limited by the incidence

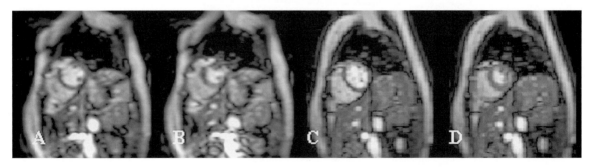

Fig. 16.10A–D. Real time cardiac magnetic resonance imaging in an adult volunteer. End-diastolic (**A**) and end-systolic (**B**) frames of mid-ventricular, short-axis view of the left ventricle using fast field echo with five-shot echo-planar-imaging readout with a SENSE reduction factor of two, yielding a temporal resolution of 27 ms (equivalent to 37 frames per second) at an in-plane resolution of 4.36×2.79 mm. End-diastolic (**C**) and end-systolic (**D**) frames of mid-ventricular short-axis view of the left ventricle using balanced FFE yielding a temporal resolution of 56 ms (equivalent to 17 frames per second) at an in-plane resolution of 5.76×2.79 mm. All images were obtained with a standard five-element cardiac phased-array coil. (All images are courtesy of Raja Muthupillai, PhD, of Philips Medical Systems, and were obtained at St. Luke's Episcopal Hospital/Texas Heart Institute, Houston, Texas)

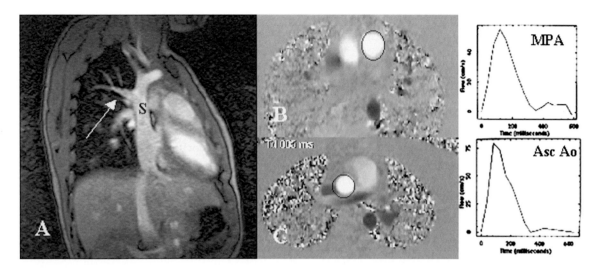

Fig. 16.11A–C. The cine phase contrast technique to estimate left-to-right shunt in a patient with partial anomalous pulmonary venous return. **A** Oblique-coronal image from a cine turbo field echo sequence showing the right upper pulmonary vein (*arrow*) draining into the superior vena cava (*S*). **B,C** Phase images of the main pulmonary artery (*MPA*) and ascending aorta (*Asc Ao*), respectively, with the plane of acquisition perpendicular to the long axis of the vessels of interest. The graphs of flow (cubic centimeters/second) vs time (seconds) show the flow pattern of both the MPA and Asc Ao in one cardiac cycle. By integrating the areas under the curves, the stroke volume of the right and left side of the heart can be estimated. In this patient, the left-to-right shunt was estimated to be 1.3

angle as in the Doppler ultrasound technique. Clinical applications of flow analysis in patients with congenital heart disease such as quantification of systemic-to-pulmonary flow ratio (Fig. 16.11), valvular regurgitation, right and left lung perfusion, and estimation of stenoses in vessels and valves have recently been reviewed by POWELL and GEVA (2000).

Unlike in adult ischemic heart disease where much of the emphasis has been on the evaluation of the morphologic left ventricle, the function of the morphologic right ventricle, in congenital heart disease, is equally as important. In many situations such as in patients with tetralogy of Fallot, the most common cyanotic congenital heart lesion (HOFFMAN 1995), MRI can provide valuable physiologic information non-invasively. MRI flow quantification is the only non-invasive means to quantify pulmonary regurgitation (REBERGEN et al. 1993a). Comprehensive non-invasive functional evaluation of the right ventricle in patients after surgical repair of tetralogy of Fallot by MRI has recently been reviewed by HELBING and DE ROOS (2000). This excellent review demonstrates the utility of MRI in obtaining physiological information, such as right and left ventricular function, including right ventricular diastolic function, ventricular mass, degree of pulmonary regurgitation, to assist in clinical problem solving in this particular cohort of patients.

The cine phase contrast technique can be applied to encode for blood flow in all three dimensions. This can generate a time-resolved three-dimensional flow pattern for further analyses. Currently, this technique remains investigational. However, interesting works have been reported where this technique has been applied to study flow patterns in the total cavopulmonary or atriopulmonary connections of patients with Fontan repair of single ventricle physiology or complex congenital heart disease. One report suggested that total cavopulmonary connection is a more hemodynamically efficient circulation (BE'ERI et al. 1998), while another study found higher shear stresses in pulmonary arteries in patients with total cavopulmonary connections and postulated that increased shear stresses may alter endothelial function and may affect the longevity of the repair (MORGAN et al. 1998).

More recently, work has been done to combine phase contrast data and real time interactive imaging. The phase contrast data was displayed with a color scale over a traditional gray-scale image in real time and the scan plane can also be changed by the operator in real time (NAYAK et al. 2000). This seems to be a promising technique; unfortunately, it is not generally available and needs to be further evaluated clinically, although it does generate enthusiasm for the potential of interactive cardiac MRI examinations in the future.

There are other techniques such as myocardial tagging and blood tagging, but quantitative analyses of these data are beyond the scope of this overview of cardiac MRI. The application of these techniques on patients with congenital heart diseases has recently been reviewed by FOGEL (2000). Finally, one other very interesting technique merits attention. WRIGHT et al. (1991) have shown encouraging data using MRI to measure the blood oxygen content, initially in the superior mesenteric vein of adults to diagnose chronic mesenteric ischemia (LI et al. 1997), and more recently in the ascending aorta and main pulmonary artery of patients with congenital heart disease in the pediatric population (NIELD et al. 2000). This technique, if it proves to be a robust technique with more clinical evaluation and in vivo validation, may have a significant impact on the functional evaluation of complex congenital heart disease, especially if one can interrogate the oxygen content in the atria and ventricles as well as vessels.

16.3
Imaging Strategies

For a cardiac MRI examination to yield useful information, the MR imager must be aware of the clinical questions to be answered. The key lies in good communication between the referring cardiologists or cardiothoracic surgeons and the MR imager. In our experience, most patients for cardiac MRI have had prior echocardiograms and/or cine cardioangiograms. There are very specific questions to be answered by the cardiac MRI examination. Therefore, the imaging strategy needs to be tailored to those questions.

In general, most examinations require both morphologic and functional information. We usually use CE-MRA and cine fast gradient echo sequences to obtain the morphologic information. If there is a need for better definition of vessel walls or size of trachea (as in work-up of vascular rings), then we will use an ECG-triggered T1-weighted sequence. In general, the morphologic data can be obtained in 30 min or less and the rest of the examination time can be spent acquiring functional data such as ventricular function and flow quantification. For example, in patients with transposition of the great arteries which has been surgically corrected by an arterial switch operation in the neonatal period, MRI can be the imaging modality of choice. Echocardiogram, due to its poor acoustic window, cannot fully evaluate the relevant anatomy; cine cardio-

angiography may be considered too invasive, especially when cardiac MRI is available. In these patients, one can easily evaluate the aortic and pulmonary anastomoses and the appearance of the proximal right and left pulmonary arteries with a combination of CE-MRA (see Fig. 16.4) and cine TFE sequences. Then, one can compare flow across the right and left pulmonary arteries with a cine phase contrast sequence, and access the biventricular function with cine TFE sequence prescribed along the short axis of the left ventricle from base to apex. Finally, one can evaluate the coronary anastomoses and the proximal coronary arteries by using one of the many techniques of coronary MRA, such as 3-D TFE with ECG-triggering and adaptive respiratory navigators, now available thanks to the tremendous efforts of numerous centers working on MRI of ischemic heart disease in the adult population (DUERINCKX 1999; LORENZ and JOHANSSON 1999). Thus, one can use a combination of pulse sequences to design a comprehensive cardiac MRI examination that will provide both morphologic and functional data to answer the specific clinical questions relevant to an evaluation of patients with congenital heart disease.

16.4
Conclusion

MRI is an extremely powerful non-invasive imaging tool for the evaluation of both morphology and function in patients with congenital heart disease. It should be the modality of choice for the imaging of extra-cardiac vascular anatomy in the thorax, especially when echocardiography cannot fully evaluate all the anatomy due to a limited acoustic window. Cardiac MRI has also been shown to yield important physiologic information in terms of ventricular function and flow quantification analyses. Patients, who in the past would have needed invasive cine cardioangiograms in order to obtain certain anatomic information which the echocardiogram could not provide, can now undergo a non-invasive cardiac MRI examination instead. Although cardiac MRI cannot yet provide all the physiological information that can be obtained by cardiac catheterization, there are selected cases in which cardiac MRI can be a substitute for catheterization. With the steady advances in MR technology in cardiovascular imaging and functional imaging, there may be a day in the future where cardiac MRI can take the place of diagnostic cardiac catheterization in patients with congenital heart diseases.

References

Bailes DR, Gilerdale DJ, Bydder GM et al (1985) Respiratory ordered phase encoding (ROPE): a method for reducing respiratory motion artifacts in MR imaging. Comput Assist Tomogr 9:835–838

Be'eri E, Maier SE, Landzberg MJ et al (1998) In vivo evaluation of Fontan pathway flow dynamics by multidimensional phase-velocity magnetic resonance imaging. Circulation 98:2873–2882

Bloomgarden DC, Morris GR, Valentine J et al (1999) Improved ECG triggering with the T-wave Terminator. Proc Int Soc Magn Reson Med 7:1995

Bogren HG, Klipstein RH, Firmin DN et al (1989) Quantitation of antegrade and retrograde blood flow in the human aorta by magnetic resonance velocity mapping. Am Heart J 117:1214–1222

Brenner LD, Caputo GR, Mostbeck G et al (1992) Quantification of antegrade and retrograde blood flow in the human aorta by magnetic resonance imaging. J Am Coll Cardiol 20:1246–1250

Caputo GR, Kondo C, Masui T et al (1991) Right and left lung perfusion: in vitro and in vivo validation with oblique-angle, velocity-encoded cine MR imaging. Radiology 180:693–698

Chia JM, Fischer SE, Wickline SA et al (2000a) Performance of QRS detection for cardiac magnetic resonance imaging with a novel vectorcardiographic triggering method. J Magn Reson Imaging 12:678–688

Chia JM, Fischer SE, Wickline SA et al (2000b) Arrhythmia rejection using a VCG-based triggering algorithm. Proc Int Soc Magn Reson Med 8:201

Chung KJ, Simpson IA, Newman R et al (1988) Cine magnetic resonance imaging for evaluation of congenital heart disease: role in pediatric cardiology compared with echocardiography and angiography. J Pediatr 113:1028–1035

Chung T, Powell AJ, Geva T (1998) Initial clinical experience with 3-D magnetic resonance angiography in the evaluation of patients with congenital heart disease (abstract). Circulation 98:2533

Chung T (2000) Assessment of cardiovascular anatomy in patients with congenital heart disease by magnetic resonance imaging. Pediatr Cardiol 21:18–26

Dimick RN, Hedlund LM, Herfkens RJ et al (1987) Optimizing electrocardiography electrode placement for cardiac-gated magnetic resonance imaging. Invest Radiol 22:17–22

Duerinckx AJ (1999) Coronary MR angiography. Radiol Clin North Am 37:273–318

Evans AJ, Iwai F, Grist TA et al (1993) Magnetic resonance imaging of blood flow with a phase subtraction technique. In vitro and in vivo validation. Invest Radiol 28:109–115

Firmin DN, Nayler GL, Klipstein RH et al (1987) In vivo validation of MR velocity imaging. J Comput Assis Tomogr 11:751–756

Fischer SE, Wickline SA, Lorenz CH (1999) Novel real-time R-wave detection algorithm based on the vectorcardiogram for accurate gated magnetic resonance acquisitions. Magn Reson Med 42:361–370

Fletcher BD, Jacobstein MD, Nelson AD et al (1984) Gated magnetic resonance imaging of congenital cardiac malformation. Radiology 150:137–140

Fogel MA (2000) Assessment of cardiac function by magnetic resonance imaging. Pediatr Cardiol 21:59–69

Fogel MA, Weinberg PM, Chin AJ et al (1996) Late ventricular geometry and performance changes of functional single ventricle throughout staged Fontan reconstruction assessed by magnetic resonance imaging. J AM Coll Cardiol 28:212–221

Frank E (1956) An accurate, clinically practical system for spatial vector-cardiography. Circulation 13:737–749

Frayne R, Steinman DA, Ethier CR et al (1995) Accuracy of MR phase contrast velocity measurements for unsteady flow. J Magn Reson Imaging 5:428–431

Helbing WA, de Roos A (2000) Clinical applications of cardiac magnetic resonance imaging after repair of tetralogy of Fallot. Pediatr Cardiol 21:70–79

Helbing WA, Bosch HG, Maliepaard C et al (1995) Comparison of echocardiographic methods with magnetic resonance imaging for assessment of right ventricular function in children. Am J Cardiol 76:589–594

Helbing WA, Niezen RA, Cessie SL et al (1996) Right ventricular diastolic function in children with pulmonary regurgitation after repair of tetralogy of Fallot: volumetric evaluation by magnetic resonance velocity mapping. J Am Coll Cardiol 28:1827–1835

Herfkens RJ, Higgins CB, Hricak H et al (1983) Nuclear magnetic resonance imaging of the cardiovascular system: normal and pathologic findings. Radiology 147:749–759

Hernandez RJ, Aisen AM, Foo TKF et al (1993) Thoracic cardiovascular anomalies in children: evaluation with a fast gradient-recalled-echo sequence with cardiac-triggered segmented acquisition. Radiology 188:755–780

Hoffman JI (1995) Incidence of congenital heart disease I. Post-natal incidence. Pediatr Cardiol 16:103–113

Hundley WG, Li HF, Lange RA et al (1995) Assessment of left-to-right intracardiac shunting by velocity-encoded, phase-difference magnetic resonance imaging. A comparison with oximetric and indicator dilution techniques. Circulation 91:2955–2960

Katz J, Milliken MC, Stray-Gundersen J et al (1988) Estimation of human myocardial mass with MR imaging. Radiology 169:495–498

Keltner JR, Roos MS, Brakeman PR et al (1990) Magnetohydrodynamics of blood flow. Magn Reson Med 16:139–149

Kondo C, Caputo GR, Semelka R et al (1991) Right and left ventricular stroke volume measurements with velocity-encoded cine MR imaging: in vitro and in vivo validation. Am J Roentgenol 157:9–16

Lee SY, Cho ZH (1988) Fast SSFP gradient echo sequence for simultaneous acquisitions of FID and echo signals. Magn Reson Med 8:142–150

Li KC, Dalman RL, Chi'ien IY et al (1997) Chronic mesenteric ischemia: use of in vivo MR imaging measurements of blood oxygen saturation in the superior mesenteric vein for diagnosis. Radiology 204:71–77

Lorenz CH, Johansson LO (1999) Contrast-enhanced coronary MRA. J Magn Reson Imaging 10:703–708

Lorenz CH (2000) The range of normal values of cardiovascular structure in infants, children, and adolescents measured by magnetic resonance imaging. Pediatr Cardiol 21:37–46

Lorenz CH, Walker ES, Morgan VL et al (1999) Normal human right and left ventricular mass, systolic function and gender differences by cine magnetic resonance imaging. J Cardiovasc Magn Reson 1:7–22

Marx GR, Geva T (1998) MRI and echocardiography in children: how do they compare? Semin Roentgenol 3:281–292

Meaney JFM, Saysell M, Ridgway JP et al (1999) Timing of 3-D abdominal MRA using single slice fluoroscopic imaging with real time complex subtraction and real time display. Proc Int Soc Magn Reson Med 7:1206

Morgan VL, Graham TPJ, Roselli RJ et al (1998) Alterations in pulmonary artery flow patterns and shear stress determined with three-dimensional phase-contrast magnetic resonance imaging in Fontan patients. J Thorac Cardiovasc Surg 116:294–304

Nayak KS, Pauly JM, Kerr AB et al (2000) Real-time color flow MRI. Magn Reson Med 43:251–258

Nayler GL, Firmin DN, Longmore DB (1986) Blood flow imaging by cine magnetic resonance. J Comput Assis Tomogr 10:715–722

Nield LE, Qi XL, Yoo SJ et al (2000) MRI-based blood oxygen saturation measurements in infants and children with congenital heart disease (abstract). Circulation 102 [Suppl II]:457

Pattynama PMT, Lamb HJ, van der Velde EA et al (1995) Reproducibility of magnetic resonance imaging-derived measurements of right ventricular volumes and myocardial mass. Magn Reson Imaging 13:53–63

Pelc LR, Pelc NJ, Rayhill SC et al (1992) Arterial and venous blood flow: noninvasive quantitation with MR imaging. Radiology 185:809–812

Pelc NJ (1995) Flow quantification and analysis methods [Review]. Magn Reson Imaging Clin North Am 3:413–424

Powell AJ, Geva T (2000) Blood flow measurement by magnetic resonance imaging in congenital heart disease. Pediatr Cardiol 21:47–58

Powell AJ, Maier SE, Chung T et al (2000) Phase-velocity cine magnetic resonance imaging measurement of pulsatile bloodflow in children and young adults: in vitro and in vivo validation. Pediatr Cardiol 21:104–110

Prince MR, Yucel E, Kaufman J et al (1993) Dynamic gadolinium-enhanced three-dimensional abdominal MR arteriography. J Magn Reson Imaging 3:877–881

Pruessmann KP, Weiger M, Schiedegger MB et al (1999) SENSE: sensitivity encoding for fast MRI. Magn Reson Med 42:952–962

Rebergen SA, Chin J, Ottenkamp J et al (1993a) Pulmonary regurgitation in the late postoperative follow-up of tetralogy of Fallot. Volumetric quantitation by nuclear magnetic resonance velocity mapping. Circulation 88:2257–2266

Rebergen SA, Ottenkamp J, Doornbos J et al (1993b) Postoperative pulmonary flow dynamics after Fontan surgery: assessment with nuclear magnetic resonance velocity mapping. J Am Coll Cardiol 21:123–131

Rebergen SA, Helbing WA, van der Wall EE et al (1995) MR velocity mapping of tricuspid flow in healthy children and in patients who have undergone Mustard or Senning repair. Radiology 194:505–512

Roest AA, Helbing WA, van der Wall EE et al (1999) Postoperative evaluation of congenital heart disease by magnetic resonance imaging. J Magn Reson Imaging 10:656–666

Sakuma H, Fuijita N, Foo TK et al (1993) Evaluation of left ventricular volume and mass with breath-hold cine MR imaging. Radiology 188:377–380

Sieverding L, Jung WI, Klose U et al (1992) Noninvasive blood flow measurement and quantification of shunt volume by cine magnetic resonance in congenital heart disease. Preliminary results. Pediatr Radiol 22:48–54

Sodickson DK, Manning WJ (1997) Simultaneous acquisition of spatial harmonics (SMASH): ultra-fast imaging with radiofrequency coil arrays. Magn Reson Med 38:591–603

Sodickson DK, Griswold M, Jakob PM (1999) SMASH imaging. Magn Reson Imaging Clin North Am 7:237–254

Sodickson DK, McKenzie CA, Li W et al (2000) Contrast-enhanced 3D MR angiography with simultaneous acquisition of spatial harmonics: a polit study. Radiology 217:284–289

Steffens JC, Bourne MW, Sakuma H et al (1994) Quantification of collateral blood flow in coarctation of the aorta by velocity encoded cine magnetic resonance imaging. Circulation 90:937–943

Weber OM, Eggers H, Spiegel MA et al (1999) Real-time interactive magnetic resonance imaging with multiple coils for the assessment of left ventricular function. J Magn Reson Imaging 10:826–832

Weiger M, Pruessmann KP, Boesiger P (2000a) Cardiac real-time imaging using SENSE. SENSitivity Encoding scheme. Magn Reson Med 43:177–184

Weiger M, Pruessmann KP, Kassner A et al (2000b) Contrast-enhanced 3D MRA using SENSE. J Magn Reson Imaging 12:671–677

Wright GA, Hu BS, Mascovski A (1991) 1991 I I Rabi award. Estimating oxygen saturation of blood in vivo with MR imaging at 1.5 T. J Magn Reson Imaging 1(3):275–283

Yang PC, Kerr AB, Liu AC et al (1998) New real-time interactive cardiac magnetic resonance imaging system complements echocardiography. JACC 32:2049–2056

Subject Index

List of Contributors

RONIT AGID, MD
Department of Radiology
Hadassah Medical Organization
Clinical Instructor, Faculty of Medicine
The Hebrew University
P.O. Box 12000
91120 Jerusalem
Israel

JACOB BAR-ZIV, MD
Professor and Chairman
Department of Radiology
Hadassah Medical Organization
Kiryat hadassah, PO Box 12000
91120 Jerusalem
Israel

ALAN S. BRODY, MD
Department of Radiology
Children's Hospital Medical Center
3333 Burnet Avenue
Cincinnati, OH 45229-3039
USA

AMPARO CASTELLOTE, MD
Department of Pediatric Radiology
Hospitals Vall d'Hebron
Ps. Vall d' Hebron, 119-129
08035 - Barcelona
Spain

TAYLOR CHUNG, MD
Edward B. Singleton Department of Diagnostic Imaging
Texas Children's Hospital
6621 Fannin St.
MC 2-2521
Houston TX 77030-2399
USA

PEDRO AUGUSTO DALTRO, MD
Instituto Fernandes Figueira
Fiocruz and Clinica de Diagnóstico por Imagem
Barrashopping
Av. Ataulfo de Paiva
226 Leblon
Rio De Janeiro, RJ 22440-030
Brasil

LANE F. DONNELLY, MD
Department of Radiology
Children's Hospital Medical Center
3333 Burnet Avenue
Cincinnati, OH 45229-3039
USA

HUBERT DUCOU LE POINTE, MD
Service de Radiologie Pédiatrique
Hôpital d' Enfants Armand-Trousseau
26, avenue du Dr. Arnold Netter
75012 Paris
France

GEORG F. EICH, MD
Division of Pediatric Radiology
Kantonsspital
5001 Aarau
Switzerland

GOYA ENRIQUEZ, MD
Department of Pediatric Radiology
Vall d' Hebron Hospitals
Ps. Vall d' hebron, 119-129
08035 - Barcelona
Spain

DONALD P. FRUSH, MD
Department of Radiology (1508-D)
Duke University Medical Center
Box 3808
Durham NC 27710
USA

PILAR GARCIA-PEÑA, MD
Department of Pediatric Radiology
Vall d'Hebron Hospitals
Ps. Vall d' Hebron, 119-129
08035-Barcelona
Spain

DAVID GILDAY, MD
Department of Nuclear Medicine
Hospital for Sick Children
555 University Ave.
Toronto ON M5G 1X8
Canada

LENA GROVER, MD
Department of Radiology
Long Island College Hospital
339 Hicks Street
Brooklyn, NY 11201
USA

JACK O. HALLER, MD
Department of Radiology
Beth Israel Medical Center
16th Street & First Ave.
New York, NY 10003
USA

SUE KASTE, MD
Department of Diagnostic Imaging
St. Jude Children's Research Hospital
332 N. Lauderdale
Memphis TN 38105-2794
USA

CHRISTIAN J. KELLENBERGER, MD
Division of Pediatric Radiology
The University Children's Hospital
Steinwiesstrasse 75
8032 Zürich
Switzerland

BENJAMIN Z. KOPLEWITZ, BSc, MD
Department of Radiology
Hadassah Medical Organization
Clinical Instructor, Faculty of Medicine
The Hebrew University
P.O. Box 12000
91120 Jerusalem
Israel

JAVIER LUCAYA, MD
Director, Division of Diagnostic Imaging
and Institute of Diagnostic Imaging
Vall d'Hebron Hospitals
Autonomous University of Barcelona
Ps. Vall d' Hebron, 119-129
08035 - Barcelona
Spain

JOSEP M. MATA, MD
UDIAT, Servei de Diagnòstic per la Image
Corporació Parc Taulí, s/n
08208 - Sabadell
Spain

KIERAN McHUGH, FRCR, FRCPI, DCH
Department of Radiology
Great Ormond Street Hospital for Children NHS Trust
Great Ormond Street
London WC1N 3JH
UK

ELOÁ NUNEZ-SANTOS, MD
Instituto Fernandes Figueira
Fiocruz
Rua Almirante Guillobel
93-402 Lagoa
Rio De Janeiro, RJ 22471-150
Brasil

XAVIER SERRES, MD
Department of Radiology
Hospital General de Granollers
Avda. Francesc Ribas, s/n
08400 - Granollers
Spain

JANET L. STRIFE, MD
Radiologist-in-Chief
Children's Hospital Medical Center
3333 Burnet Avenue
Cincinnati, OH 45229-3039
USA

ULRICH V. WILLI, MD
Division of Pediatric Radiology
The University Children's Hospital
Steinwiesstrasse 75
8032 Zürich
Switzerland

MEDICAL RADIOLOGY
Diagnostic Imaging and Radiation Oncology

Titles in the series already published

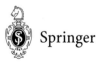

Springer

MEDICAL RADIOLOGY
Diagnostic Imaging and Radiation Oncology

Titles in the series already published

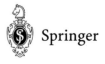

Springer